THE COMPLETE BOOK OF
massage and
aromatherapy

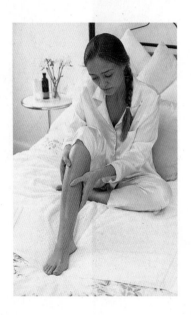

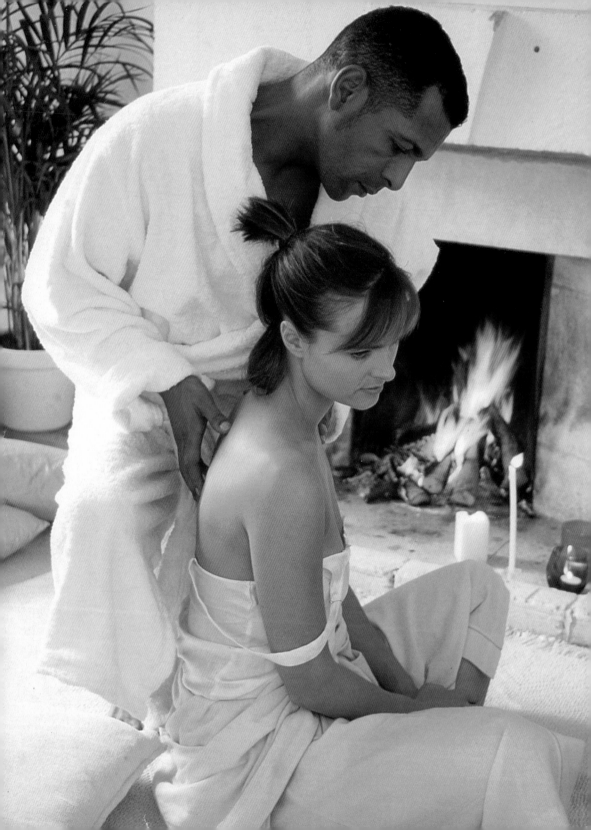

THE COMPLETE BOOK OF
massage and aromatherapy

A PRACTICAL ILLUSTRATED STEP-BY-STEP GUIDE TO ACHIEVING RELAXATION
AND WELL-BEING WITH TOP-TO-TOE BODY TREATMENTS AND ESSENTIAL OILS

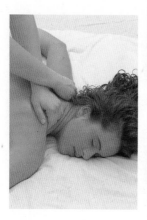 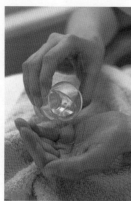 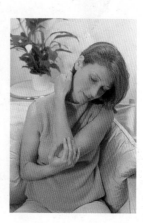

CONSULTING EDITOR: **CATHERINE STUART**

southwater

This edition is published by Southwater, an imprint of Anness
Publishing Ltd, Blaby Road, Wigston, Leicestershire LE18 4SE;
info@anness.com

www.southwaterbooks.com; www.annesspublishing.com

If you like the images in this book and would like to investigate using
them for publishing, promotions or advertising, please visit our website
www.practicalpictures.com for more information.

Publisher: Joanna Lorenz
Editorial Director: Helen Sudell
Project Editors: Ann Kay, Joanne Rippin
Jacket Design: SteersMcGillan Design
Design: Nigel Partridge and Design Principals
Illustrator: Sam Elmhurst
Editorial Reader: Rosanna Fairhead

Previously published in two separate volumes, *Total Body Massage*
and *Reiki Healing*.

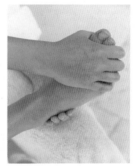
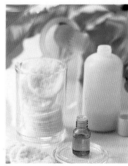

Contents

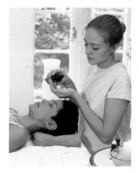
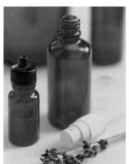

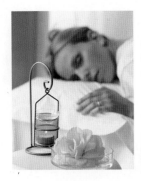
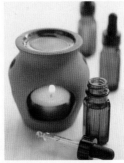
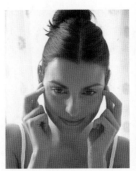
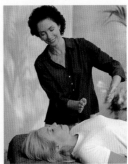

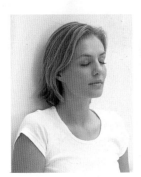
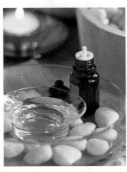
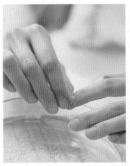
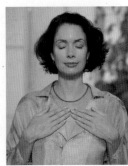

Introduction

Massage is a touch therapy that is not only a wonderfully pleasurable and relaxing experience, but also brings countless health benefits. A massage treatment can relieve tension in the body, calm the mind and nourish the soul, bringing healing on a number of different levels simultaneously.

approaches to massage

In general terms there are two main approaches in massage: those that are "energy"-based, and those that are more concerned with muscular physiology, though the trend is towards increasing integration. Energy-based approaches are influenced by ideas from the East, where it is widely believed that a universal life force runs through the body. In India, energy centres known as "chakras" are believed to run down the centre of the body, each affecting a different aspect of life. In the Far East, life energy is believed to be channelled along "meridians" that run through the body. Energy-based techniques such as shiatsu use thumb or finger pressure at points along the meridians to help release blocked energy, enabling it to flow freely. Reiki is a therapy in which the practitioner channels a form of healing life-force energy for the highest good of the recipient.

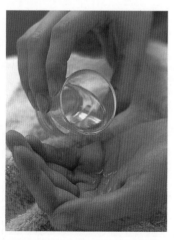

◁ Using a massage medium such as oil or cream will help the massage to flow and be more soothing for the recipient.

In the West, there is more of a tradition of muscular-based massage. This approach is more concerned with physiology and focuses on the muscular-skeletal system. It is generally a fairly firm style of massage, and sports massage has grown out of this tradition.

head massage

With its origins in India, head massage is a relatively new addition to the different types of massage therapy available in the West, yet it is a newcomer that has very rapidly gained popularity.

Head massage is quick to receive, and does not involve undressing or necessarily using oils. It is mess-free, convenient and possible to do almost anywhere. Head massage is also effective in dealing with a range of physical and emotional complaints, especially those that are stress-related, while it can also form an essential part of body-care routines.

body massage

The fast pace of modern life, combined with a sedentary lifestyle and an emphasis on mental activity, puts the whole body under a great strain. Body massage involves a flowing sequence of soothing and stimulating strokes combined to bring a harmonious state of relaxation and invigoration. Massaging much larger areas of the body can bring greater relief to body systems, and can be used to work on specific problems and stresses, as well as improving energy levels.

foot massage

A foot massage can be highly therapeutic, particularly for those of us who spend much of our lives on our feet and they tend to take a huge amount of stress. Massage

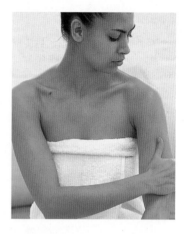

△ Learning the techniques of self-massage pays dividends at the end of a hard day, especially after a relaxing bath.

techniques for the feet are similar to those used elsewhere on the body, but need to be adapted for maximum effectiveness. Massage is equally good for relaxing and invigorating feet, especially when specific aromatherapy oils are used, while there are also routines for the feet and legs that improve circulation and general well-being. For a complete foot workout, massage may be used alongside reflexology and acupressure, which aim to free blockages in vital energy pathways, easing everything from a headache to a sluggish immune system.

aromatherapy

Increasingly, essential plant oils are used in massage for specific therapeutic effects. Known as aromatherapy, this is a lighter style of massage and focuses on introducing the aromatic oils into the body via the skin. This type of massage is popular for its "feel-good" factor, as well as being effective in treating emotional or mental problems.

Increased synthesis between the approaches of East and West has resulted in many massage therapists using energy work and meditation in their practice.

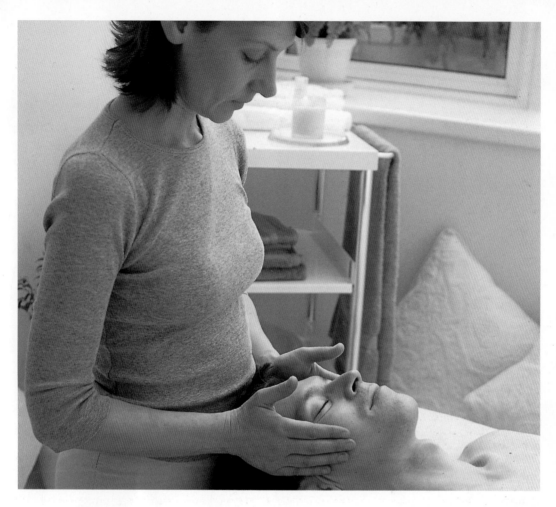

△ While the hands relax and soothe the body and mind, the oils work their intrinsic aromatic magic, to uplift the spirits and balance the whole system.

about this book

This book begins with an overview of the history of massage and goes on to explain the power of touch and how massage affects our body systems. It shows how massage can be used to treat the symptoms of stress – at home and at work – or to alleviate common conditions such as asthma, insomnia and headaches.

Clear information is given on the basic massage strokes, and by following the step-by-step instructions you are guided through massages for every part of your body from head to toe.

Each section is divided into chapters on techniques, the massages and therapeutic treatments. Some step-by-step sequences are also included for self-massage, as well as shorter, stress-busting treatments that can be used throughout the day.

This book makes massage accessible and easy to integrate into your everyday life. By including chapters on energy-based systems, such as reiki and shiatsu, as well as a chapter on meditation, its aim is to encourage a truly holistic approach to caring for ourselves and others. As you work on the body with sensitivity and awareness, changes can be effected throughout the

body's systems, engendering relaxation and peace of mind, and harmonizing body and soul.

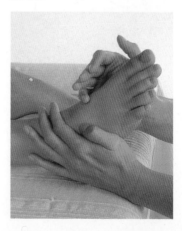

▷ A foot massage can be simply relaxing, or you can use reflexology techniques to help balance the body and clear energy blockages.

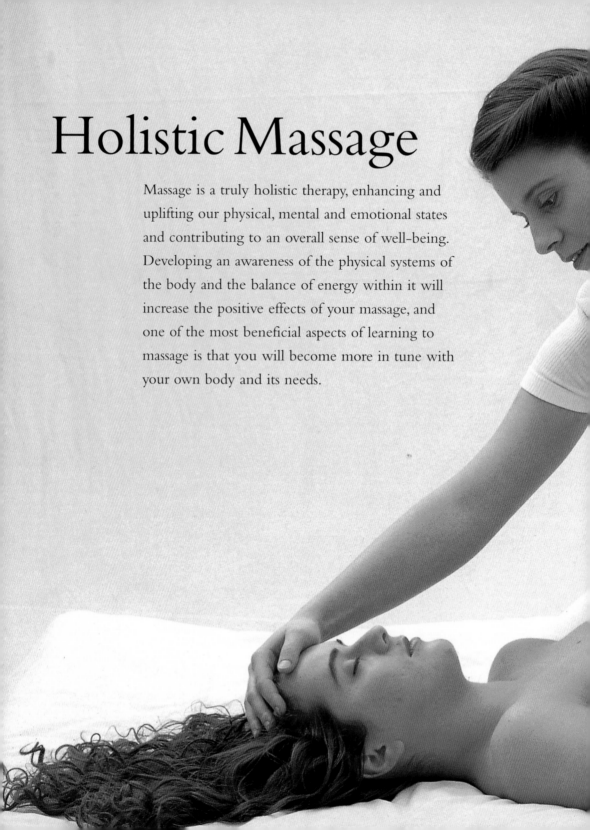

Holistic Massage

Massage is a truly holistic therapy, enhancing and uplifting our physical, mental and emotional states and contributing to an overall sense of well-being. Developing an awareness of the physical systems of the body and the balance of energy within it will increase the positive effects of your massage, and one of the most beneficial aspects of learning to massage is that you will become more in tune with your own body and its needs.

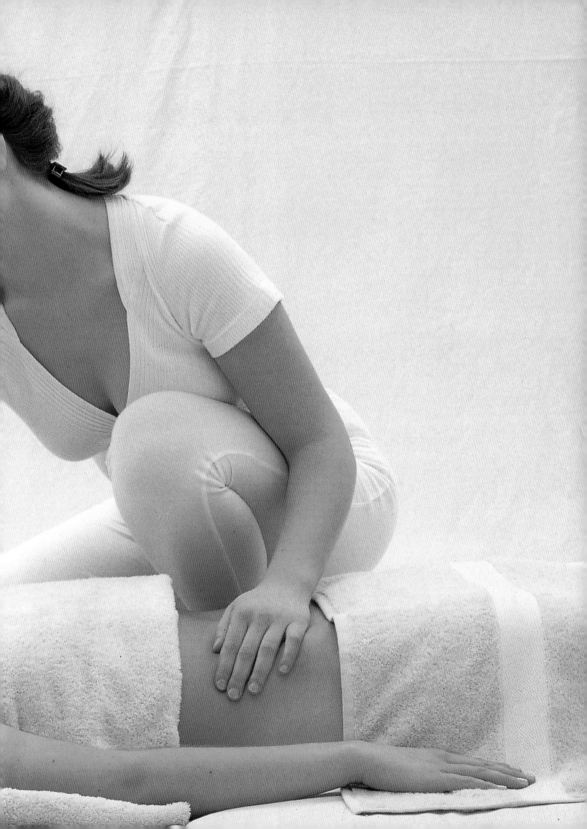

Massage in history

Massage is one of the oldest therapies in the world, and to discover its precise origins is almost impossible. The use of touch for grooming, stroking and rubbing is a behaviour that we share with many animals. Touch is instinctive, and from here it is a small step to develop this natural ability into a healing art. There is evidence that every culture throughout the world has used massage in some form or other, and every language, ancient or modern, has a word for massage. In the East the tradition of massage has always been unbroken, although its practice has been more staggered and erratic in Western cultures.

the ancient and classical world

Ancient Chinese medical texts, dating back some 5,000 years, advocate stroking the body to "protect against colds, keep the organs supple and prevent minor ailments".

Another text contains information that is akin to the passive limb movements used in modern Swedish massage. In India, Ayurvedic scripts from around 4,000 years ago also recommend rubbing the body to treat and prevent disease. Since then massage has been inextricably linked with Indian culture. For instance, it is customary for a bride and groom to receive a massage before their wedding day, and most Indian mothers are taught how to massage their newborn babies and young children.

In ancient Egypt, *bas-relief* carvings dating back more than 4,000 years show Pharaoh Ptah-Hotep receiving a leg massage from a male servant, while centuries later, Queen Cleopatra is recorded as enjoying a foot

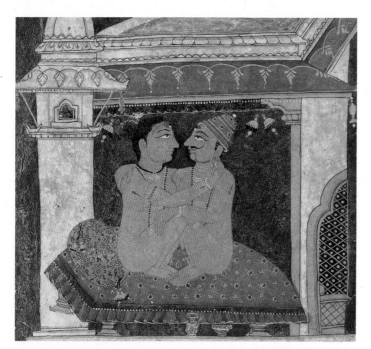

▽ The Kama Sutra and ancient Ayurvedic scripts contain many references to sensual massage, which was used for pleasure, spiritual practice and general health and well-being.

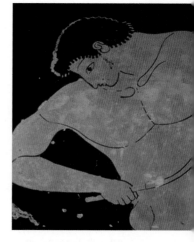

△ The Greeks used oil to cleanse themselves before bathing and massage. Here an athlete in a gymnasium removes the oil from his body.

massage during dinner parties. However, enjoyment of massage was not restricted to the wealthy. Ancient records show that even the lowliest Egyptian workers were paid in wages of body oil sufficient for daily use.

For the ancient Greeks, the pursuit of physical excellence was paramount, and massage played an intrinsic part in their exaltation of the body. Their famous medical centres, or gymnasia, contained open-air training rooms, sports grounds and massage rooms. In ancient Greece, massage was highly recommended for treating fatigue, sports or war injuries, as well as illness. Writing in the 5th century BC, Hippocrates, the reputed "father of modern medicine", stated that a successful physician must be experienced in the art of "rubbing", and prescribed a scented bath followed by a daily massage with oils as the pathway to good health and fitness.

The Romans were equally fond of massage and incorporated it into their bathing rituals. For the wealthy, it was

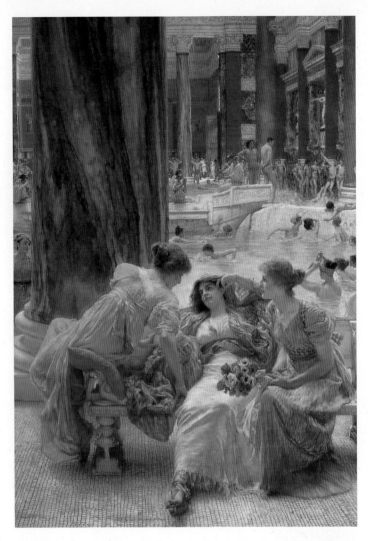

▷ The Roman Empire placed great value on bodily pleasures and rituals, including massage and cleansing, which were practised in the ubiquitous Roman baths.

customary to attend the baths and have stiff muscles rubbed with warm vegetable oil. This was followed by a full body massage to awaken the nerves, get the circulation going and mobilize the joints. The routine was completed as fine oil was liberally applied all over the body to nourish the skin and keep it fine and smooth. Physicians also promoted the therapeutic benefits of massage. One of the most famous of these was Galen (AD130–201), who wrote books on massage, exercise and health. He also classified different massage strokes, and used massage in the treatment of many diseases.

the Middle Ages and beyond

After the decline of the Roman Empire, the Arab world became the centre of learning and culture. The works of Hippocrates, Galen and other famous physicians were translated into Arabic, preserving the medical knowledge built up since antiquity. Avicenna (980–1037), one of the greatest Arab physicians, added to this knowledge and went on to describe the use of healing plants, spinal manipulation and various forms of massage in great detail.

Meanwhile, in Europe, touch became associated with "carnal pleasures" in the eyes of the Catholic Church, and massage was denounced as a highly sinful activity. Its practice was consigned to the realm of folklore, and knowledge was passed down through the female line – the local "wise woman" or midwife – along with knowledge of herbs and other healing remedies. This information was regarded with suspicion and could lead to persecution as a witch.

The Renaissance saw a revival of interest in classical medicine, and massage gradually became more respected by mainstream society. Ambroise Paré, a 16th-century physician to the French court, used massage in his practice. European journeys of exploration also revealed how other cultures valued massage. Captain Cook described

how massage cured his sciatic pains in Tahiti, and in the 1800s there are records of the Cherokee and Navaho peoples of North America using massage on their warriors.

towards the modern age

However, it was at the end of the 19th century that a Swedish gymnast, Per Henrik Ling (1776–1839), restored to favour therapeutic massage in Europe. Having cured himself of rheumatism, Ling developed a system of massage that was based on physiology, gymnastic movements and massage. Receiving royal patronage for his work, Ling's methods laid the foundation for modern physiotherapy with the

establishment in 1894 of the Society of Trained Masseurs. A few years later, St George's Hospital in London opened a massage department, and "Swedish" massage therapy soon became part of mainstream medical practice.

This emphasis continued unchecked until the 1960s, when personal growth centres, notably the Esalen Institute in California, adapted massage therapy into a holistic treatment that could balance mind, body and emotions, rather than simply relieving muscular aches and pains. This holistic approach is now widely used alongside mainstream medicine to complement conventional medical treatments.

The power of touch

Touch is a basic human instinct and it has the power to comfort and reassure on many levels. It can relax the body, calm the mind and encourage healing and well-being.

a natural impulse

To touch others or to be touched is one of our most instinctive needs. The sense of touch is the first to develop in the embryo, and babies require and thrive on close physical contact with their mothers and fathers. The caring, loving touch of another is fundamental to the development of a healthy human being. This need to be touched does not stop as childhood ends, yet as we grow to adulthood many of us become afraid to reach out and touch one another. Mistrustful of our instinctive loving impulse, we have lost touch with ourselves and with the wisdom of the body. One of the most appealing aspects of practising therapeutic touch techniques is that we can begin to re-establish contact with ourselves – and others – in a way that is safe, caring and non-intrusive.

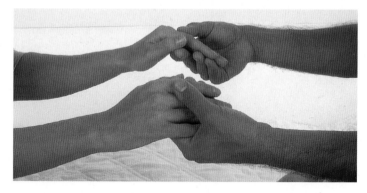

△ It is a natural reaction to reach out and touch, very often with the intention of soothing and comforting, so it is not surprising that the hands have come to be seen by many as the focus and centre for healing energies.

benefits of touch

Awareness of the therapeutic value of touch is growing and many touch therapies are widely used in conventional healthcare to treat pain, ease discomfort and to improve the functional workings of the body. Given the pressures of modern-day living and the increased incidence of stress-related illness, touch therapies also have an important part to play in everyday life. Aching backs and shoulders after a tiring day at work hunched over a computer or spending most of the day on your feet, strained leg muscles after excessive exercise, or circulatory problems from a sedentary lifestyle are some of the occupational hazards of adult life. Through the healing power of touch we can learn to

take better care of ourselves. Taking time to channel healing energy or enjoy a soothing foot massage can ease some of the day-to-day tensions of life and put us back in touch with ourselves and our priorities, to feel relaxed and at home in our bodies.

touch therapy

Working on both physical and psychological levels, massage has the ability to relax and invigorate the person receiving it. While the

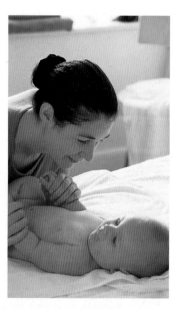

◁ For a baby, being touched, washed, held, carried, caressed and dressed is a fundamental part of existence, and touch is essential for healthy growth and development, both physical and emotional.

▷ Most of us, almost unconsciously, rub tense, aching muscles to bring comfort and relief.

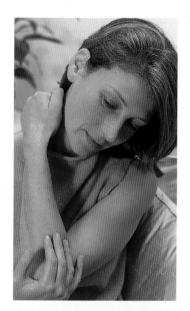

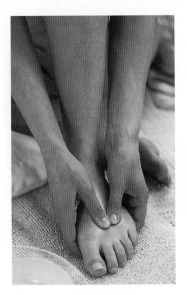

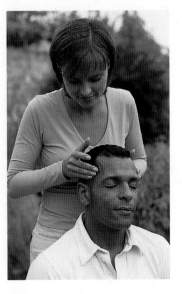

◁ Our hands are a vital tool in daily body care. Touch can help us identify problem areas, as well as keeping skin healthy and smooth.

▷ Massage contributes to our minimum daily touch requirements, now recognized as fundamental to good health and well-being.

emotional health

Massage provides a safe and neutral situation in which to receive loving touch and stimulation of the skin senses, which are so important for emotional health and self-esteem. Touch is fundamental to the development of a healthy human being, and touch deprivation in the early stages of life is known to inhibit the emotional and physical growth of a child. Since touch is so bound up with the emotions, it can also lead to feelings of vulnerability, so massage needs to be practised in a safe environment, with great care and sensitivity. A loving touch can heal, share empathy, and comfort, and massage should combine skilful techniques with loving touch, so that as the hands stroke the body, they unlock not only the physical tensions trapped in muscles, but also acknowledge, with complete acceptance, the essence of the

techniques and strokes of massage can ease pain or tension from stiff and aching muscles, boost a sluggish circulation, or eliminate toxins, the nurturing touch of the hands on the body soothes away mental stress and restores emotional equilibrium at the same time. As tensions dissolve there is an ensuing integration between the physical body and underlying emotions, which breaks the vicious cycle of tension between mind and body.

soothing hands

Massage allows time for the replenishment of innate resources of vital energy. This is particularly relevant in a modern world when stress is known to be the root cause of many serious physical and mental conditions. Stress is a natural factor of life, and moderate levels of stress can be beneficial for certain activities. However, if stress is not discharged appropriately, or is suffered for a prolonged period of time, it robs the body of health and energy. Stress can also lower the natural defences of the body's immune system and its ability to fight disease. When a person is constantly exposed to the adverse effects of stress, anxiety, depression, lethargy, insomnia, and panic attacks can result. Increasingly, both the medical profession and the public recognize the benefits of massage as a successful treatment of symptoms arising from stress.

person within. While massage itself is active, the underlying quality of the touch is one of stillness and calm, a sense of being totally present with that person. For all these reasons, massage is a highly beneficial therapy, because it helps the person receiving it to feel safe enough to relax completely and unwind from the deepest parts of the mind.

▽ Throughout life, touch has the power to comfort, reassure and relax.

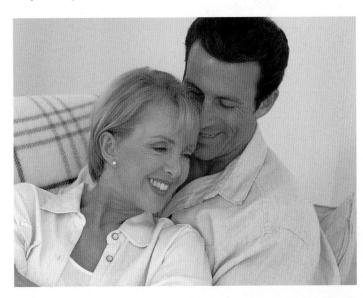

How massage works

On a physiological level, massage affects all the body systems, resulting in improved general functioning, as well as relieving specific conditions. It can also assist with self-esteem, release emotional blocks, increase mental clarity, and help you to connect with your "inner light". Having a massage is simultaneously relaxing and refreshing. It is about taking time out to restore harmony and well-being so that you feel ready to take on the world again.

body systems
The skin is the body's largest sensory organ. When it is touched, thousands of tiny nerve receptors on its surface send messages to the brain via the central nervous system. The brain interprets these messages and returns them to the muscles. Stroking can trigger the release of endorphins (the body's natural painkillers) and send messages of calm and relaxation. More vigorous massage works on the body's underlying muscles, easing tension and stiffness.

▽ A soothing self-massage of tired legs and feet can relieve muscle tension, improve circulation and calm and relax the whole body.

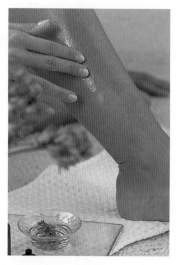

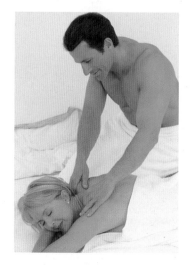

physical benefits
A sound circulatory system is vital for the healthy functioning of the whole body. Massage causes breathing to deepen and the blood vessels and capillaries to dilate, which boosts the circulation and helps oxygenate the blood. Improved circulation also means that vital nutrients are carried around the body more effectively, while temporarily

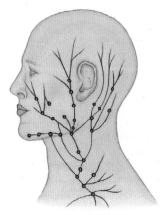

△ Lymph nodes and ducts in the face and neck help eliminate toxins. Massage stimulates the effectiveness of this cleansing action.

◁ Regular massage is a good immunity booster. Research has shown that it can have a protective effect on the body for up to a week after a single treatment.

reducing blood pressure and pulse rate and so relaxing and calming the body and mind. Massage stimulates the functioning of the skin's sebaceous and sweat glands that work together to moisturize, clean and cool it. Massage also has an exfoliating action, helping to eliminate dead skin cells and thus resulting in a fresher appearance to the skin. Boosting the circulation improves the supply of necessary nutrients needed for healthy hair, nails and skin, and can also help relieve a range of problems including headaches and digestive disorders.

Massage also has a direct benefit on the body's muscular structure. By relaxing and stretching muscles that have become contracted and shortened with tension, massage helps the body to regain its flexibility as the elasticity and mobility of the body tissues is restored. These actions can help to ease painful muscles and improve posture by helping to bring the body's musculature back into a more balanced position. It can also help to restore muscles that have become weak and flaccid through underuse. The physical action of massage also works directly on the lymphatic system, helping the body eliminate lactic acid and other chemical wastes that contribute to pain and discomfort in the joints and muscles. Many lymphatic nodes are situated in the neck, back of the head, face and jaw.

As a massage treatment progresses and the body relaxes more deeply, there is a gradual switching over in body functioning towards the parasympathetic nervous system. This system operates outside of our conscious control and is related to the hidden work of general maintenance and repair, and essential functions such as digestion and elimination. We are often in

▽ Blood is transported around the body by a complex network of arteries (shown in red) and veins (shown in blue). Massage increases peripheral circulation and assists blood flow through the system.

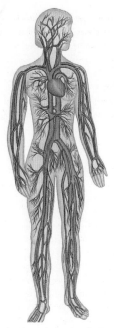

▽ Movement in the body is produced by the action of muscles. It is these skeletal muscles that register discomfort, or ache when we get tired or put them under strain. Massage works directly on these key muscle groups.

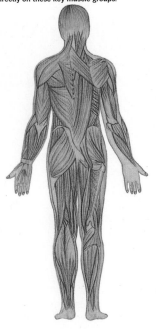

▽ Messages are transmitted between the brain and receptors and nerves through the body's "wiring system", which runs via the spinal cord. These include messages of relaxation from massage action.

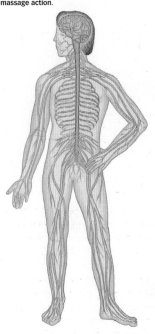

so much of a rush that we don't give our bodies enough time for this important work. Massage is a good way of giving the body a "pit stop", where it can attend to its inner workings.

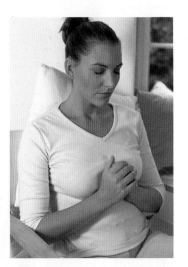

mind and emotions

An extensive body of research supports the therapeutic claims of massage, with growing evidence that it can contribute to the relief of conditions such as stress, depression and anxiety. Head massage in particular has a significant impact on a mental level. The physical release of muscular tension and the increased blood supply to the head results in improved mental functioning and a greater sense of clarity. There is a reduction in mental exhaustion, feelings of irritability or being overwhelmed and a corresponding increase in alertness, mental agility, concentration and insightfulness.

Massage is also valued for its "feel-good" factor. As the body releases tension, a weight is lifted, leading to an increased sense of lightness and happiness. These emotional shifts correspond to the hormonal changes

◁ Glowing hair and skin, relaxed muscle tone and an upright, balanced posture are some of the visible benefits of massage.

that occur in the body during a massage treatment. Research indicates that the level of stress hormones such as cortisol falls during massage, while the level of feel-good bonding hormones, such as oxytocin, significantly increases. Stress hormones have a weakening effect on the immune system.

nourishing the soul

Massage can also work on the energetic balance of the body through the chakra system, which centres around its spiritual dimension. By aligning body and soul through massage, a deep sense of peace, calm and balance can be achieved. The sense of lightness that people often feel after a treatment can also bring an increased awareness of their spiritual identity or inner light. After a massage, people often feel more at one with themselves. Some people report an improved perspective on life, the return of their sense of humour, or say that they are simply more relaxed and comfortable within their own bodies.

Energy work

There is more to the body than meets the eye. As you approach another person, they may be able to sense your presence before you touch them. That is because you have entered their "energy field" or aura, the invisible vibrations that radiate from our bodies. The stronger and healthier we are, the bigger and more expansive our aura; when we are tired or sick, this field is smaller and closer to the body. The chakra system is part of this energy field and some understanding of it is useful in massage. Although you may not be able to see it, you will be affecting the way it functions through your touch.

health and the chakras

The chakras represent energy points in the body. The word *chakra* means "wheel" in Sanskrit, indicating that the chakras are like

▽ Spiritual awareness is part of Eastern culture, and in India it is commonplace to see the "third eye" marked by wearing a bindi.

spinning vortexes, receiving energy from the universe and transforming it to be utilized by the body. In energy-based medicine, the first signs of ill health are believed to show up as blockages or disturbances in the chakras. If these imbalances are not sorted out then the issue will eventually show up as a physical problem. Keeping the chakras working effectively is important for good health.

the chakra system

There are seven major chakras, each having its own characteristics and correspondences. They are found at points that run up the body from the base of the spine to the top of the head, and can be located on the front and back of the body. Each chakra is associated with different organs and systems of the body and with a different colour, although there are some variations according to which chakra system you are using. It is a dynamic and ever-changing interaction of energies.

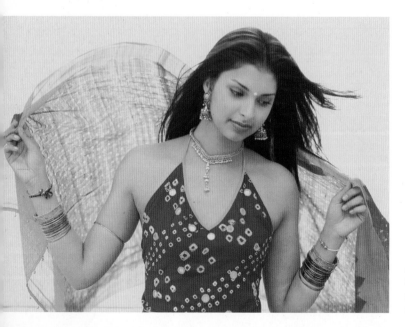

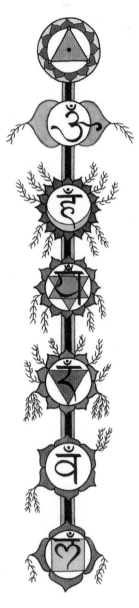

△ The seven major chakras are energy centres for accessing and distributing *chi* or *prana* or life force around the body through the system of meridian channels.

to the thyroid, ears, nose and throat, the neck and teeth. Physical release points are in the neck, shoulders, fingers and toes.

The "third eye" chakra is located in the middle of the forehead or the brow. Its energy release points are in the eyes, temples, forehead and at the base of the skull. It is concerned with the development and deepening of intuition and soul knowledge. It regulates the energies of the pituitary and nervous systems, as well as the brain, head, eyes and face.

The crown chakra is located at the top of the head. Its energy release points are in the head, hands and feet. It is concerned with higher consciousness and spirituality.

working with the chakras

As you massage, you can become aware of these energy centres, especially when working near the areas of the body where they reside. At the end of a treatment, when your partner is still, you could experiment by using "holds" over one or two chakras. To do this, place one hand gently over the other and let them rest lightly over a chakra spot for a few moments. Follow your intuition when choosing each spot. For instance, if you sense your partner needs comfort and reassurance, then you may feel drawn to the heart chakra in the middle of the upper back. Or if your partner has communication issues, then a gentle holding on the throat chakra at the back of the neck may be helpful. As you "hold" imagine healing energy flowing from your heart chakra down your arms and out of your hands into your partner, and intend that it goes where it is most needed.

When you have finished, take your hands away slowly and carefully. See if you can feel your partner's energy field and notice the point at which your hands finally leave it. It is likely that after a treatment their energy field will have expanded, as the chakras have become more balanced and their energies are flowing more efficiently.

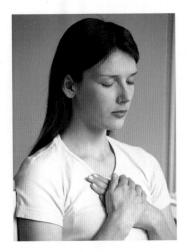

△ Resting your hands over your heart centre and breathing into the hold will help you feel your own heart energy through which love and healing forces flow.

the seven chakras

The base chakra, at the base of the spine, is related to the testicles or ovaries in some systems, and in others to the adrenal glands.

The sacral chakra is located in the lower abdomen and is associated with emotions and sensuality.

The solar plexus chakra, found at the front of the body between the bottom of the ribcage and the navel, is related to personal energy and power. It is associated with the adrenal glands and the pancreas.

Roughly halfway up the spine, the heart chakra corresponds to unconditional love, compassion and friendship. It relates to the thymus, heart, lungs, bronchial tubes, upper back and the arms. Physical release points are in the shoulders, the intercostal muscles of the ribs, the upper arms, under the chin and at the base of the skull.

The throat chakra is located at the base of the neck where it connects to the shoulders. It is concerned with all forms of communication and self-expression. It relates

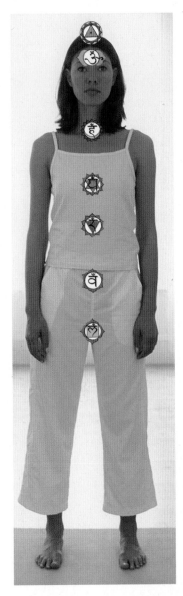

△ The chakras are located in key areas and these energy centres nourish, and have correspondences with, the physical and emotional dimensions of the whole person.

Massage systems

There are various approaches to the art of healing through touch, massage, and bodywork. Some systems focus directly on the physiology of the body, and others on the release of emotional tension. Others work more subtly on energy levels within the body. These days, many touch therapies combine ancient and modern techniques drawn from both the East and the West. What they all have in common is the aim to bring harmony and well-being to the recipients by releasing tension and congestion, thereby allowing the restoration of natural vitality.

soft tissue massage

This system makes use of a variety of techniques to stroke and manipulate the skin and the superficial muscles and tissues in order to alleviate pain and tension. The strokes themselves help to boost the circulatory system and increase the exchange of tissue fluids. Variations such as Swedish massage, sports massage, physiotherapy and lymphatic massage are particularly beneficial for these purposes, as they work directly with the anatomy and physiology of the body to restore vitality and a state of relaxation.

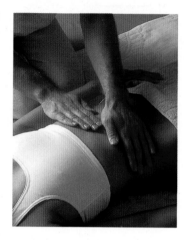

◁ Soft tissue massage uses a variety of techniques to stroke and manipulate the skin and the superficial muscles and tissues to alleviate pain and tension, and restore vitality.

Holistic massage also works with the body's soft tissue, but is generally more concerned with psychological relaxation. Soporific strokes predominate, lulling the mind, calming the nervous system, and restoring a sense of equilibrium, thereby producing an inner release of tension. A nourishing touch and the delivery of massage in an atmosphere of loving care is seen as the main medium of transformation. A holistic session can also combine the strokes of therapeutic and remedial massage, but its main emphasis always remains on relaxing the body and mind.

deep tissue massage

The aim of deep tissue massage is to restore structural alignment and balance within the body by releasing chronic tensions, formed by deep muscular tension, which inhibit postural ease and movement. It works mainly on the body's connective tissue, or fascia, which wraps, binds, supports and separates all the internal structures, including the skeletal muscles, bones, tendons, ligaments and organs. This muscular "armour" in the body may be the result of injury, habitual bad posture, or the repression of emotions.

Connective tissue is present throughout the entire internal structure of the body, and is best recognized by its shiny white fibres, which are formed mainly from a type of protein called collagen. When the body is free of trauma (injury) and tension, the fascia is generally elastic, but if the system is sluggish or inactive, or muscular armour has formed in the body, the fascia can become rigid and immobile. Since connective tissue envelops and connects every internal structure, tension in one area can have a detrimental effect on the whole system.

Deep tissue massage strokes manipulate the fascia by the action of friction and stretching, releasing blocks that impede the flow of energy and life force throughout the whole body. This is a skill that requires a professional training and a thorough

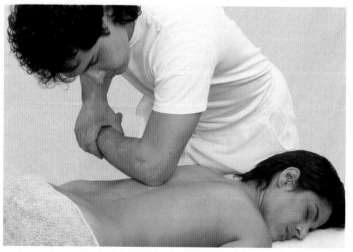

◁ A deep tissue massage may involve applying pressure from the elbow or forearm to sink into the connective tissue before stretching and manipulating it.

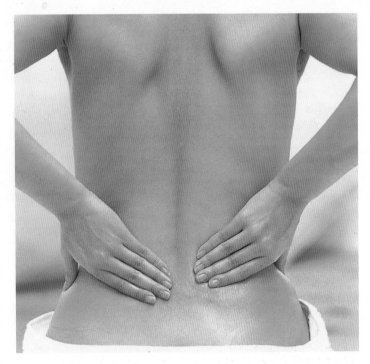

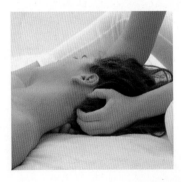

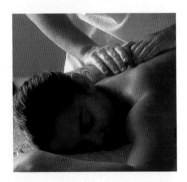

▷ Self-massage can give you a physical and a psychological boost. It is also invaluable for gaining confidence to treat others by practising massage techniques on your own body.

knowledge of anatomy and physiology. While the strokes penetrate the body at a deeper level than in soft tissue massage, the practitioner's hands must work with great sensitivity and patience, and the client must be willing to release tension. Causing undue pain in the attempt to free the body from tension is counter-productive, as the neuro-muscular response of the tissues will be to contract in defence.

Deep tissue massage is usually based over a series of at least 10 sessions, so that the whole structure of the body can be balanced and realigned. In the process of breaking down chronic tensions, breathing becomes deeper and the body regains its vitality and feeling. Emotions and memories that have been repressed within the body by the muscular armour may be released. It is important, therefore, for a deep tissue bodyworker to be aware of the psychosomatic link between the emotions and physical tension, and to understand that behind the most defended areas of the body there is a great deal of vulnerability.

A deep tissue practitioner may use the thumbs, fingers, knuckles and forearms to stretch and manipulate the fascia. Pressure is applied slowly, and in conjunction with the client's awareness and breathing.

▽ Rolfing can appear to be quite rough, as the connective tissue is manipulated using deep tissue massage techniques.

The tissue is then stretched and moved in specific directions, depending on its location in the body. By ungluing and freeing the fibres, the tissue becomes warm and revitalized, and returns to its natural fluidity. When the whole body is treated systematically in a series of sessions it is able to regain its vitality, structural alignment, and ease of movement.

There are a number of schools of deep tissue bodywork. The most established of these is rolfing, also known as structural integration, which was founded in the United States by Ida Rolf. Rolf pioneered many new techniques in her work with connective tissue, and it is her profound understanding of its role in the body's structural balance that has laid the foundations for the ensuing development of connective tissue massage.

head massage

For centuries, head massage has played an essential part in Ayurvedic medicine, widely practised throughout India and some parts of Asia. In India it is still a regular aspect of daily life, and head massage is frequently practised on street corners. However, this ancient art is also highly practical and relevant to the Western world.

Head massage combines energy-based pressure-point techniques with more traditional massage strokes such as rubbing and stroking, thus working on the body's energy system as well as its physical structure. In addition to focusing on the head, it also targets the upper back, shoulders and neck area – significant places in the body where we store tension.

▽ Head massage is particularly helpful for relieving tension commonly found in the upper back, shoulders and neck areas.

foot massage

Like head massage, foot massage has become increasingly popular in recent years because it is simple, fast and effective, as it focuses on a relatively small area of the body.

The feet are highly sensitive and very responsive to touch: they contain more than 14,000 nerve endings between them. Foot massage uses a combination of the energy-based pressure-point techniques of acupressure and reflexology and more traditional massage strokes aimed at relaxing and soothing as well as improving circulation. A foot massage can be carried out as a quick-fix soother, using an appropriate aromatherapy blend, after a busy day's shopping. Combined with the principles of reflexology it can also be used to treat a range of problems and disorders.

reflexology

A reflexologist believes that energy is channelled through the body along specific paths, or meridians. When a person is

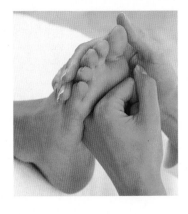

△ Foot massage is easy to learn and quick to apply. A soft-tissue massage using a relaxing oil blend and soothing, flowing strokes can be highly therapeutic.

healthy, energy moves freely along these channels. However, if the energy is impeded or blocked through tension, congestion, imbalance, or sluggishness within the system, then all those organs and internal structures that lie in the energy path have the potential to succumb to disease.

Reflexologists maintain that an individual's health can be restored when pressure is applied to certain points on the body, generally the feet and sometimes the hands. This helps to unblock the energy channel, thereby having a revitalizing effect on all the organs, glands and other structures that lie within its zone.

Reflexologists divide the body into 10 vertical zones, 5 on each side of the medial line that runs from the top of the head to the tips of the fingers and toes. Although the pressure-point therapy can be applied on the hands, the treatment is usually more effective when used on the feet.

The technique involves applying pressure to the reflex points on the sole or palm, sides, and top of each foot or hand in turn, for up to three seconds – using the top or side of the thumb or finger to apply pressure – before walking, or inching, the digit to its next position. The foot or hand must be securely held and supported, and leverage applied by the fingers or thumb opposing the movement.

While no scientific explanation, as yet, can be given to explain exactly how reflexology works, it is widely accepted as a successful treatment for a number of ailments. When applied skilfully the techniques can help to relax and invigorate the entire physiology of the body, stimulating the nervous system and the blood circulation, and boosting the elimination of toxins, in addition to clearing congestion within the organs. Reflexology is now firmly established as a complementary healing art.

acupressure

An ancient Chinese therapy, acupressure is based on very similar principles to acupuncture. In common with acupuncture and reflexology, it is based on the belief that the body's energy flows through channels called meridians.

Acupressure uses the same points as acupuncture, but instead of using needles, it uses the fingers to apply gentle but firm pressure on the key points. This pressure stimulates the flow of energy and helps to release blockages, thus alleviating many common complaints and disorders and restoring harmony and balance to the body, mind and spirit.

▽ A qualified reflexologist will be able to detect or locate a disorder in a corresponding body part because of tenderness or the accumulation of granular deposits at certain points of the foot.

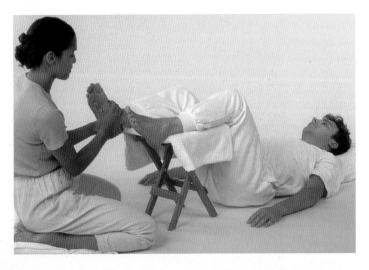

▽ The bladder meridian is the largest in the body and runs down each side of the spine to the back of the pelvis. In acupressure, a steady thumb pressure applied on the sacral points can relieve sciatica and lower-back pain.

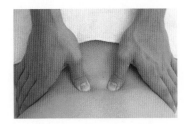

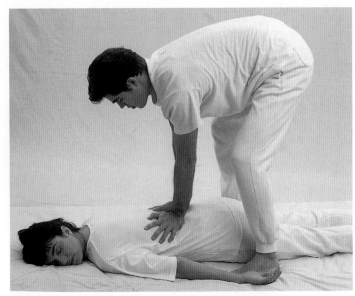

▷ The shiatsu therapist also uses the palms and heels of the hands to press firmly but gently. Here the focus is on the bladder meridian points.

shiatsu

A relatively modern Japanese body therapy, shiatsu derives its principles from the ancient wisdom of Chinese medicine. It operates on the belief that health is restored when a balance is reached between the energetic forces of yin and yang within the body, mind, and spirit. Yin is feminine and passive, yang is masculine and active. Shiatsu helps to bring a harmony between the yin and yang energies of the body and its internal organs. In shiatsu there are 14 energy meridians, and pressure is applied to key points along those pathways where the energy, or ki (chi), is blocked or over-stimulated. The word "shiatsu" translates literally as "finger pressure", although the practitioner can use the hands, elbows, knees, and feet to apply pressure on specific meridian points to stimulate or massage them. Shiatsu can also incorporate the passive movements of Western osteopathy to stretch and manipulate the joints and ease tension from the major segments of the body, thereby helping to clear congestion in the energy pathways. The aim of shiatsu is to restore a balance in the flow of ki as it interconnects the vital organs.

▷ Passive stretch movements increase the effects of shiatsu treatment by relaxing joints and unblocking congested energy meridians.

Shiatsu works on our ki or life force, which maintains and nurtures our physical body and so also affects our mind and spirit. The flow of ki can be disturbed by external trauma such as injury or internal trauma such as anxiety or stress.

The shiatsu practitioner assesses the client's health through observation, or by taking a case history. Steady weight is then applied to the key points of the relevant meridian for up to 10 seconds before slowly releasing the pressure. A whole body session can be given as a maintenance treatment or to detect an imbalance between the organs.

Ancient and modern techniques drawn from traditions of the East and the West can be combined to provide truly holistic massage therapy for body, mind and spirit.

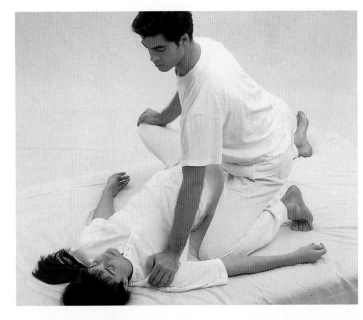

Body awareness and visualization

Massage is an ongoing process of learning about the human body in all its holistic aspects, and the best place to explore the relationship between mind, body and spirit is within your own body.

If you are giving massage on a regular basis it is important that your body is strong and flexible. Exercise regularly to relax and strengthen your muscles and, in particular, to provide support for your spine and back. Visualizations will help you contact your energy resources and cleanse and relax your body, mind and spirit.

exercises for strength, flexibility and energy

The following exercises will help you to learn how to breathe deeply and synchronize your breathing with your movements, so that your strokes become fluid and you remain energized. The more you learn about your own body, the better able you will be to pass on that knowledge through your massage to help others.

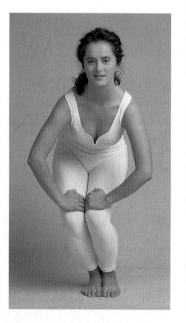

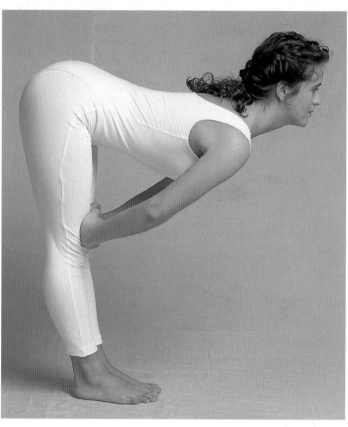

creating a stable foundation

Your legs help you to maintain a balanced and stable posture as you massage. They provide a firm but flexible foundation to support your body weight and to connect you to the ground, so that you can release tension away from your spine and back as you work. This exercise helps you gently to warm and loosen the ankle and knee joints, areas that are vital to structural support.

◁ **1** Rest your hands on your knees without straining your shoulders. Place your feet together and, bending your knees, rotate them in circles, first in one direction and then in the other. Begin with small circular movements and gradually make larger ones as your joints and muscles warm up.

△ **2** Straighten the knees slowly and gently press your abdomen down in the direction of the floor to create a stretch in the hamstrings at the back of your legs. Alternate this step with the knee circles carried out in step 1, repeating them two more times.

warming up

You will probably not have time to do all these exercises before every massage session, but it is a good idea to combine at least one or two of the sequences as a warm-up and to focus your mind.

breath and movement

The next exercise is a series of continuous flowing movements adapted from the t'ai chi form, a Chinese martial art. It helps to create stability and strength in the legs, while making pushing movements with the arms and hands. The complete motion is made in conjunction with your cycle of inhaling and exhaling. This makes the exercise particularly appropriate when learning how to apply long effleurage strokes with a graceful posture and synchronized breathing.

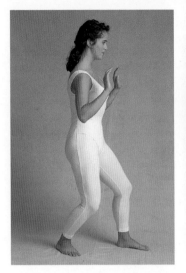

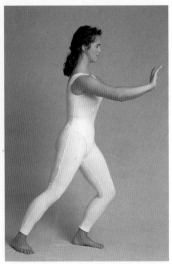

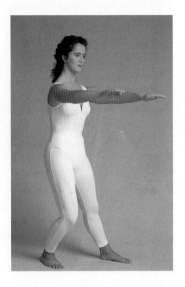

△ **1** Begin with the basic stance of good posture, keeping both feet parallel and the knees slightly flexed. Step forwards with the front foot and turn the back foot out at an angle of 45 degrees. As you breathe in, bend your elbows and draw both hands to chest level, palms facing outwards.

△ **2** Keeping both feet flat on the floor and the spine erect, transfer your weight to the front foot and push your hands away from your body while you exhale. Your torso should be facing in the direction of your front foot.

△ **3** As you inhale, move your weight to the back foot, allowing your body and arms to swing around to face the same direction. Draw your hands back to chest level. Continue breathing in as you turn towards the front foot to repeat the full movement again. Repeat 10 times before changing the position of your legs and repeating the full flowing cycle from the other side.

swinging the torso

Limbering up the spine and torso prevents strain and tension from gathering in the back while giving massage. It keeps the body supple, enabling it to turn easily while performing some of the longer strokes. The key to the following exercise is to transfer weight from one foot to the other as you swing around, leaving the other foot feeling "empty" and weightless. Flex both knees so your height never changes during the exercise, and your head rests comfortably on top of your spine. This gentle spinal twist will relax your muscles and nerves and stimulate your breathing.

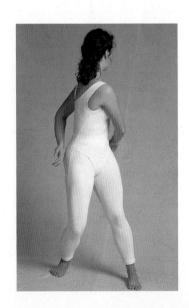

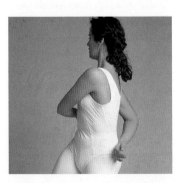

▷ **1** Begin the exercise with your feet parallel, and more than the width of your hips apart. Transfer your weight on to one foot, leaving the other weightless. Swing your torso and arms around to face the "empty" foot, letting your arms flop against the sides of your body.

◁ **2** Swing your torso back to the other side as you transfer your weight across to the other foot. As you turn, relax the gaze of your eyes so they take in a moving picture of your surroundings without fixing on any point.

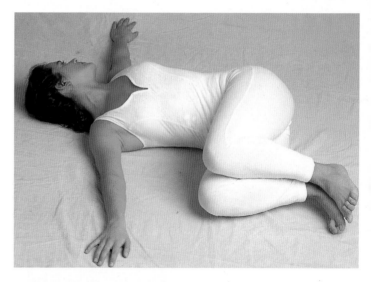

strengthening abdominal muscles

The abdominal muscles flex and support the spine, and it is important to strengthen them in order to safeguard your back while giving massage. A firm but relaxed abdomen will allow tension to sink away from the upper back and shoulders, while stabilizing the lumbar region. The belly is also the source of power and vital energy. These exercises will bring it strength and relaxation, helping you to gain stamina. Perform them slowly and carefully to avoid strain, and gradually build up to 10 complete movements for each exercise.

▷ **1** Lie on your back with your knees bent towards your chest and your feet flexed. Begin to make circles in one direction with your knees, making certain you keep them together. Gradually enlarge the circles, keeping the middle and base of your back in contact with the floor at all times, as this will activate the abdominal muscles. Remain lying down on your back and spread your arms to the sides of your body, palms facing downwards. Bend your knees towards your chest and flex your feet. Breathe in.

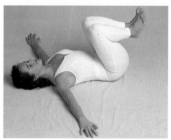

△ **2** Breathe out as you take your knees to one side of the body as far as they will comfortably go, keeping them close together. At the same time, roll your head in the opposite direction. As you inhale, return both head and knees to their original position. Repeat the exercise, moving your head and knees to the other side of the body.

visualizations for healing energy

Visualization is a powerful tool frequently used in healing work. It allows an intuitive use of the imagination to bring about subtle and beneficial changes in the body and mind. Within massage and body awareness work, imagery combined with "good intention" can be used in relaxation exercises as a means of directing the movement of energy within the body, or to "see" and heal its internal structure and physiology.

tuning in to light and energy

When massage is performed with a relaxed posture and breathing, the experience can be equally as nourishing and invigorating for both people involved. If you believe, however, that you are using up all of your own energy while giving a massage, then the experience can sometimes leave you feeling tired or drained. This visualization exercise helps you to replenish your vital resources by opening you up to the idea of a constant stream of energy, or light, that passes through you to your partner. You can practise this during the massage, with or without a partner; it is an excellent way to start or finish a session.

▷ Stand with your feet apart and with your arms slightly out in front of your body, palms facing downwards. As you breathe in, imagine a white light descending through the crown of your head and filling your body with vital energy. Breathe out and visualize the light flowing out of your arms and through your hands to the person beneath them, or towards the ground. As you continue to inhale and exhale, repeat this visualization several times.

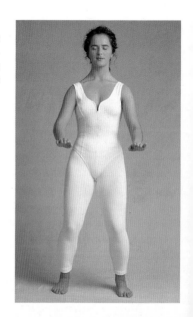

bone breathing

During massage, your hands are mainly in touch with the body's skin, soft tissues, and superficial muscles. However, it is also beneficial to gain a sense of the skeletal structure, which is vital to the body's support and locomotion. Try this exercise to provide a mental image of the bones, and to encourage a sense of relaxation into the core of the physical body.

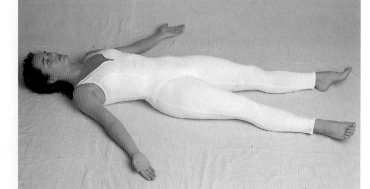

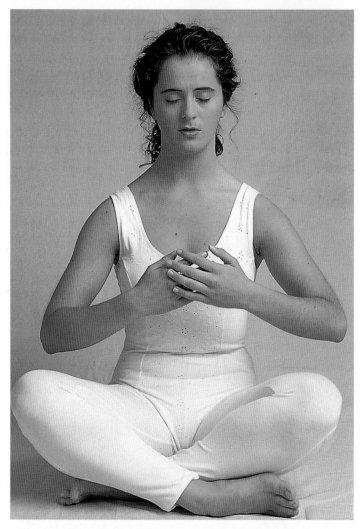

△ Lie on your back. As your breathing deepens, focus your attention on your right leg and consciously relax the muscles from the foot up to the hip. Then try to visualize the bones as they link together from the toes, through to the ankle and knee joint and up to the hip socket. Now imagine that the bones are hollow, so that as you breathe in, a white light is drawn in through the toes and is pulled up through the bones to the top of the leg. As you breathe out, the light returns via the same pathway and out of the body.

Repeat this visualization several times with the right leg before repeating the exercise with the left leg. Finally, breathe in deeply and draw the white light up the right leg and into the belly. Hold your breath for a few moments and breathe out, before sending the light down through the left leg. Reverse the imagery so that you draw the light from the left to the right side of the body. The same visualization can now be applied to the arms and chest.

opening the heart centre

Just as it is essential to connect through breath and awareness to your abdomen during massage – in order to work from your source of power and vital energy – it is also important to allow your heart and feeling centre to open and expand. This allows the essence of life to flow to your hands, enlivening them with a nourishing and healing quality of touch. In this visualization, you imagine that your heart is like the bud of a flower. As you focus your breath towards your heart, allow the flower to open its petals until it fills the whole of your chest.

◁ To help you connect with the heart centre, sit and close your eyes while breathing, holding your hands just in front of your heart.

Cautions and contraindications

Although the massages in this book are well-established, safe techniques for working on the body, as with any therapy, it is important to be aware that there are certain situations where you should be particularly careful or where a treatment may be contraindicated. If you are in any doubt, always ask a doctor or professional therapist for advice before giving any treatment.

At the beginning of the session make sure you have time to ask your partner how they are feeling, and find out if they have any medical conditions and/or are taking any medication. You should also check for any recent injuries, fractures or surgery. If your partner is feeling unwell, it is best to postpone the treatment, as it could aggravate

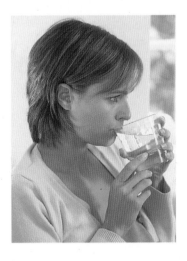

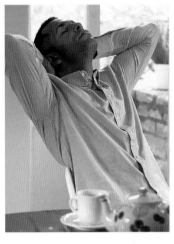

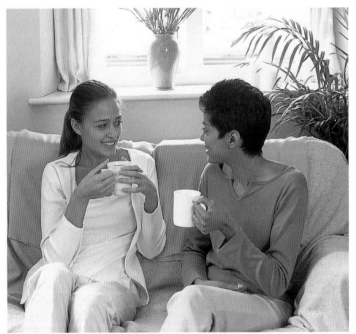

▽ Make sure you take enough time to talk through the massage with your partner to establish a rapport and sort out any concerns he or she may have about the treatment.

△ Drinking a glass of water is a good way to begin and end a massage treatment, as it is cleansing and grounding for the system and will aid the elimination of toxins from the body.

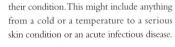

△ If your partner is particularly tense, and their muscles are sore and tender, always make sure you massage with caution in order not to aggravate their discomfort.

their condition. This might include anything from a cold or a temperature to a serious skin condition or an acute infectious disease.

skin conditions

Be aware of any cuts, bruises, open sores, blistering, redness or swelling. These areas will be painful when touched and could become infected, so are best avoided. Any contagious skin conditions, such as ringworm, impetigo, scabies or herpes (cold sores), should also be avoided to prevent the risk of you picking up the infection.

Large areas of bruising on the skin may indicate internal injuries, so massage could be extremely dangerous.

Ringworm is a fungal infection. It begins as small red papules that spread to form red, itchy, shiny circles under the skin over the body. Impetigo is a highly contagious bacterial skin condition, usually found around the mouth, nose and ears, in which raised, fluid-filled sores seep and leave honey coloured crusts on the skin. Scabies is

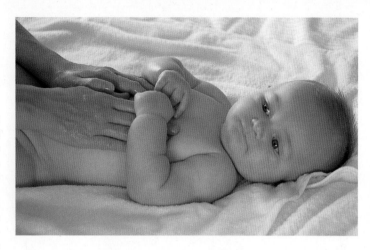

▷ For babies, gentle body and foot massage can be soothing and nurturing. However, as babies' skulls are so delicate, due to the unfused fontanelles, massaging the head is not advisable.

identified by small reddish marks around the wrist and between the fingers, and is very itchy. Herpes is a viral infection that erupts in sores around the mouth and nose, particularly after exposure to the sun or during times of stress.

Eczema and psoriasis may look unsightly, but they are not contagious, and unless the skin is broken, they are not contra-indicated for massage. However, it is best to check with your partner that they find it comfortable to be touched in these areas.

Scalp conditions to be aware of include head lice (nits), ringworm and folliculitis. The latter is a bacterial infection with swelling and pain around the hair follicles.

the skeleton

Conditions relating to the bones and the skeleton, which include brittle bones, osteoporosis and spondylitis, are clearly contraindicated for massage because of the high risk of injury to your partner. Bone diseases, congenital problems and habitual poor posture can cause spinal weakness. In such cases it is advisable to massage only after you have sought medical advice.

You should also be aware of any head, neck or shoulder injuries, such as whiplash. Massage could make these conditions worse, so check with a doctor.

circulatory problems

With high blood pressure there could be a risk of clotting, so always seek medical advice. When this is related to high stress levels, massage can be effective in reducing stress triggers, but do seek medical advice first. Low blood pressure increases the likelihood of feeling faint so make sure your partner gets up slowly after the massage. Recent haemorrhages, a history of thrombosis and embolisms are other blood disorders that can cause problems. Anyone with any of these conditions should not be massaged in the absence of medical supervision. Although massage can be helpful in boosting circulation, varicose veins should be treated with great care and no pressure should be applied to affected areas.

epilepsy

This condition requires medical advice before carrying out any treatment. Epilepsy is normally controlled and stabilized by medication, but it is thought that stimulating massage, particularly to the head, can trigger an attack.

cancer

Massage is contraindicated with cancer, but it is increasingly recognized as having a supportive role in palliative care. Always seek medical advice first. It is not advisable to massage immediately after chemotherapy or radiation treatment.

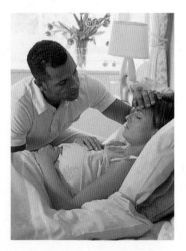

pregnancy

Massage can be helpful during pregnancy but remember that you are treating two people, not one, so be particularly sensitive. Avoid the abdomen, and use a lighter pressure than normal, and this is particularly crucial during the first trimester.

Head massage is an ideal treatment during pregnancy, as it is possible to remain sitting rather than lying down, which can be awkward and uncomfortable.

children and the elderly

The rule of working lightly also applies to children, the frail and the elderly. Adjust your pressure to the energy of the person you are massaging. Even when treating robust-looking older children, it is advisable to work lightly until you are both familiar with massage. If it is done too strongly it can stimulate a rise of energy that is too much for your partner's young body and could cause them to faint.

emotional response

People can have emotional reactions to massage such as feeling tearful or upset. This is because the effect of massage can be to release pent up feelings. In these situations, be sensitive in your response and check if your partner would like you to continue or to pause for a while before carrying on with the massage.

◁ During illness it is not advisable to massage deeply, although a tender loving touch can be comforting and healing – to give and to receive.

Head Massage
Principles

It is not difficult to learn how to practise Indian head massage. By mastering a few basic strokes and techniques you will soon be on the way to becoming a proficient masseur. However, although the strokes are important, they are not the only elements of a good massage. How you give the massage is equally important. Your ultimate aim is to give a treatment in which all the strokes and techniques blend together, each flowing seamlessly from one to the next. To achieve this level of mastery takes practice.

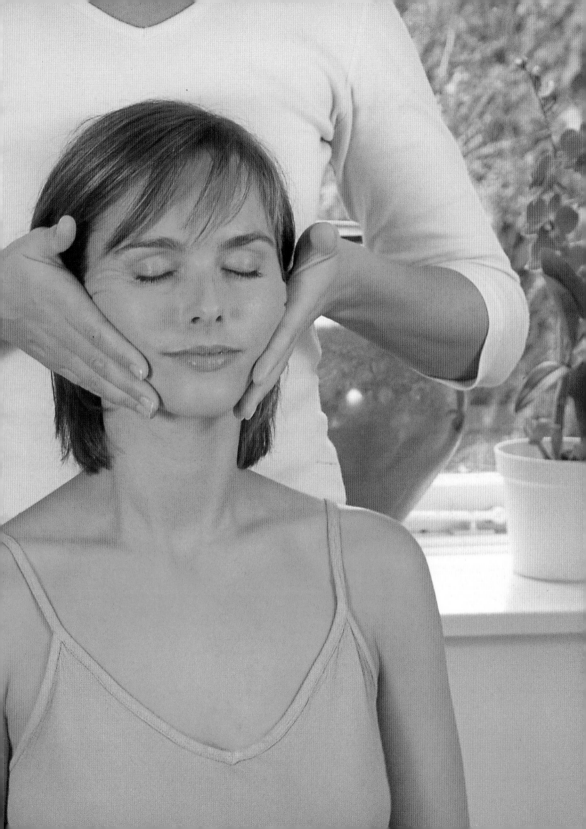

The history of head massage

Unlike many other healing traditions, Indian head massage is as widely practised today as it was thousands of years ago. It has its roots in Ayurveda, one of the oldest healthcare systems in the world. Dating back more than 4,000 years, Ayurveda is grounded in the philosophical and spiritual traditions of India. It offers comprehensive and practical guidelines for how to achieve health and well-being, and covers many different aspects of daily life.

the science of longevity

Ayurveda is known as the "science of longevity". It is based upon the holistic principle that illness or disease is created when we are out of balance. It describes three energy forces (known as the *doshas*), namely *vata*, *pitta* and *kapha*, each having its own characteristics and purpose. All physical, emotional and mental functions are controlled by the *doshas*. When they are balanced and working in harmony, we feel vibrant and enjoy good health.

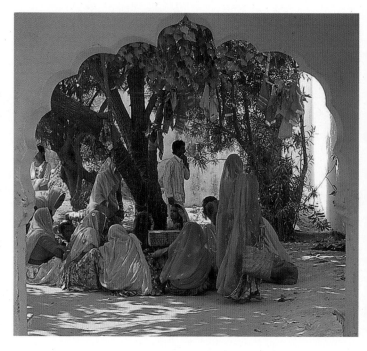

△ An Indian wedding is about to begin. The ritual of preparing the bride and groom for the ceremony will have included head massage.

▽ Indian women have been admired throughout history for their long, lustrous, thick black hair that is traditionally nourished, maintained and groomed with oils and by head massage.

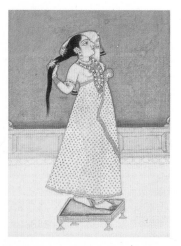

The Ayurvedic healthcare regime is comprehensive. It covers diet and exercise, yoga and meditation, detox and herbal remedies, as well as regular massage treatments using essential oils. A weekly head massage is highly recommended as a way of restoring and maintaining balance in the body's systems. Specific oils and herbs are used with head massage to help to stabilize the *doshas*. For instance, a *vata*-type imbalance may manifest as dry skin and hair, in which case sesame oil, with its strengthening and nourishing properties, would be recommended.

touch culture

The healing power of touch to restore and maintain well-being is deeply embedded in the culture of India, and head massage has to be seen within this context. Massage plays an important part in many major life events, such as marriage and pregnancy, or in

looking after babies and children. It is customary to give massage to both the bride and groom before they get married. This involves ritual and the use of specially blended herbs and oils designed to strengthen, beautify and bless the couple in preparation for marriage.

The practice of baby massage is also widespread. Even at the poorest level of society, where people live on the streets, and deprivation and hunger are rife, mothers can be seen oiling and massaging their babies every day, regardless of the traffic, dogs, pedestrians and street sellers all around them. In India, massage is not seen as a luxury, but as one of life's essentials. Daily massage continues until the child is about three years old, when it is reduced to twice a week. From the age of six, children then take part in a weekly massage ritual with other members of the family, even learning to exchange massage with one another.

male and female traditions

Historically the practice of Indian head massage is carried through both the female and male line, each having a different emphasis. The female line is primarily concerned with grooming, bonding and nurturing. Every week, head massage is carried out in the family home, where mothers nourish and condition their children's hair with oils and scalp rubs. For daughters and women, the weekly ritual is elaborate and time-consuming, involving lengthy preparations. That is because in India a woman's hair carries great status, so taking

▽ *Shirodhara*, the sensual ritual of running warmed sesame oil on to the middle of the forehead, is a relaxing and therapeutic part of traditional Ayurvedic practice.

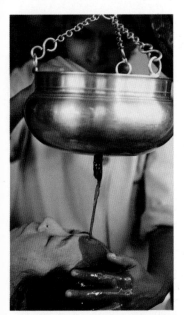

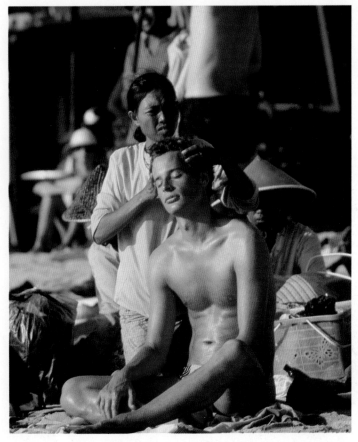

care of it is extremely important. There are many different traditions and ways of doing this. In the villages, it is usually a communal outdoor activity. Women of all ages get together once a week and sit in the sunshine to indulge in head massage and brush and groom each other's hair. The heat of the sun allows the oils to penetrate into the hair shaft, nourishing and conditioning it. The ritual is very much a social activity that gives the women involved a chance to talk and relax with one another.

Men also enjoy a tradition of head massage, which is practised by barbers. Treatments take place in shops, in the home, and also on many street corners. It is a more vigorous style of massage than for women, designed to energize and stimulate. Sometimes manipulation is also involved. As with the women's tradition, different kinds of oils are used at different times of the year and to treat a range of different

△ In India head massage is traditionally practised on the streets by male masseurs. In areas frequented by tourists, however, women have taken up this public work.

conditions. Because of its cooling properties, coconut oil is often used in the summer, for example, while mustard oil may be preferred in the winter because it is warming. Being a head masseur is a fully recognized profession, and there is even a special caste attributed to it, in which the skills and expertise are handed down from father to son through each generation.

Experiencing an Indian head massage usually leaves the recipient feeling relaxed and unburdened. Some people even report a deep feeling of peace, such as may be experienced after meditation. Perhaps this is because the practice has its roots in India, where spirituality is so much an integral part of everyday life.

Combining the traditions

Traditional Indian head massage is somewhat different from the style of head massage that is generally practised in the West today. There are a number of reasons for this, although both styles of massage are equally effective and appropriate to the culture in which they are enjoyed.

head massage in India

Traditional Indian head massage is carried out in the context of a culture where social etiquette dictates that the masseur and recipient should be the same sex as one another. In India, a woman's hair is one of her most valuable beauty assets, and a great deal of time is devoted to cultivating the long, lustrous well-oiled locks that are so highly prized. The pace of life is unhurried, and it is quite possible to spend several hours a week enjoying massage and beautifying rituals as a regular social activity. Personal grooming is carried out either in the home or the community, an excuse for friends, family and neighbours to gather together to exchange stories and catch up with

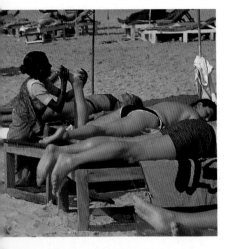

▽ Massage is part of the everyday culture in Indian society, and its benefits are increasingly appreciated by tourists.

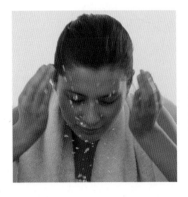

△ The trend in the West towards a faster lifestyle has meant that there is less time available for lengthy grooming procedures.

one another. Even when life is fast, the therapeutic value of massage is so much a part of everyday life that people still seem to find enough time to enjoy its simple and sensual pleasures.

the Western tradition

It is not so long ago in the West that practices such as hair-washing or bathing would also have taken up a large chunk of time each week. Today, however, the pace of life demands that grooming practices be as fast and practical as possible. In the Western world, the last fifty years or so has seen the accelerated development of a lifestyle based on speed, quantity and production. Showers, hairdryers and special beauty products, such as shampoos and conditioners "in one", are designed to cater for our overriding need for speed and convenience, and a more perfunctory "wash-and-go" attitude towards personal maintenance has taken over.

redefining our values

This emphasis on speed and convenience means our primal need for touch is largely unmet, and there is a danger that living life in the fast lane is at the expense of a real

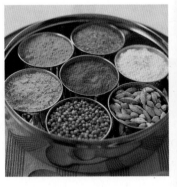

△ Traditional Indian head massage uses Ayurvedic oils from spices and plants, such as mustard, sesame, cinnamon, and cardamom.

quality of life. Stress-related conditions are on the increase, and despite our material abundance many people experience a sense of emptiness. This has caused many Westerners to look for ways to discover their inner values and a more fulfilling lifestyle. The growing wave of interest in holistic

▽ The daily practice of yoga is part of the holistic Ayurvedic system of health, of which head massage is an integral component.

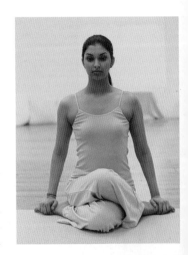

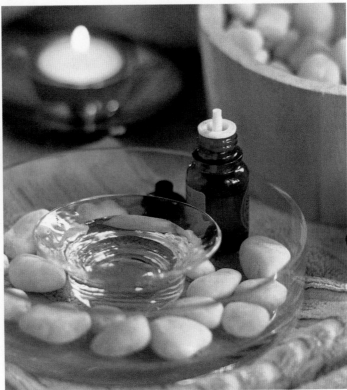

▷ A relaxing bath fragranced with essential oils will round off a head massage. Alternatively, it will help you to fully unwind at the end of a long and tiring day.

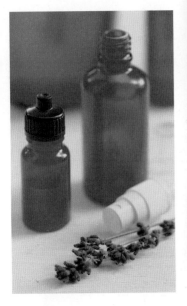

△ Lavender oil is the most popular essential oil in the West because of its wide variety of uses for both young and old alike.

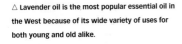

essential oils

You can choose an essential oil, or a blend of several oils, on the same basis as for any aromatherapy treatment – each oil has distinctive properties, as well as contributing to the pleasure of the experience. However, certain oils are particularly useful in head massage, and the following are all recommended. Remember that essential oils should never be used undiluted.

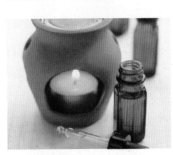

lavender One of the most universal of all the essential oils, lavender's relaxing and balancing properties make it useful for stress, insomnia, anxiety and depression. It is useful for treating dandruff, hair loss and lice and blends well with geranium and rosemary.

rosemary The refreshing and stimulating properties of rosemary oil have a head-clearing effect, so it is useful for periods of mental work. Rosemary is also a good treatment for greasy hair and skin, dandruff and hair loss, as well as restoring the shine to dark hair. It blends well with lavender.

sandalwood This oil's woody, haunting aroma quiets the mind and relaxes the nervous system, making it useful for stress-related conditions. Its softening and soothing action is good for dry skin and scalp conditions, while its aphrodisiac properties

◁ Using essential oils in a burner will enhance the ambience of the space you work in and help transport you to another dimension.

are well suited to sensual massage. Sandalwood blends well with bergamot, cedarwood, jasmine, palmarosa, vetiver or ylang ylang.

frankincense This has calming and relaxing properties for body, mind and soul. Because it deepens and slows down breathing, frankincense is good for respiratory conditions such as asthma, blocked sinuses, coughs or colds. Its moisturizing properties make it especially nourishing for older skin. Frankincense has a tradition of use in sacred ceremony and is helpful for inner journeys or a process of change.

geranium A light floral fragrance with a refreshing and balancing action, it is used to normalize very dry or very greasy skin and hair conditions by bringing them back into balance. Emotionally it is calming, restoring, uplifting and useful for anxiety or depression. It is an oil to use if you are uncertain which to choose. It blends well with lavender, sandalwood, rose, bergamot, marjoram, lemon or orange.

Working with oils

Oils are messy to work with so you need to make sure your partner is not wearing anything that could be spoiled – an old t-shirt is ideal. Keep a couple of towels specifically for this purpose, and drape one around your partner's shoulders. Have a good supply of tissues to hand and gather together all your oils, plus a suitable spoon and mixing bowl. Put the equipment on absorbent paper to soak up any accidental spills. You will also need a shower cap or silver foil to wrap your partner's hair up in when you've finished. If your partner has long hair, it is best to apply oil in sections over the head, in which case you will also need a comb, tinting brush and hair clips.

using essential oils

The head is a sensitive area, so essential oils should be used sparingly. As a rule, they should be blended with a carrier oil at a ratio of 2 drops to every 10ml (2 tsp) – weaker than for a body massage. Exceeding

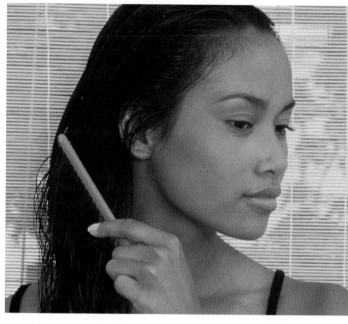

△ Leaving the oils in your hair after an oil massage is a holistic treatment and helps leave your hair and scalp in excellent condition.

the recommended dose could result in toxicity. Sometimes essential oils can cause allergic skin reactions. If you are using an oil for the first time, it is a good idea to do a patch test by dabbing a little of the blended oil on the inside of the wrist or elbow. Wait for 24 hours to see if there is any adverse reaction before using the oil.

Because of their potent effect, do not use essential oils with babies, young children or in pregnancy. When treating older children or the elderly, it is best to halve the dilution to 1 drop essential oil to every 10ml (2 tsp) carrier. If you are in doubt, consult a qualified aromatherapist.

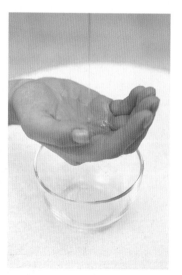

△ Warm the oil up in the palm of your hand or on a radiator before applying it, as heated oil is more easily absorbed and feels nicer.

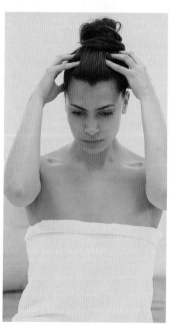

▷ Applying nourishing oils to your hair as part of your weekly beauty routine can be combined with a relaxing head massage.

oils for the hair and scalp

Choose from the following recipes to give your hair and scalp a nourishing conditioning treatment.

normal hair

carrier oils: sweet almond, coconut, jojoba
essential oils: rosemary, lavender, geranium

dandruff

carrier oils: jojoba, olive, coconut, sweet almond
essential oils: rosemary, lavender, eucalyptus, geranium

greasy hair

carrier oils: sweet almond, sesame, jojoba
essential oils: rosemary, lavender, sandalwood, lemon

thinning hair

carrier oils: sesame, olive
essential oils: rosemary, lavender, geranium

dry or chemically-treated hair

carrier oils: sesame, coconut, jojoba, sweet almond
essential oils: lavender, rosemary, geranium, sandalwood

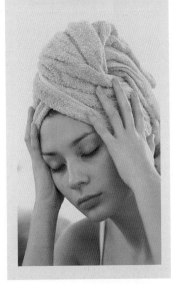

hair and scalp treatments

Mixing up your own blends of oils for your treatments is both very satisfying and beneficial. It is empowering, and you can also ensure that the ingredients you are putting on your hair and scalp are fresh and potent (all the oils have a limited shelf life) and are of a high quality. Because you are choosing the raw ingredients, you can guarantee that the blend you make is appropriate and of nutritional benefit to your body. Choose a carrier oil and an essential oil or two from the category on the left that best describes your hair. As a rough guide, 10ml (2 tsp) carrier oil should be sufficient for short hair, 15ml (1 tbsp) for medium length hair, and 30ml (2 tbsp) for long hair. The amount of oil you will need will also depend on the texture and thickness of the hair.

Measure the carrier oil into the mixing bowl. You may use more than one carrier oil if you wish, but mix them well together. Next add your chosen essential oil(s). Try not to make up more than you think you'll need, as it is best to work with a fresh mix each time. If you do have any left over, you could rub it into areas of rough skin, such as the elbows or heels. To get the most from the treatment, leave the oils on the hair for as long as possible, from a minimum of 30 minutes to up to 12 hours.

treating head lice

Head lice (nits) are a common problem among school-age children, and they can be difficult to eradicate. Using essential oils is becoming a popular treatment, as it offers a natural rather than a chemical approach to the problem. When treating lice it is essential that the whole family is treated to prevent the risk of cross-infection, and that all bedding, clothes, combs and brushes are washed to remove the eggs.

The quantity given below is sufficient for one complete treatment for one person. It comprises three separate applications, so you will have to store the remainder of the mixture in a sealed dark glass jar or bottle. It will keep for up to 12 months.

Use 30ml (2 tbsp) coconut or almond oil (or a combination of the two if you prefer). Add 5 drops lavender, 5 drops geranium and 5 drops eucalyptus oil. Apply the mix all over the head and hair, massaging it in well. Cover the head and leave the oils in for a minimum of 4 hours, although overnight is better. To remove the oil, massage the shampoo well into the hair before applying water. Wash and rinse as normal. Comb through the hair with a lice comb. Repeat the whole process after 24 hours and again after 8 days. This will give you the opportunity to treat any lice that have hatched since the first treatment and to ensure the head is clear.

▽ Oil treatments can be therapeutic, and the treatment of head lice with oil blends is very effective, toxic-free and pleasant.

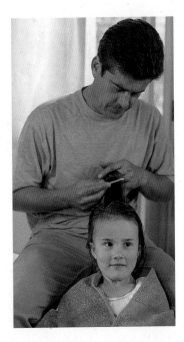

How to apply oils

The tradition of anointing the head with oil dates back to antiquity. There are many references to the practice throughout the Bible, while it has always played an important part in Ayurvedic medicine. In India, the practice of putting oil on the head begins at birth when a piece of soft cloth soaked in oil is placed over the fontanelle (the "soft spot") on a newborn baby's head. There are also complex ritual procedures within Ayurveda for applying oils to the head. Today traditional methods for applying oils have been integrated into a style more suited to a Western approach. Oil can be applied with your partner lying on a couch or sitting upright on a chair. Whichever method you use, warm the oil first. Warm oil not only feels nicer but it is more easily absorbed by the hair and scalp. To warm the oil, place it in a bowl on top of a radiator, or in a pan of hot water. Make sure the oil is not too hot before putting it on your partner's head. Take some time to discuss with your partner which oils and aromas they prefer, let them sniff the bottles and together work out a mix that will suit their state of mind and preferences.

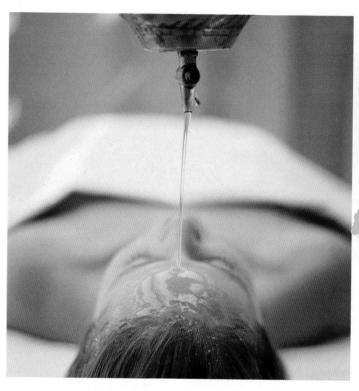

△ In Ayurvedic medicine the calming treatment of slowly and steadily pouring warmed oil over the forehead soothes and uplifts the spirit.

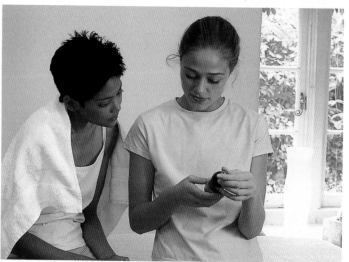

◁ Choosing which oils to use is part of the session and it is a good idea to discuss any preferences with your partner before starting.

lying-down method

Cover the surface of a couch or bed with suitable towels and have your partner lie down with their head near the edge. It's also a good idea to put a towel on the floor immediately below your partner's head.

Pour a little of the warmed oil directly on to the crown of your partner's head – it is a wonderful feeling as the oil seeps across the scalp. If you prefer, you may find it easier to pour some oil into the palm of your hand

▷ Make sure you have assembled everything and that it is to hand before you begin working with oils, as they can be messy.

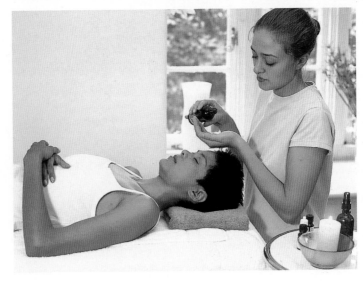

and put it on top of your partner's head like that. Work the oil into the scalp, applying more oil should you need to.

Pour more oil into your palm and massage up from the sides of the head towards the top. Put some more oil in your hand and apply it to the front of their head and work it upwards towards the middle. Then apply oil to the back of the head. Make sure that you have covered the whole head with oil. You can use this method with your partner sitting in a chair, too. You are then ready to proceed with the head massage routines described in the following section. The strokes are the same; the only difference is the presence of the oil.

▽ Use your hands to apply a little oil into the hair at a time, working it well into the hair and scalp for a nourishing treatment.

sectioning method

This method applies the oil in sections and works well for longer hair. You will need hair clips and a comb.

Divide the head into eight or so sections, clipping the hair out of the way. Starting at the front of the head, take down a section and comb the oil through, beginning at the roots and working down to the hair ends. Working with one section at a time, continue until the whole head is covered, then proceed with your head massage sequence.

▽ The sectioning method ensures that the oil is evenly applied all over the head and hair.

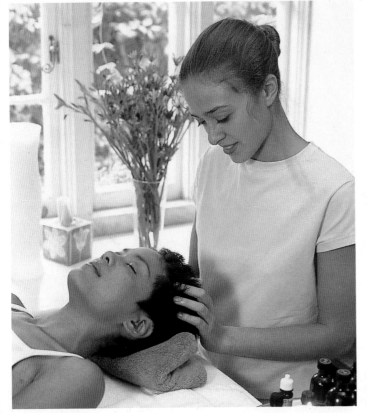

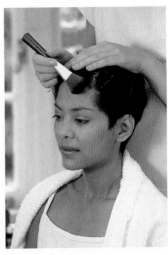

leaving and removing oils

To get the most out of an oil treatment the oils are best left on the head for some time. This maximizes their beneficial effects, giving them a chance to sink into the hair shaft and nourish it at a deep level. They will also be absorbed through the skin and enter the bloodstream where they will work their benefits through the whole body. Oils can be left on the hair from anything from 20 minutes to 24 hours. When it is time to remove them, there are a few guidelines for leaving your hair grease-free.

leaving oils on the hair

Once you have put the oils on, you will need to cover up your head. This will trap body heat and help the oils sink further into the hair and scalp. It may also feel more comfortable, particularly if you have long hair. You can do this by wearing a shower cap or by covering the head with silver foil, and bending it round at the corners to form a cap. You can then wrap a towel round your head to keep warm.

If you are keeping the oils on for an evening, then the treatment can be made part of a general pampering session combining self- or partner massage and other "feel-good" treats, such as a relaxing aromatherapy bath. Alternatively, leaving the oils in overnight will provide your hair and scalp with a deep conditioning treatment.

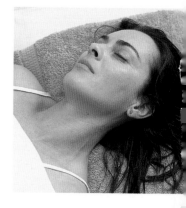

△ For a really deep conditioning treatment, oils can be left on overnight and can continue working while you recharge with a restful sleep.

▽ Leaving oils on your hair gives them a chance to sink in and deeply condition while you relax and take some quality time out.

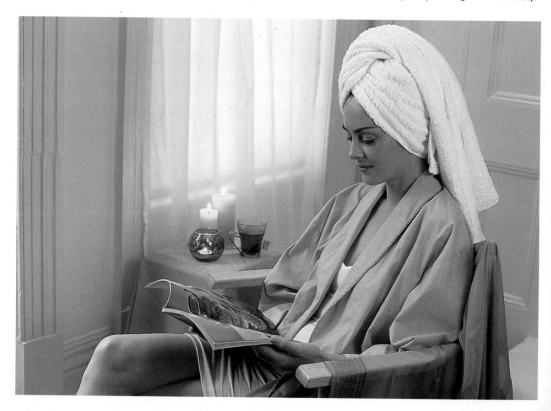

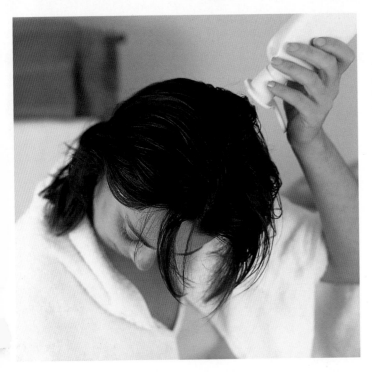

◁ When removing oils, always apply liberal quantities of shampoo directly onto the hair itself and work it repeatedly into the hair shafts and scalp before rinsing.

in, shampoo again for a third time, working it in as before. When this stage is finished you are ready for rinsing.

Using warm water (once again the temperature will help break down any residual oil), thoroughly rinse out the shampoo. For a final time, shampoo your hair again. Your hair should be a mass of lather and soapsuds by now, so you should only need to use a little shampoo for this final wash. Rinse out as usual. Your hair is now ready for your usual drying and styling.

aftercare

To maintain the good you've just done to your hair, follow some of the advice suggested in the section on hair care. Particularly, try to leave your hair to dry naturally if you have the time. If you only have a little time to spare, and need to use a hairdryer, remove any excess water from the hair by towel-drying it first. This reduces the drying effects of a hairdryer.

▽ Your hair should be free of oil and full of foamy suds by the end of the oil-removing session. It should be in tip-top condition.

If you plan to leave the oils on overnight, then you may find it more comfortable to have the hair loose and use old towels or sheets to protect the bedding.

removing oils

When it comes to removing the oil from your hair, it is vital to use lots of shampoo at the start.

Do not wet your hair, but put the shampoo on first. If you put water on your hair it will interfere with the break down of the oil molecules and will make the oil harder to remove – it's the same principle as using oil paint and then trying to clean your brush with water. On the other hand, shampoo without water emulsifies with the oil, making it easier to rinse out later. You will probably need to use a lot of shampoo, but don't be alarmed at the amount you are using as it will take a lot to get the oil out of the hair. It is unlikely at this stage that you'll notice any lather. Once you have thoroughly shampooed your whole head, begin the whole process again as if you were starting from scratch.

Still without water, shampoo over your whole head and hair, working it well into the hair fibres. If you have long hair, take a handful and rub it between your hands as if you were scrubbing. At this point, it is likely that you will begin to see some lather. This is a good sign and indicates that you are well on the way to being able to wash out the oil successfully. Work your way round the whole head, rubbing your hair between your hands. When this is all worked

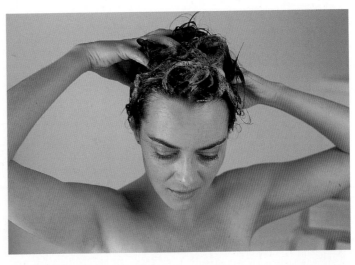

Getting started

One of the beauties of Indian head massage is that it can be performed almost anywhere and doesn't need a lot of equipment. The essentials are a suitable chair, a pair of hands, a willing heart and knowledge of what to do. To get the most out of it, a few preliminaries will help put you and your partner in the right frame of mind. These include getting all your equipment together, scene setting, and preparing yourself and your partner for a treatment.

seating

The best chair is one without any arms and a relatively low back to give you easy access to your partner. Cushions or pillows can be used to soften or raise seating or to provide comfort or support. However, you can always adjust the massage according to the situation. For instance, if you can't get to your partner's arms easily then just stroke them gently. If your partner is too tired to sit up, they could sit astride the seat and lean

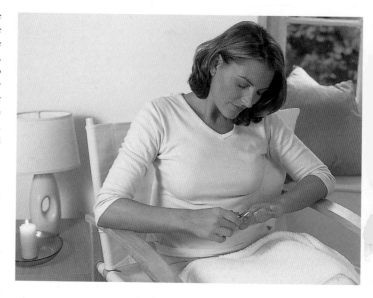

▽ Make sure that you prepare a relaxing space and have everything to hand before you begin so that your massage will go smoothly. A low backed chair without arms is ideal.

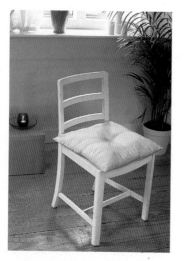

over the back of the chair, supported by cushions. The most important thing is for them to be comfortable.

preparation

Clean and tidy the room to create a harmonious space that is easy to work in. Make sure that it is warm, and eliminate as many potential distractions as you can. Unplug the phone, turn off any mobiles, and put a "do not disturb" sign on the door.

Next think about mood setting. Sound, lighting and fragrance can all be used to help create a particular ambience and turn the room into a healing space. Candles give a soft and subdued light, while certain types of music can help you relax. Burning incense or vaporizing essential oils will fragrance the air, as well as helping to clear impurities. If you want to use music and/or scent, choose something that both you and your partner will enjoy.

Make sure that you are wearing loose comfortable clothes, and take a few moments to make the following preparations. You also need to take a few

△ Remove your watch, and any rings or bracelets, and wash your hands. File your nails so that they are short and smooth to the touch.

▽ Make sure your hair is tied back or clipped up so that it does not fall over your face as you massage, as this is distracting.

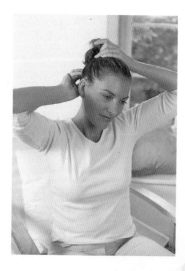

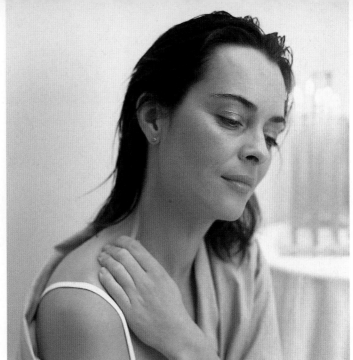

▷ For a truly nourishing experience, use oils to help you massage away tensions and knots and to help create a greater sense of ease within your own body.

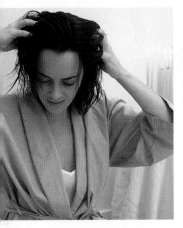

△ Release tension in the head and discharge mental stress and worries by working them out through massage with oils. Then you can wash them all away.

To continue working with oil you can follow the basic self-massage sequence outlined earlier in the book. However, because of its slippery nature there will be more "give" with oil, and you will have less of a grip than with dry massage, so the experience will feel very different. With oils your strokes are likely to be smooth, gliding over the skin in a continuous movement.

After you have finished with your hair, you may want to use up any remaining oil on your face and neck. Place your hands on your face and gently smooth the oil into the skin with small circular strokes, being particularly careful around the eyes. Move to your neck and glide your hands up and out to the sides. You can leave the oil to soak in or wipe it off with a tissue.

Remember that when giving self-massage you are both the giver and the receiver. As the giver you are your own therapist, so be sympathetic and understanding to how you feel inside. As you massage you could inwardly thank the different parts of your body for serving you

so well each day. You may also notice how your thoughts stray away or become negative, worrying or busy. When this happens, bring your attention back to the self-massage. As the receiver, you have the opportunity for self-empowerment and healing. If it hurts, you can instantly lighten the depth of your touch. Alternatively you can apply pressure for much longer than is conventional if it feels good to you. You also know exactly where it hurts and can find the precise location of any knotty and painful spots.

As you massage, make sure that your strokes give you pleasure, adjusting the pace so that it is faster, slower, deeper, or more loving. Be responsive to your own needs and be flexible in your approach. A basic guideline is to recognize that the body has a wisdom of its own and that if something feels good, it is likely to be doing you good.

▽ Relieve tension in your face with an oil facial that will leave you feeling good and your skin soft, smooth and glowing.

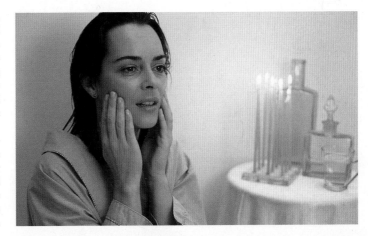

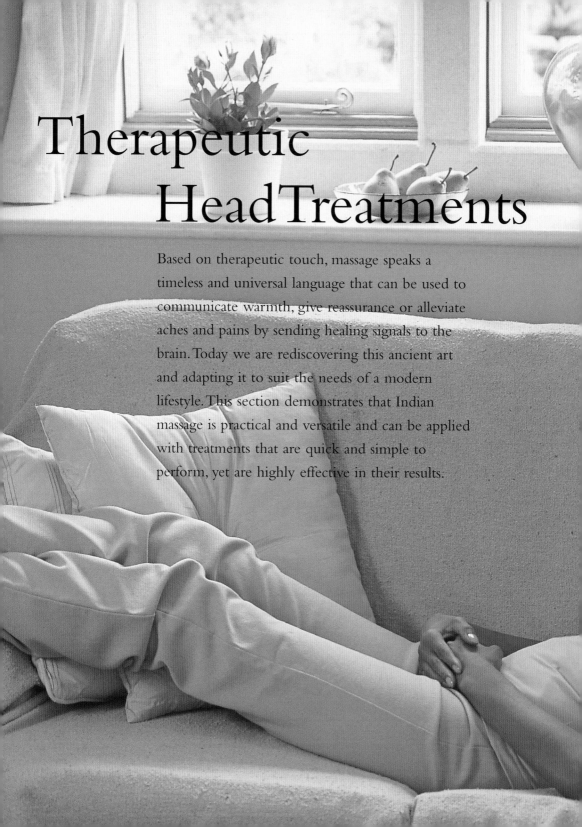

Therapeutic HeadTreatments

Based on therapeutic touch, massage speaks a timeless and universal language that can be used to communicate warmth, give reassurance or alleviate aches and pains by sending healing signals to the brain. Today we are rediscovering this ancient art and adapting it to suit the needs of a modern lifestyle. This section demonstrates that Indian massage is practical and versatile and can be applied with treatments that are quick and simple to perform, yet are highly effective in their results.

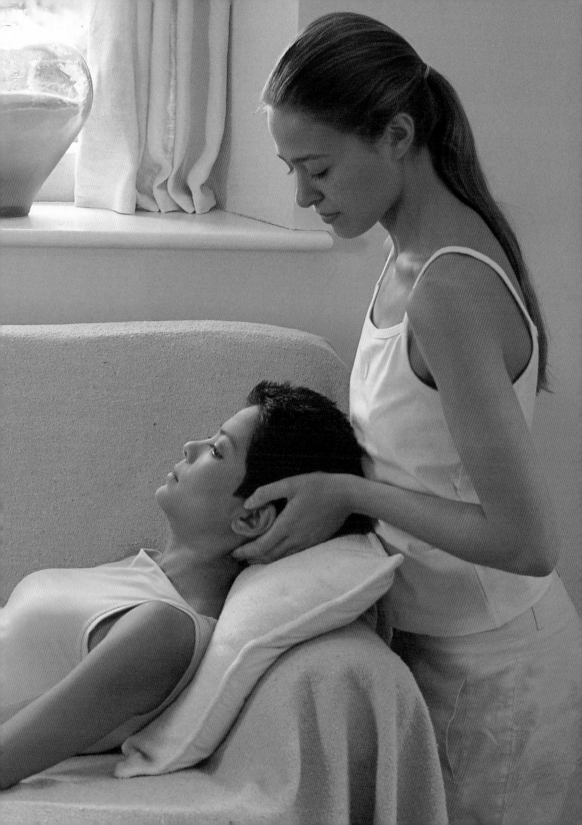

Relieving stress at work

Technological advances have revolutionized our working patterns. Many of these changes are associated with computers and an increase in sedentary jobs, which in turn is leading to a build-up of tension in the body and an increase in emotional stress. This is because our bodies are designed for movement, and our muscular structure functions most effectively when it is used in a whole, active and dynamic way. Increasingly this is not the case. We move in limited ways and hold our bodies in relatively static positions for extended periods of time. This is creating a range of common problems. It is in this context that massage becomes such a valuable tool for relieving stress in the workplace.

work stress

A typical office worker is likely to hold their back, neck, shoulders, arms and eyes in static positions for long periods of time. This causes the muscles to "freeze" into an almost permanent state of tension, in which they no longer work efficiently. The flow of nutrients, oxygen and blood supply is restricted, reducing the efficient circulation of blood to the brain and throughout the body. This leads to tiredness and irritability, as well as poor concentration and difficulties with decision-making. If the muscles are not released through movement or manipulation, they contract and toxins build up in the muscle tissue. This reduces mobility and causes all manner of aches and pains, while specific work-related conditions, such as repetitive strain injury (RSI) and carpal tunnel syndrome, are becoming increasingly common.

On top of the physical stress, many people experience psychological stress at work, which usually makes the physical discomfort worse. Time limits, dealing with frustration or feeling pressurized to perform can all literally become "a pain in the neck" if emotional pressures are not discharged at some point.

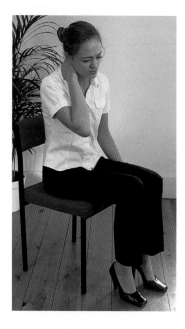

△ Sitting down working at a desk or computer for long periods of time often causes tension and pain in the neck and shoulders.

self-help measures

Current thinking says that for every hour that you spend working at a computer screen, you should take a ten-minute break. During this time you should do something active to help discharge physical tension. This could include self-massage, stretch and release exercises or massage with a co-worker. Done regularly, such measures will help discharge tension, particularly from the upper body. They will also help to keep body and mind relaxed and alert during the whole working day.

releasing neck tension

With one hand, grab a handful of flesh from the back of your neck. Squeeze it as hard as feels comfortable and hold the pressure, slowly nodding your head up and down at the same time. Mentally say the word "yes"

to yourself as you do this. Keep breathing as you repeat this movement a couple of times. Swap hands, and this time shake your head from side to side, mentally saying "no" inside your head.

neck and shoulder stretch

This stretch helps to release tight neck and shoulder muscles and can be done standing or sitting. Lift one arm and bend it so that your hand is facing palm down on your upper back. Take your other arm and bend it so that your hand reaches up your back with the palm facing outwards. Move both hands towards each other so that the fingers meet and clasp together. If the hands do not reach one another, then rest them as close together as possible. Hold for 15 seconds, maintaining a steady breathing rhythm. Change hands and repeat the stretch on the other side, again holding it for 15 seconds while breathing steadily.

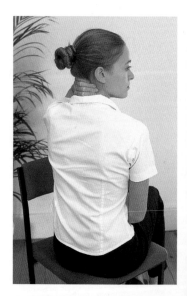

▽ Taking regular breaks to release taut neck muscles with self-massage contributes greatly to preventing the gradual build-up of chronic tension.

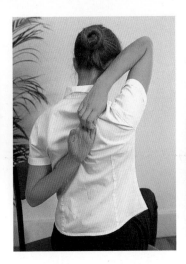

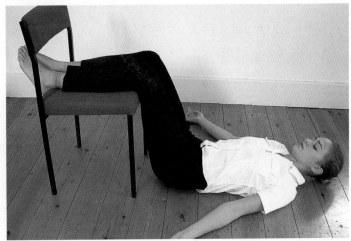

△ Stretching breaks help release and promote deeper breathing, which oxygenates the body and brain, increasing brain functioning.

resting the eyes

Our eye muscles get surprisingly tired from focusing for long periods on a fixed plane of vision, such as a computer screen. This simple palming exercise will give your eyes a rest and help to release taut eye muscles. Vigorously rub your hands together so that they become warm and energized, then place them over your eyes, your fingers

▽ It is important to rest your eyes following periods of concentrated work, as this helps to prevent strain and stress, which contribute to headaches and impaired vision.

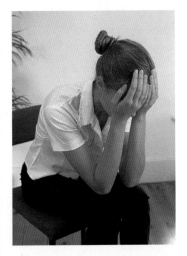

resting on your forehead. Close your eyes. Hold for a few minutes while your eyes rest in the darkness of your hands. Use the time to tune in to your breathing and focus on letting go of tension as you breathe out.

back, neck and shoulder release

The following exercise should help release tension in the upper back, neck and shoulders. It encourages the effective flow of blood back to the head and brain and is ideal after an extended period of deskwork, such as at lunchtime. If you cannot do it at your own desk, you may be able to find another suitable place such as an unused conference or meeting room.

Sit on the floor at right angles to a chair. Then swivel around so that you are facing the chair and put the lower half of your legs up. Your feet and calves should be resting flat on the chair and your knees should be bent at right angles with the floor. Let your arms fall out to the sides with palms facing upwards. Wriggle your back and adjust your position so that your spine is as flat as possible on the floor. It is best if you can close your eyes and rest in this position for at least five minutes.

Gently breathe in and out and use your imagination to visualize the fresh flow of oxygen, blood and nutrients flowing up through your back, shoulders, neck and head to your brain and then down again. This will help to replenish and recharge your upper body and head.

△ Lying down so that your spine can be supported by the ground gives it a chance to decompress and rehydrate, leaving you feeling refreshed and alert.

co-worker massage

Massage between work colleagues can create a much happier atmosphere. This is a very quick and easy routine. Sit your partner in front of you and gently rest your forearms on their shoulders. Ask them to take a deep breath in and on the out breath, press down on their shoulders. Then use the whole of your hands to rub briskly over their shoulders and upper back.

▽ Making co-worker massage part of your work culture makes a noticeable difference in terms of increased creativity and efficiency.

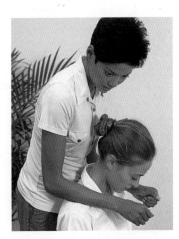

Asthma management

Asthma is a breathing disorder that affects one in seven of the population. It can occur at any age and involves inflammation of the bronchial tubes, excess mucus production and the contraction of muscles in the chest area. This narrowing of the air passages restricts the flow of oxygen and leads to breathing difficulties. These can range from a mild tightening in the chest to restrictions that are so severe that they require urgent hospital treatment. Regular massage to the neck and shoulder area can help reduce both the number and severity of asthma attacks. Massage can also be used to alleviate the symptoms of a mild attack.

a typical asthma profile

Asthma sufferers tend to be highly sensitive and particularly prone to stress and anxiety. Their breathing is rapid, shallow and restricted, with a tendency to breathe through the mouth rather than the nose.

pressure points on the back

The lung-associated acupressure point, situated on either side of the spine between the scapulae, is associated with relieving the symptoms of asthma and reducing muscle spasms in the shoulders and neck. Massage in between and around the shoulder blades can therefore help relax the muscles and give some relief during an asthma attack.

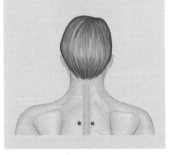

useful essential oils

These are some of the essential oils that help to open up the breathing, relax bronchial spasms and calm anxiety during a mild asthma attack. Use 3–5 drops essential oil added to 10ml (2 tsp) massage oil or lotion, and use as a chest rub. Alternatively, vaporize the oils in a burner.

• eucalyptus or juniper: opens up the airways, encourages expulsion of mucus
• frankincense or marjoram: helps to calm and relax
• rosemary or peppermint: reduces general breathing difficulties

They are especially liable to hold tension in the neck, upper back and shoulders. Constriction in these areas inhibits the full expansion of the diaphragm, which in turn restricts lung capacity. Releasing tension in the neck and upper back through massage can help to open up the breathing. It can also help to calm anxiety and help the person to relax.

healthy breathing

Research has shown that there are some basic breathing principles that are especially helpful for asthmatics. The first is to develop the habit of breathing through the nose and not the mouth. Breathing through the nose helps to regulate and slow down the breathing. It also means that the air is warmed in the nasal passages before it enters the lungs. Cold air entering the lungs changes the chemical balance and can make the internal environment more susceptible to an asthma attack. Second, it is advised to try to breathe from the abdomen rather than the upper chest. This will help to slow down and deepen the breathing, which helps to stave off an oncoming attack.

causes and effects of asthma

Some types of asthma are triggered by an allergic response to dust, pollen and animal hair, as well as certain foodstuffs, such as dairy products. Other causative factors include stress and exposure to tobacco smoke and high levels of environmental pollution. There can also be cases where a genetic factor may also be involved.

During an asthma attack, the constricted bronchial passages cause wheezing, coughing, and feelings of panic, which serve to exacerbate the symptoms.

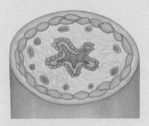

△ Bronchial passages contract during an asthma attack as the surrounding muscles exert pressure on them, restricting breathing capacity.

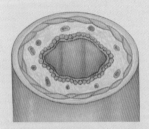

△ When the attack has subsided and the muscles have relaxed, the airways can expand once more, allowing air to pass through unrestricted.

massage for asthma

Have your partner sit at a table so they can lean forwards if they want or need to.

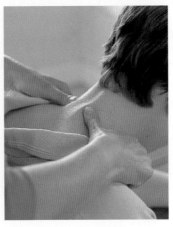

△ **3** Stand behind your partner and hold their shoulders, positioning your thumbs at the base of the neck. With both thumbs working together, make small firm circular strokes across the base of the neck (avoiding the spine), moving a little down into the upper back and a little up into the shoulders.

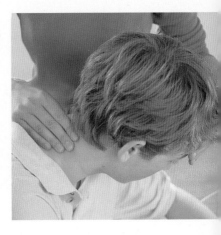

△ **4** Move to the left of your partner. Support their forehead with your left hand. Place your right hand at the base of the neck and, with a wide span, grasp and pull back the neck muscles. Sweep up to the middle and then to the top of the neck, using the same movement. Repeat three times.

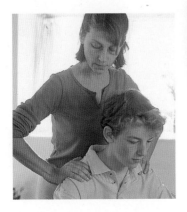

△ **1** Gently place your hands on your partner's shoulders. Ask them to breathe in through their nose and then out for as long as possible. Do it with them. Ask them to take a second deep breath. On the out breath, gently press down on their shoulders, encouraging them to soften.

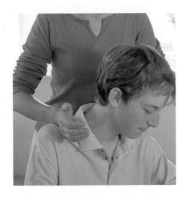

△ **2** Move a little to the left of your partner and anchor your left hand on their left shoulder. Holding your right hand loose and open, use a zigzag rubbing motion with the side of your hand, working along the top of your partner's right shoulder and then down around the shoulder blade into the back. Work the muscles that run between the shoulder blade and the spine itself. Change sides and repeat.

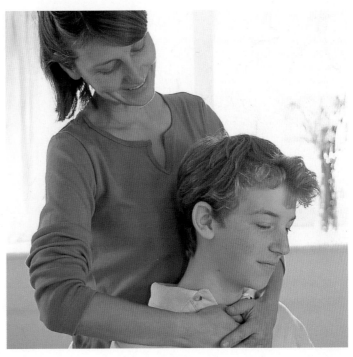

△ **5** To finish the massage, put your hands on the front of your partner's chest just below the collarbone. Using a sweeping stroke, brush outwards and upwards towards the shoulders. Have a sense of your partner's chest opening and expanding as you work. Repeat three times. Come to a rest, putting your hands on your partner's shoulders, and take a deep breath in and out together.

Massage for anxiety

It is more or less impossible to go through life without ever feeling anxious. Any change constitutes some level of stress. Positive life events, such as marriage, the birth of a child or a new job, as well as the more obvious negative ones like divorce, bereavement or redundancy, are fairly common situations, which put us to the test. Sometimes however, anxiety can become a more chronic condition. This happens when we have more stress in our lives than we feel able to cope with and are living in a perpetual state of fear and worry. Massage is an excellent treatment for anxiety. It can reassure and help discharge many unpleasant symptoms.

symptoms of anxiety

Anxiety has a way of pervading the personality so that the symptoms seem to take over. This can show up as someone who is short-tempered, over-reactive, preoccupied and restless, or alternatively as someone who feels overwhelmed, tearful and unable to cope. Anxiety also affects the body. Muscular tension, shallow, rapid breathing, palpitations and aching muscles can all be symptoms of anxiety. Similarly signs of general unease, such as butterflies in the stomach, feeling light-headed or else permanently exhausted are signs that the body is under too much stress.

the benefits of massage

Anxiety is linked with fear and insecurity so the gentle touch of another person can be especially reassuring, helping to alleviate negative symptoms in a safe, supportive environment. A treatment can help the anxious person to relax, leaving them feeling stronger and more able to cope with anxiety-provoking situations. To help with the

▽ Take time at the beginning of the session to chat with your partner to make sure you have an accurate idea of how they are feeling.

releasing process, it can help to encourage your partner to sigh as you work, but only do this if you both feel comfortable with it. Other signs that your partner is releasing tension and anxiety during a treatment include reactions like yawning, laughing, shivering or even shuddering. Sometimes they may feel upset and start to cry.

friction strokes

Firm, fast action friction strokes are very effective for cutting through tension. By vibrating the muscle fibres together, they access the deeper muscle layers and nerve bundles and encourage them to relax. It is a little like shaking a bowl of sand, where all the bigger grains and stones are brought to the surface as you shake.

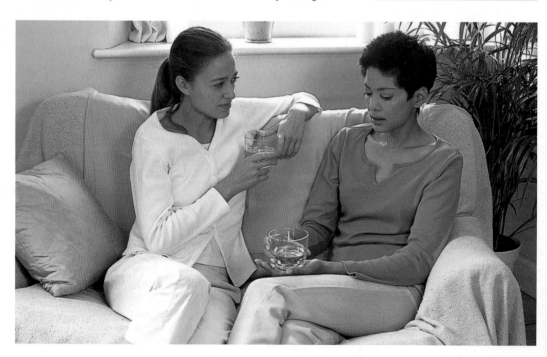

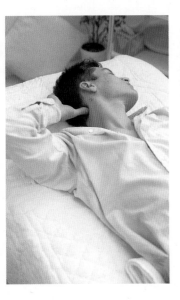

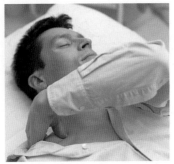

△ **6** With your left hand on your right shoulder, place your thumb in the hollow behind the collarbone and the remaining fingers over the top of the shoulder. Squeeze your thumb and fingers together, and on the out breath pinch this muscle and hold for as long as you can. Release and repeat at intervals along both shoulders till you have pinched both three times.

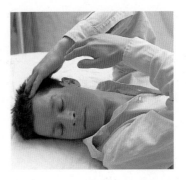

△ **8** Run your fingers across your scalp as if you were combing and lifting your hair away from your head. Flick your fingers away as they come off the ends of the hair. You can either do this stroke softly and slowly for a relaxing effect, or firmer and faster for an energizing clearing effect. Work over the whole of your head three times.

△ **4** Move your head back to the left and press your right thumb into the bony ridge behind the ear. Press, hold and release. Continue working in this way along the edge of the skull towards the middle. Aim for comfortable pressure, repeat twice and swap sides.

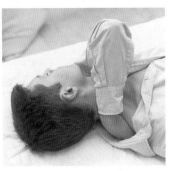

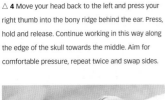

△ **5** With your head on the left, hook your left hand over your right shoulder, resting the heel on top of the shoulder with the fingers pointing down the back. Dig your fingers into the muscle, grab some flesh and drag it up until your fingers slide over your shoulder. Continue finding tight spots along both shoulders. Repeat three times on both sides.

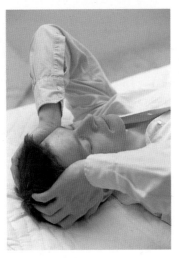

△ **7** Place the heels of your hands on your temples and, using medium to firm pressure, press while simultaneously making circles. Make at least six big slow circles and work into areas of tension. If you wish, you can extend this circling action to include the whole head and scalp, using the heel of your hands or your fingers.

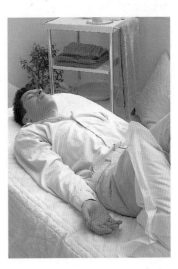

△ **9** To finish, take a deep breath in and out from your belly as in the beginning. Rest for a few moments, covering yourself with a blanket, if you wish. Imagine stale energy and stress leaving your body as you breathe out, and fresh energy revitalizing your body and mind as you breathe in. When you are ready, roll on to one side and get up slowly.

Relieving tension from driving

Driving is an integral part of a modern sedentary lifestyle. We use our cars to make short journeys around town, as well as for longer trips, and we spend a lot of time behind the steering wheel. For most of us, our cars are indispensable, yet driving can also create stress and tension in the body. To minimize this, we can cultivate some good driving habits. These include improving and adjusting our driving posture, taking breaks during long journeys and using some stretching and self-massage treatments to ease out tense muscles.

improving posture

How you sit at the wheel is a key to body tension. Bad habits include craning your neck to peer over the driving wheel or overextending your back by leaning too far backwards. The body's muscles then become tired and stressed, leading to aches and pains. If the back's lumbar region is not supported, it can have a tendency to sag and slump. This pulls on the muscles and puts a strain on the rest of the spine.

▽ **Driving in poor conditions, a hurry or heavy traffic can all contribute to poor posture and can have the effect of making it worse.**

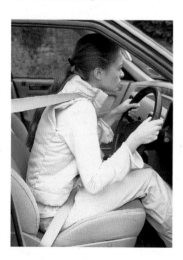

Good posture supports the body's musculature and helps keep its energies flowing. Make sure that you sit up straight and that your seat supports you. You can use cushions to adjust your position, or buy the special back supports now available. Have enough headroom between your head and the roof of the car, otherwise you may slouch to fit yourself into the available space. Adjust all the mirrors so you can see them without straining. Hold the middle of the steering wheel, keeping your arms relaxed. Don't twist your feet. They should be in line with your legs and facing forwards.

Sitting for prolonged periods in the same position impairs circulation and causes the body to stiffen up. This can lead to aches and pains in your neck and back, arms and wrists, or legs and ankles. It can also result in eyestrain and headaches, as well as lower levels of mental alertness.

To avoid freezing in the same position, make little postural adjustments as you drive. For instance, you can wriggle yourself further back into your seat, or if you are stuck in traffic, try relaxing your shoulders by lifting and releasing them. As you drive check periodically that your jaw is relaxed, your shoulders stay soft and that you are breathing from your abdomen.

▽ **Sitting in an upright position with a supported back can help make driving safer and minimizes the build-up of tension.**

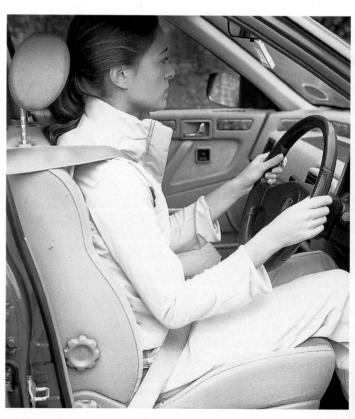

body stretches

On long journeys it is very important to take regular breaks to have some fresh air and a chance to stretch. This will help to release tension, improve circulation and restore concentration, making you a more relaxed and effective driver. Research now shows that taking regular massage and stretch breaks while driving has a beneficial effect on improving driver concentration and on reducing the number of road accidents. It has been shown to be much more effective than coffee breaks.

These stretches and massages are easy to do wherever you take a break from driving. Do each one a number of times. The stretches mobilize the spine, lower back, arms and shoulders.

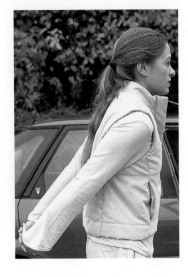

△ **2** Clasp your hands together behind your back. As you breathe out, bring them up slowly as far as possible. Hold and release slowly as you breathe in. Release your arms and let them drop down. Repeat at least three more times. This helps relieve tightness in the shoulders and between the shoulder blades.

self-massage tension relievers

You can also try this quick-fix self-massage during a driving break or when you get home. It will help to ease out tension in the head, neck, and shoulder areas.

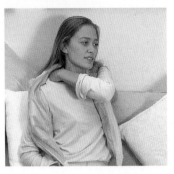

△ **1** Sit with your back well supported and place one hand over the opposite shoulder. Make small circular strokes across the shoulder using your fingertips. Work your way down into the upper back and along the edge of your shoulder blade as far down as you can. As your hand returns up your back, massage the muscles between your shoulder blade and spine.

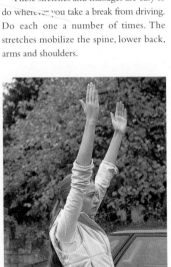

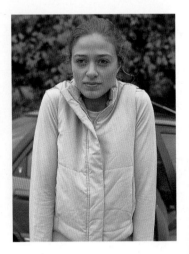

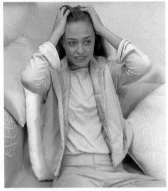

△ **1** Stand with your feet together and facing forwards. Breathe in and stretch your arms up above your head, lengthening up through your spine. On the out breath, bend your knees, tuck your chin in and roll your spine down, vertebra by vertebra, slowly bending forwards as far as is comfortable. Bring your arms down as you do this movement and let them swing gently backwards and forwards. On an in breath, bring your arms forwards and lengthen up through your body to come up to standing.

△ **3** Take a deep breath in and slowly begin to lift your shoulders up as far as they will comfortably go. Hold them up tightly as near your ears as possible. As you breathe out, let your shoulders drop abruptly in a release. You can extend this stretch by lifting and rolling your shoulders forwards as slowly as possible. Then change directions so that you roll your shoulders backwards. It can help if you try to imagine your shoulder blades meeting together in the middle of your back as you circle them.

△ **2** Using your fingertips, rub back and forth across the top of your shoulder, following the muscles up into the side of your neck. Continue the movement up to your head, working around the whole head with this rubbing motion.

Sensual massage

Touch is the language of lovers and enjoying massage with your partner adds another dimension to your relationship, becoming part of your intimate exchange and a special way of spending time together. Head massage can be given in such a way that it becomes a sensual experience. Although some of the strokes in a sensual head massage are different from those in the standard routine, the key feature is the sensual quality of your touch and the blending of your energies together. It can be done with or without oils.

mood setting

To set the scene for a romantic and intimate space, think soft and warm. Candles, cushions and an open fire are traditional favourites for creating the right atmosphere; if you don't have an open fire, turn up the heating. Use your creative flair to beautify the space with flowers, fabrics and background music. You could also light

some incense or vaporize essential oils in a burner. Many fragrances have sensual, aphrodisiac qualities – some of the most popular include sandalwood, jasmine, ylang ylang, rose and patchouli. Have plenty of towels and warm coverings to hand and a comfortable surface to work on. A duvet, futon, blankets or soft sheepskins make a well-padded surface. Finally, wear something loose and comfortable and appropriate to the romantic occasion.

giving sensual massage

If you are tense it will be difficult for your partner to relax, so make sure you keep your jaw and shoulders soft and breathe from your belly. Focus on giving pleasure to your partner by tuning in to their breathing and being sensitive to their changing responses. Enjoy making your strokes long and lingering or firmer and more stimulating, using your judgement and spontaneity as you work. The massage can be done sitting up or lying down.

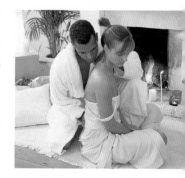

△ **1** This stroke stimulates the release and flow of sexual energy from the sacrum at the base of the spine. Place one hand on your partner's shoulder and the other at the base of the spine. Using your fingertips and very light pressure, make circular strokes in a clockwise direction around the sacrum. Build up a smooth rhythm and make the circles larger till the whole back is circled, each time returning to the sacrum. Gradually decrease their size, finishing at the sacrum.

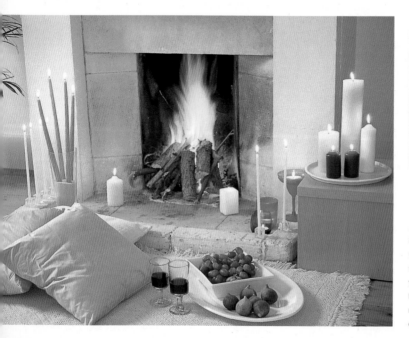

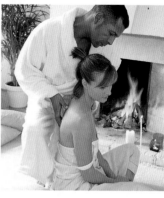

△ **2** With one hand on your partner's head, gently draw the fingers of your working hand up their back to the base of the neck. From here, gently stroke up the back of the neck a couple of times. If you wish you may also blow soft circles of warm air on the back of the neck. Both of these actions stimulate the nerve receptors in the skin and should send shivers of pleasure up your partner's spine.

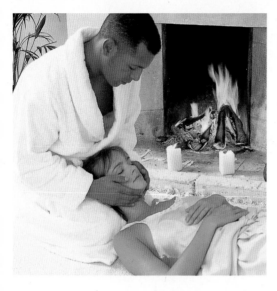

△ **3** For work on the face, your partner may prefer to lie down. Find a comfortable position with their head cradled on your lap or on a cushion. Place your hands at the bottom of their face so that you are cupping their chin. Slowly and gently draw your hands up over the face, up to the forehead and then stroke back down the sides to the chin. Repeat five times. To extend this stroke, use one finger to trace the features of your partner's face, beginning at the lips, and moving up around the nose, cheeks, eye sockets and eyebrows. Trace each feature three times.

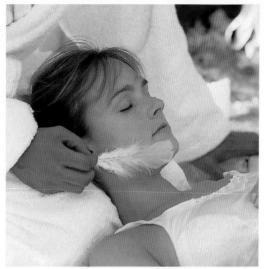

△ **5** Use a feather (or your own hair if it is long enough) for this stroke. Beginning at the chin, slowly trail the feather up the side of the face with slow luxurious strokes. Return to the chin and repeat several times and then switch sides. You can also stroke across the cheekbones and brow, working from the middle out towards the hairline each time. Imagine you are caressing away all cares and tensions as you lovingly stroke. Repeat several times. Should your partner find this ticklish, substitute the feather with some lingering finger-stroking up and across the face.

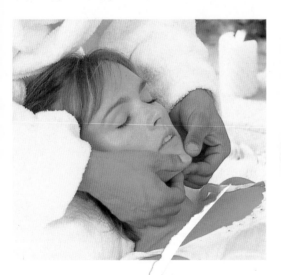

△ **4** Place both thumbs in the middle of your partner's chin, with the index fingers curled underneath. Make small circles with your thumbs on the chin, underneath the mouth and a little out into the lower cheeks, using your fingers underneath for support. As you work, make the circles slightly bigger to include the lower lip. Then gently use your thumbs to pull the lower lip down so that the lips are slightly open. To extend this stroke, continue to make small circular strokes with the pads of your fingers all over the face and forehead. Use a light touch and avoid the eye area.

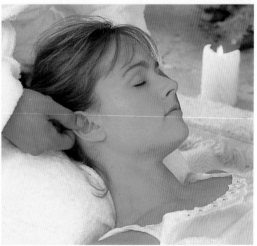

△ **6** Holding your partner's earlobes between your thumb and fingers, gently massage the ears by squeezing and rolling, moving up along each ear's outside edge and then down on the inside edge. Continue working round the ears until you have completed three laps. Then, using your ring finger, trace round each ear's outside and top edge as well as its inside surface. This is a highly delicate area, but done sensitively it can feel very intimate and sensual. Finish by gently pulling down on the earlobes a couple of times.

Body Massage Principles

There are many different schools of body work and massage, but holistic body massage has become one of the most popular. At its core is the idea that caring touch in itself is a powerful agent for the healing process. When combined with skills and techniques drawn from both ancient and more modern approaches to the science of massage, it can bring about many beneficial changes within the body, mind and spirit of the whole person.

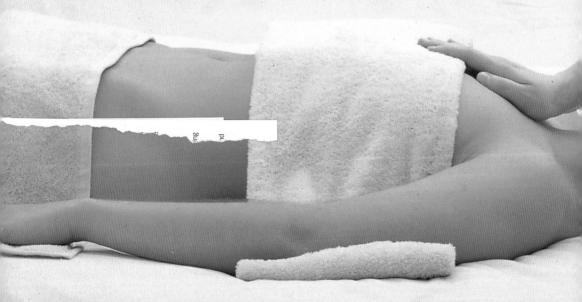

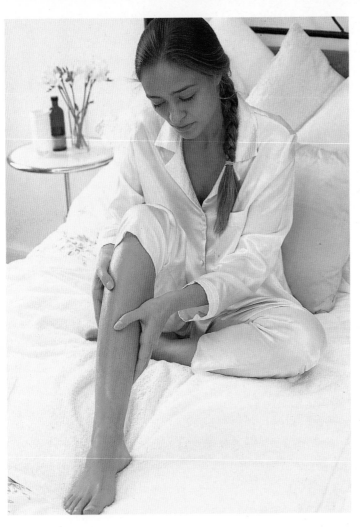

◁ Taking time out to relax is essential for maintaining good health and well-being. Self-massage is a nurturing way to do this, requiring you to sit down quietly.

extent that you may enter a very deep state of relaxation, akin to meditation, in which mind, body and soul are recharged.

food and drink

Our diet can either help or hinder our ability to cope with stress. Stimulants such as caffeine, alcohol and smoking deplete our nutritional store and contribute to stress levels. Sugary snacks and most processed foods stimulate the release of the stress hormone cortisol, leading to swings in blood sugar and energy levels. Opt instead for "slow release" energy found in whole foods – fresh fruits, vegetables, pulses and grains, seeds and nuts. Substitute herbal teas for tea and coffee and drink plenty of water to keep the body hydrated. Under stress the body uses up its nutrients more quickly, particularly the B vitamins, vitamin C, calcium and magnesium, so it's worth considering a multi-vitamin and mineral supplement to correct any deficiencies.

▽ Eating raw foods and drinking water helps reduce stressful thought patterns and is the best way to keep your body and skin hydrated.

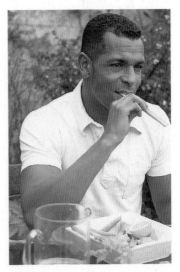

faced with a stressful situation, the body's instinctive reaction is to prepare for immediate "fight or flight" by pumping out adrenalin. This is nature's way of increasing our levels of alertness and ability to respond to danger – whether real or perceived – and causes physiological changes, such as rapid breathing, increased heartbeat, sweating and muscle tension. If the adrenalin that has been produced is not then utilized or discharged in some way, it remains in the body, leading to high levels of anxiety and frustration, as well as disturbances in thought processes and perception.

It can take a long time for the body to return to normal after having been aroused in this way, and ongoing stress can result in exhaustion. At this stage, we may be continually tired and experience a range of unpleasant and frustrating physical and psychological symptoms.

relaxation and sleep

Being able to relax and enjoy a good night's sleep is one of nature's best stress cures. While we are under stress we need more sleep, but this is when we are most likely to experience sleep problems. Pursuits such as singing or painting, enjoying a long, warm aromatic bath, or eating delicious food, are all good ways of switching off in the evening. Massage is also excellent for relaxing body and mind. During a massage the brain waves can slow down to such an

Body work

Holistic body massage uses the basic strokes of Swedish massage but tends to work in a softer and slower way, with emphasis on relaxing the client psychologically and emotionally as well as physically. The focus on relaxation applies to the practitioner as well, so that the experience has a calm and meditative quality for both people concerned. While the strokes and techniques remain important to the treatment, the caring and loving quality of the touch is fundamental to the holistic principle.

the art of massage

Correct breathing and posture are crucial in massage. It is essential to know how to relax your own body in order to pass the same vital message on to another person through the medium of your strokes. An awareness of breathing and posture helps you to remain energized and comfortable while giving a massage, so that the massage experience is wholly beneficial for both you and your partner. Particularly when massaging larger areas of the body, it will help you to perform fluid strokes and allow you to remain relaxed throughout the session, without tiring yourself or straining your own body. The following sequences introduce you to the fundamental techniques of good posture and full and easy breathing.

posture

A good posture, the way you hold and move your body, enables the whole physical structure to achieve graceful and flexible motion. This ease and grace within you will be imparted through your hands, carrying the message of relaxation to the person on whom you are working.

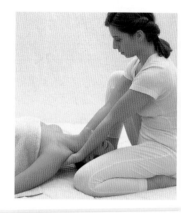

△ While massaging at floor level, kneel with one foot on the ground so you can ease your body back and forth with the longer strokes. This will allow movement from the lower body, so your torso, spine, neck, and head remain relaxed.

coordinating breathing and movement

This simple exercise helps you to deepen your breathing and to synchronize it with your movement, with each breath lasting for the length of each movement. This practice will allow you to remain calm but energized while giving a massage, increasing the vitality in your hands and bringing fluidity to your strokes. Repeat the cycle of movement and breathing up to ten times.

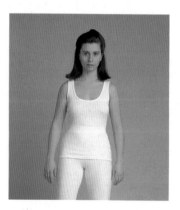

△ **1** Stand with your feet parallel and a hip-width apart, your knees slightly bent and arms loose. Lengthen your spine, keeping neck and head balanced lightly above it and away from your shoulders.

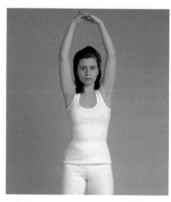

△ **2** As you inhale, let both arms float smoothly out from the sides of your body. Raise them slowly until they meet above your head, then clasp your fingers lightly together.

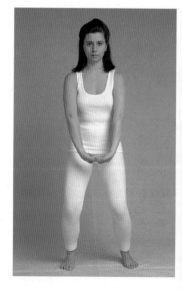

△ **3** As you slowly exhale, press your palms down towards the floor until your arms are straight. Unlock your fingers, and repeat the cycle of breathing and movement.

There are several main points to remember about posture while giving a massage. Always establish a good, firm contact with the ground, whether you are kneeling or standing during a session. This means letting the lower half of your body, your pelvis, legs, and feet, support your weight and movement. Ease your body back and forth with your strokes by using your leg muscles. Keep your knees flexed and tip forward from your hips, so that your spine is straight and extended upwards. Try to keep your neck and head in line with your spine so they don't hang forward.

Constantly remind yourself to relax your shoulders so there is width in your chest, and let your arms hang loosely downwards so that your shoulders, elbows, and wrists are flexible at all times. Keep a space between your arms and your body to avoid hunching in your shoulders. Each time your hands apply strokes to ease tension from a certain part of your partner's body, check that the same area is relaxed in your own body.

breath

Deep and easy breathing assists in bringing oxygen to the cells of your body and allows tense muscles to open and relax. Breath is the basic fuel of your vital life force, and will constantly replenish your energy. Full and easy breathing will allow you to be more present and attentive in your massage, bringing a vitality to your hands and your strokes. It will also enable you to be more connected with your feelings, thereby enhancing the loving quality of your touch.

Synchronizing your breath with your strokes will deepen the effects of the massage, so that it flows over the body like a wave of energy. The ease of your breathing and the relaxed vitality that it brings to you will transmit itself to your partner, enabling the release of tensions, and fuller, deeper breathing.

breathing and stamina

This exercise is more complex than the previous one and is adapted from the Chinese martial art form chi kung. It helps you to build up stamina and vital energy, while controlling and deepening your flow of breath. It also brings you in contact with your *ki*, the source of vital life energy in your belly, which is the centre of gravity in your body. Practice will help you to maintain a relaxed strength while giving a massage.

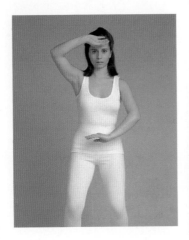

△ **1** Begin with the basic stance, but place one hand, palm facing outwards, at the front of your forehead, and the other hand, palm facing downwards, in front of your navel. Let both hands remain relaxed.

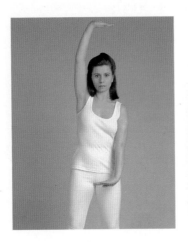

△ **2** As you breathe in, straighten your knees and push up with one hand and down with the other hand, until both arms are vertical to the body.

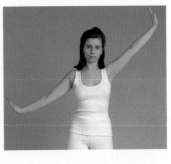

△ **3** Continue with this long inhalation of breath as you rotate your arms like a windmill to move into the opposite direction.

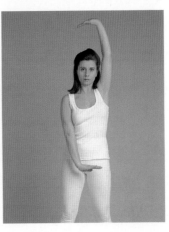

△ **4** Once you have switched the positions of your arms, flex your wrists and flatten your palms, pushing one hand up towards the sky, and the other hand down towards the ground.

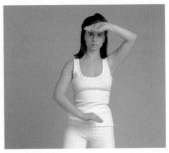

△ **5** Now slowly release your breath and sink your weight down into your knees, while bending your arms at the elbows so that, once again, one hand is in front of the forehead and the other is in front of the navel.

Body massage basics

The following sequence introduces the basic techniques of body massage, which will help you to build up a flowing sequence of strokes to bring harmony, relaxation and invigoration to your partner. From soothing effleurage strokes to more invigorating friction and pressure strokes, these basic sequences can be practised and combined together to achieve an effective massage.

effleurage

The first and main stroke of massage, effleurage prepares the body's soft tissues and warms the muscles for all deeper movements. It is also used to follow up more vigorous strokes such as kneading and friction, in order to soothe and relax an area that has just been massaged. Effleurage simply means "stroking", and is a free-flowing, continuous movement made with the flat of one or, more usually, both hands at a steady pressure.

Effleurage strokes have a calming and almost hypnotic effect on the body, allowing a sense of trust to develop so that the recipient can relax both physically and psychologically. The strokes can be applied with a light to medium pressure, with the whole hand in contact with the skin. When applied in a movement up towards the heart these strokes benefit the cardiovascular system (the heart and blood vessels) and the lymphatic system (the lymph vessels) by boosting the circulation of blood and lymph around the body. A lighter movement has a calming effect on the function of the nervous system.

The hands should be completely relaxed while making the strokes, so that they mould into the body's contours and define its shape and structure.

▷ **Effleurage strokes have a soothing, fluid quality, and are an important stroke to master because they begin, and punctuate, a massage sequence. These relaxing strokes flow smoothly around the body and never finish abruptly.**

preparation

The opening massage strokes are a flowing, continuous sequence of motions to define the contours of the area you intend to massage and also to warm the muscles and prepare them for subsequent massage techniques.

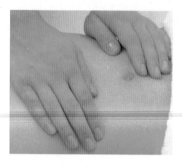

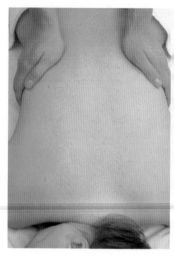

△ **1** Rub a little of the oil into the palms of your hands and spread it over the area you intend to massage with the flat of the hands, in smooth, flowing motions. This is the best method of spreading oil on any part of the body.

△ **2** It is important with effleurage to let your hands mould into the contours of the body shape. When applied as a preparatory, or integration, stroke it should be repeated three to five times for full effect.

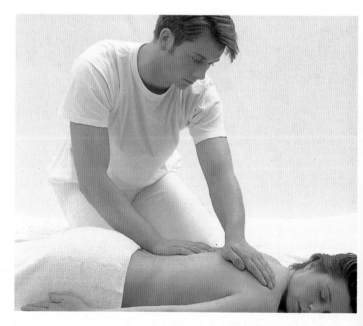

fanning

Fanning is an effleurage motion that can be applied to many areas of the body, including the back, chest, legs, and arms. It is an excellent stroke to follow on from larger preparatory movements and can be used to stretch and manipulate tension away from the muscles. Fanning can be applied either as a series of shorter movements for remedial benefit or in larger, more flowing motions for sensual and soothing effects.

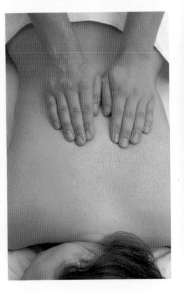

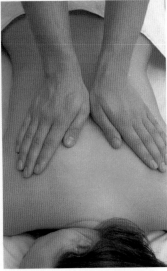

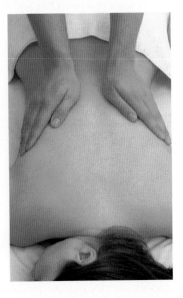

△ **1** Place the hands flat on either side of the spine, with the fingers close together and pointing towards the head. Stroke with an even pressure for about 15cm (6in) up the back.

△ **2** Let your hands flow outwards in a fanning motion, moving towards the sides of the ribcage.

△ **3** Shape your hands to the sides of the body, then draw the hands down before sliding them lightly around and towards their original position alongside the spine. Now stroke further up the back.

continuous circle strokes

Continuous circle strokes add a sensual, relaxing, and soporific element to the massage. If applied at a more vigorous pace and with slightly firmer pressure, they are excellent for warming the superficial layer of tissue and for releasing tension. These effleurage strokes can be used on any broad expanse of the body, such as the sides of the ribcage, the back, and the thighs, when they are applied in a flowing unbroken motion. Continuous circle strokes also form the main preparatory stroke on the abdomen.

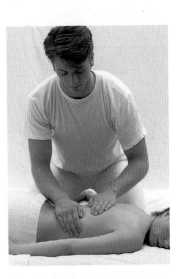

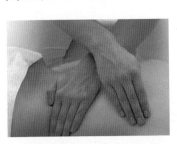

△ **1** Lay both hands parallel to each other and flat on the surface of the area you intend to massage. The hands should be both flexible and soft enough to mould into the body's contours. Begin to slide both hands in a circular motion.

◁ **2** While your left hand continues to move full circle, the right hand lifts and passes over the moving left hand.

△ **3** The right hand returns to the body to perform a half-circle stroke before lifting off again to let the left hand complete the next full circular motion.

kneading

One of the most satisfying strokes in massage both to give and receive, kneading takes hold of the muscle and moves it about, creating greater flexibility and suppleness. To knead well the hands should be dextrous and pliable; the motion is similar to the action of a baker kneading dough. Kneading is a lifting, squeezing and rolling movement that passes the flesh from one hand to the other. It has a rhythmic, circular motion and should be applied with the wrists and shoulders relaxed, and the arms held at a distance from the body.

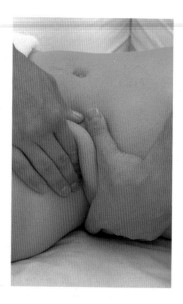

△ Kneading is an effective stroke to apply on muscular and fleshy areas such as the calves, thighs, buttocks and waist. This stroke should be applied after the muscles have been relaxed and warmed by a sequence of effleurage strokes. It benefits the muscles by releasing underlying tension, breaking down fat deposits and toxins trapped in the tissues, and aiding the exchange of tissue fluids. Always follow up kneading strokes with further effleurage sequences to soothe the area and boost the blood and lymph circulation so that releasing toxins can be properly eliminated.

friction and pressure strokes

A pressure stroke is made by leaning your weight into a particular part of your hand or arm in order to sink into muscle or connective tissue (tissue that holds organs and other structures in place). The heel of the hand, thumb pads, finger pads, knuckles and forearm can all be used. Always apply and release pressure slowly and sensitively. The grinding or stretching action can be a firm, sliding motion, circles, or a series of alternating circular motions. These deep strokes push the tissue down towards the bone and stretch it, causing friction between muscle and bone and releasing tension. Apply after kneading on fleshy areas, or after effleurage where the bone is close to the skin's surface, such as on hands, feet, face, or beside the spine.

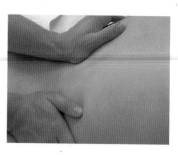

△ **1** The heel of the hand gives a broad surface to add pressure. Shift the weight in the hands to the heels and make circular motions – one hand after the other in a continuous flow. Apply pressure in the upward and outward half of the slide but lessen it in the last half, as the hands glide softly to repeat the stroke.

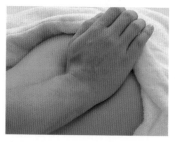

△ **2** By keeping the whole hand relaxed, but by applying direct pressure into the heel of the hand, these circular motions will ease tension from the muscles of the buttocks. These friction and pressure strokes are particularly effective in stretching and draining muscle in tight areas such as the lower back and thighs.

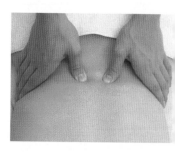

△ **3** The small surfaces of the thumb pads can penetrate areas where muscles and tendons are attached to bone, for example beside the spine. Tight spots can be eased by leaning weight into the thumbs with the hands relaxed, and then making a firm sliding motion up each side of the spine.

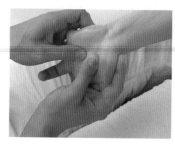

△ **4** Support the back of your partner's hand with your fingers, and use small and continuously alternating thumb circles over the palms and wrists to remove stiffness. To achieve the correct movement you must rotate the thumbs from their base joint.

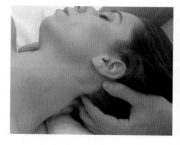

△ **5** Finger pad pressure can be applied in order to release tension from under bone, such as the ridge of the skull. The pressure should be applied gently and slowly to allow your partner time to relax. Slowly rotate your fingertips on one small area at a time. Then release the pressure gradually before moving to the next spot.

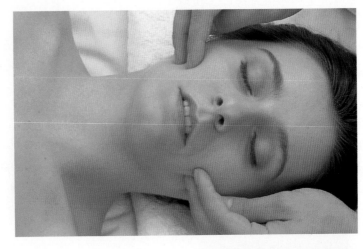

vibrating

This stroke helps to free muscle from a habitual pattern of tension. Vibration is particularly effective on small muscles such as in the cheeks of the face or those alongside the spine.

▷ Sink the fingertips into the fleshy area of the cheeks of the face and vibrate with rapid movements. Move to another spot and vibrate again. This will help the mouth and jaw to relax.

percussion

This includes a variety of invigorating movements that briskly strike fleshy and muscular areas of the body to produce a toning and stimulating effect on the skin. Percussion strokes are performed with one hand following the other in a series of rapid and rhythmic movements, helping to draw the blood towards the skin's surface and leaving it with a warm and healthy glow. The rapid action also dispels tension and rids the tissues of excess fluid and fatty deposits. To achieve the best results, keep your shoulders, wrists and hands relaxed, and bounce your hands immediately back off the skin the moment they make contact.

   The invigorating effects of percussion help to enliven the body after the euphoric effects of other massage strokes, but they may not be suitable to use if your partner is in a particularly sensitive or vulnerable mood. Percussion strokes should never be applied over varicose veins or directly on top of bone.

▷ To perform the cupping movement, form both hands into a softly cupped shape by keeping your fingers straight but bent at the lower knuckles; at the same time draw the thumbs close into the palms. This should create an airtight vacuum in the centre of your palms, which works as a suction on the skin during the rapid cupping action. Using the palms to make contact, briskly strike and flick off the skin, one hand following the other in quick succession over fleshy areas.

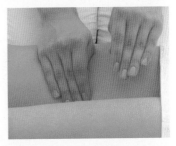

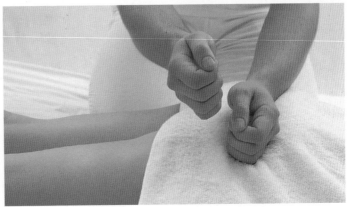

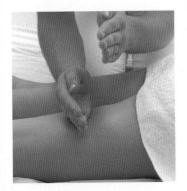

◁ Hacking uses the same fast rhythmic motion as cupping, but contact with the skin is made from the sides of the hands, one following the other in quick succession. The wrists and fingers should be relaxed, and the palms of each hand should face each other with only about 25mm (1in) distance between them. Hacking tones and stimulates all fleshy areas, and works particularly well on the buttocks, thighs, and tops of the shoulders.

△ For the pummelling stroke, keep your shoulders and wrists relaxed and make loose fists in order to pummel over the fleshy parts of your partner's body. Contact with the skin is made with the sides of the hands. Apply the stroke in the same brisk fashion as the previous percussion strokes, letting one hand after the other pummel over the area. This stroke, applied to the thighs and buttocks, is excellent for helping to break down cellulite.

applying the correct sequence of strokes

The following sequence of strokes on the calf muscles of the leg show the order in which the basic techniques of massage should be applied to create a relaxing and invigorating effect. This sequence can be used, as appropriate, on any part of the body.

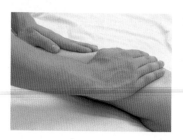

△ **1** Effleurage: Soothing strokes made with the flat of the hands will warm and loosen tense calf muscles and prepare them for deeper strokes.

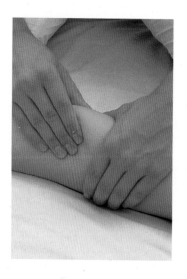

△ **2** Kneading: Knead the calf muscles to invigorate and aid the muscles to contract. Follow up with some soft strokes.

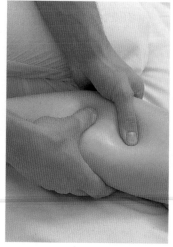

△ **3** Friction: Press your thumb pads sensitively into the muscle tissue using alternating thumb circle friction strokes. This will stretch and release a deeper level of tension. Work thoroughly over the whole area.

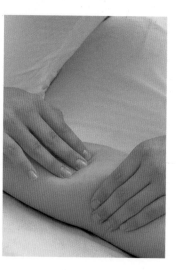

△ **4** Vibrating: Gently sink your finger tips into the calf muscle and vibrate it rapidly. Let your hands mould into the shape of the lower leg as you follow the vibrating action with flowing effleurage.

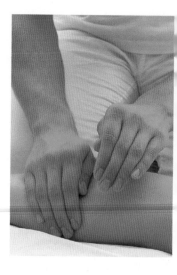

△ **5** Cupping: Cup the calf briskly to stimulate the blood circulation and tone the skin and muscles. Apply the cupping motion up and down the lower leg several times.

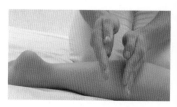

△ **6** Hacking: Use this stroke over the bulk of the calf muscles for further toning, and to aid elimination of excess tissue fluids. Do not strike the back of the knee.

▽ **7** Stroking: Gently stroke over the calf to harmonize the previous massage movements and to boost both the blood and lymph circulation towards the heart.

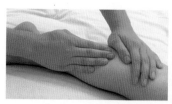

use of towels

Use warmed, fresh clean towels to cover your partner during massage. The towels are important because they prevent the loss of body heat once the oil has been applied and the person is lying still. They also ensure your partner's modesty. Move the towels as needed while applying your strokes, leaving uncovered only the area on which you are working during the massage.

▽ **1** Ideally you should use one large bath towel to cover the whole body, and two medium-sized towels to add further warmth to the upper body and the feet. Tuck the towel snugly around both feet.

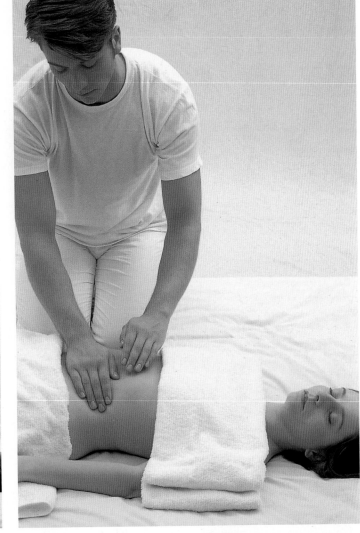

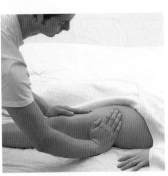

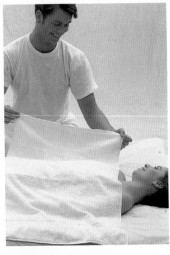

△ **2** When massaging the abdomen, peel back the large towel and cover the chest with a folded towel. Do not leave the chest exposed.

◁ **3** Once you are working on the legs, ensure that the upper body stays warm by covering it with an extra towel. Fold the large towel over so that only the leg on which you are working remains exposed.

▷ **4** When your partner turns over, hold the towel up between you both, and then let it drop softly down to cover the other side of the body.

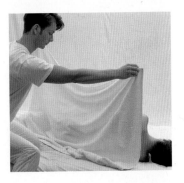

Using oils in body massage

The nurturing touch of a massage is considerably enhanced by the aroma of essential oils. A selection of blends appropriate to everyday circumstances is given below. These few suggestions are to be used as a guide. If you are already familiar with some of the essential oils and have a favourite blend, there is no reason why you should not use it.

carrier oil basics

Choosing the right vegetable carrier oil is vital. Essential oils dissolve easily in a carrier oil to make a blend that makes it easier to move the hands continuously on the skin without dragging or slipping. Some oils, such as olive oil, are too sticky for massage. Peach nut oil is good for delicate skin. Avocado oil has a distinctive fruity scent, so choose essential oils with complementary fragrances. Many carrier oils have health-giving, nutritious properties of their own, but will be much more effective if combined with a another richer carrier oil more suitable for massage.

blending essential oils for massage

Experiment with different types of carrier oil to achieve the ideal blend for your massage style. Try adding a teaspoonful of another carrier oil as well as the essential oils for a highly personal mixture. It is worth remembering that even the weather affects the state of our skin, and in the winter central heating and cold temperatures will cause it to dry out. These variations can be accommodated by changing the exotic carrier oils used to enrich each blend.

Rub a little of the blend between the palms of your hands to warm it, then test the fragrance before beginning the massage. It may require slight adjustment before you are happy with the result.

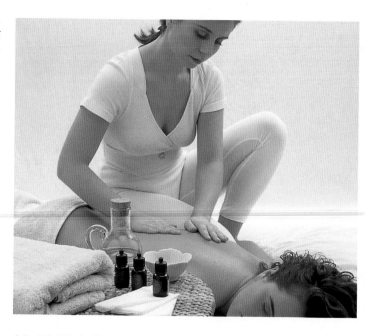

△ The right oil blend enables the hands to move smoothly and continuously over the skin, and the sensual aroma of essential oils stimulates and soothes the body and the spirit.

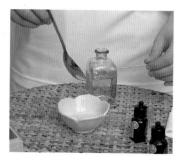

△ **1** Before you begin blending the oils, wash and dry your hands and make sure that you have all the bowls and bottles you need, and that all your utensils are clean and dry. Have your essential oils at the ready, but leave the lids on the bottles until they are required. Carefully measure out approximately 10ml (2 tsp) of your chosen carrier oil, and gently pour it into your blending bowl.

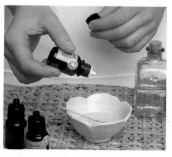

△ **2** Bearing in mind the correct ratio of essential oil to carrier oil (generally 10ml (2 tsp) base oil to 5 drops of essential oil), and the combination of top, middle and base notes required, add the first essential oil a drop at a time. Add remaining oils a drop at a time and mix gently with a clean, dry cocktail stick or toothpick, to blend.

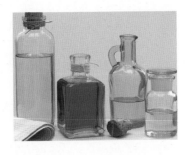

some useful blends for body massage

Choose up to four oils to add to a carrier oil to create a blend suitable for your needs.

a blend to aid relaxation Relaxation is particularly important following a stressful day at work. A massage with a blend of the following oils is an effective way to encourage relaxation: bergamot, German chamomile, clary sage, lavender, rosewood, or sandalwood. To add an uplifting note choose one of the other citrus oils, which will produce a blend that is relaxing and uplifting at the same time.

an energizing blend When everything seems grey and depressing, an enlivening massage with a blend of the invigorating oils could help turn the day around from one of gloom and despair to a more energetic one. Try a blend of three or four of the following oils: black pepper, cypress, eucalyptus, fennel, ginger, grapefruit, jasmine, juniper, lemon, nutmeg, peppermint, rosemary, tea tree.

a blend for stiff muscles Everyone suffers from minor muscular aches and pains from time to time. They may be brought on by unusual physical exercise – from gardening or dancing to sporting activities – or simply by remaining in an uncomfortable position too long. At such times the warming oils that bring blood back into the aching muscles are the most helpful. Choose your oils from the following list: benzoin, black pepper, clary sage, eucalyptus, ginger, grapefruit, jasmine, juniper, lavender, lemon, marjoram, nutmeg, orange, peppermint or rosemary.

a hangover remedy If you have over-indulged in alcoholic drinks, try to drink several glasses of water before sleeping, in order to help alleviate the dehydration caused by an excess of alcohol. Drink plenty of water and orange juice at breakfast to help detoxification and, if possible, eat some wholemeal toast with a yeast spread. A gentle massage, using three or four of the following oils, may help restore normal good health after eating or drinking too much: black pepper, fennel, geranium, ginger, juniper, orange or peppermint.

a blend for raising the spirits For the days when the ordinary activities of life seem too difficult there are a number of oils that can help raise the spirits: benzoin, bergamot, cedarwood, clary sage, frankincense, geranium, grapefruit, jasmine, mandarin, nutmeg, orange, rose, rosewood or ylang ylang. A blend of three or four from this list, and a soothing massage, can give you back a zest for life.

a warming blend After struggling with bitter winds and the cold of winter the idea of undressing for a massage may seem foolish. However, there are some warming and comforting essential oils that can be very nourishing when you are feeling emotionally, as well as physically, cold. Blend benzoin, ginger, orange and rosewood together, and allow them to envelop your body in their special aroma.

a sensual blend In a long-term relationship the intimate physical bond between partners may weaken or cease to exist. A long illness, overwork, or emotional crises can also lead to a lack of sexual interest. At such times the non-sexual but loving touch of massage can play an important part in rekindling the sexual intimacy that has been missing. Essential oils that may be helpful are: black pepper, cedarwood, clary sage, fennel, frankincense, ginger, jasmine, rose and sandalwood. This is an area where it is particularly important to bear in mind each individual's personal preferences.

seasonal blends For a festive mood, use the essences of Christmas: frankincense, ginger and mandarin. You could also try blending with benzoin, neroli, and orange. Easter, occurring at the time of renewal and refreshment, is a good time to try a blend of geranium, palmarosa and rosewood.

a pre-wedding blend There is only one blend for a pre-wedding massage: jasmine and rose, respectively the king and queen of fragrances, and neroli, to calm the nerves. A luxurious blend to bring the essence of calm to the beginning of married life.

a blend to calm Frankincense, sandalwood, neroli and ylang ylang blend together to create a rich perfume of peace. This blend can bring feelings of tranquillity and reduce feelings of fragmentation. It can be valuable in helping to reconnect someone to their strong inner core. Give or receive a massage with this mixture, and help yourself regain peace in your life.

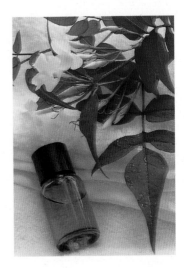

△ Jasmine, known as the king of flower oils, has a strong scent that can produce feelings of optimism, euphoria and confidence.

Getting started

In order to ensure your massage has maximum effectiveness it is important to make sure that you and your partner are in the right frame of mind. Preliminaries include making sure your equipment is ready, setting the scene and preparing yourself and your partner for treatment.

setting the mood

Creating an atmosphere of confidence and trust is an important element in giving a successful body massage. It will help your massage partner relax if it is clear that you are carefully prepared and in control. Make sure that the room is heated and all of your equipment and oils are ready. Take time to compose yourself so that your whole attention is focused on the massage. Give your partner privacy to undress, and clear directions on how to lie down on the mattress. Use the towels correctly to cover the body, both to keep it warm and to protect modesty. By following these suggestions, your partner will immediately feel safe and secure in your hands.

working at a couch

While some people prefer to kneel and give a massage at ground level, working at a specially-designed couch increases your mobility, as you can use your feet and legs to move more freely around the body. This puts less stress on your posture, enabling you to bring length to your spine and neck and a relaxed width to your shoulders. In common with the kneeling position, your movement at the couch should come from the lower half of your body, to prevent strain on your back.

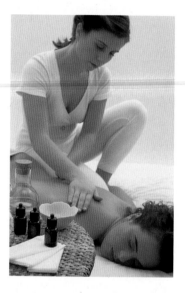

▷ A massage couch with adjustable legs allows people of various heights to use it successfully. The height can also be adjusted to suit the type of massage you are giving. In a deep tissue massage a greater degree of pressure is applied to the strokes, and so a lower height is required than would be the case for soft tissue massage.

establishing contact and applying oils

Before you begin, suggest your partner takes a moment to settle comfortably on to the mattress.

▷ **1** Establish contact with your partner by placing your hands gently on the body, so that one hand rests on the top of the spine and the other at its base.

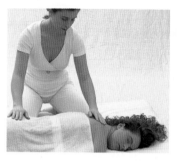

◁ **2** Fold the top towel over the lower half of the body. Pour 2.5ml (½ tsp) of blended oils into the palm of one hand, then rub your hands together to warm the oil. Apply more oil as appropriate. Using smooth and flowing effleurage strokes, spread the oil over the back. Relax your hands so they become pliable and are able to mould into the body's curves.

the body massage

The body massage usually starts on the back of the body, with special focus on main areas of tension. Once your partner has turned over, the massage moves up the entire front of the body.

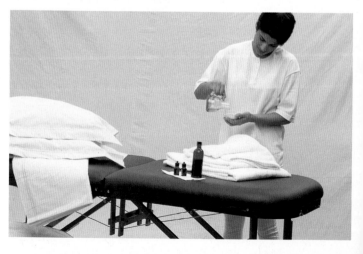

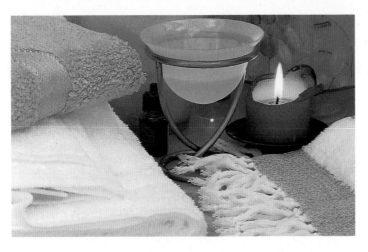

◁ When preparing for a massage it is a good idea to make sure that the room is warm and that you have all the equipment that you need to hand. It is disruptive for your partner if you have to break off half way through to replenish your massage oil blend, adjust the heating or fetch a cushion or a warm towel.

using pillows and towels to ease body tension

Postural tension remains in the body even when a person is lying down and appears to be relaxed. In fact, a prolonged period of resting on a flat surface can even exacerbate physical strain, particularly in the major joints of the body. The more you massage, the more you will be able to detect where someone is holding their tension. Once you have worked out where the problem is pillows and towels can be used effectively to support key areas of the body in order to ease tension.

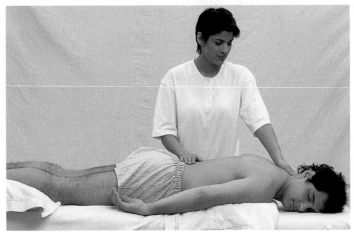

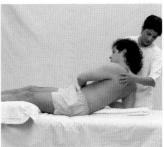

△ Lower back pain may be caused by a curve in the base of the spine, or a chronic pattern of tension in the pelvic region. A pillow placed under the abdomen can redress this imbalance during a massage, helping the lumbar region to relax under your touch.

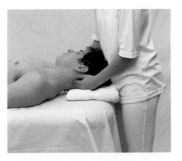

△ In a prone position, place one pillow just below the knees to relax the pelvis and lower back. A pillow under the front of the chest allows the shoulders to fall forwards opening up the upper back and creating space between the shoulder blades. This added support also helps to lengthen and relax the neck.

▷ Constriction in the muscles at the base of the skull will shorten the neck muscles, causing the head to contract backwards. Place a thin, folded towel under the skull to lift the head upwards to relieve this.

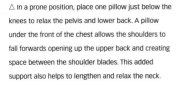

△ Tension in the chest and ribs can cause muscles to contract, pulling the shoulders forward so that they cannot rest on the table. Ease this posture by placing a towel, folded into a thin strip, under and along the spine. This helps the chest expand and the shoulders to fall back. Help your partner into position so that the towel remains in the correct place.

Body Massage Routines

The massage basics can be applied to soothe and relax the whole body. This chapter takes you step-by-step through the sequence of strokes that is needed to give a satisfying and effective body massage. Starting with the upper and lower back, which are especially prone to tension, it moves on through clearly defined and punctuated stages to the front of the body, and finally the arms and hands. A self-massage sequence and a sensual massage are also included.

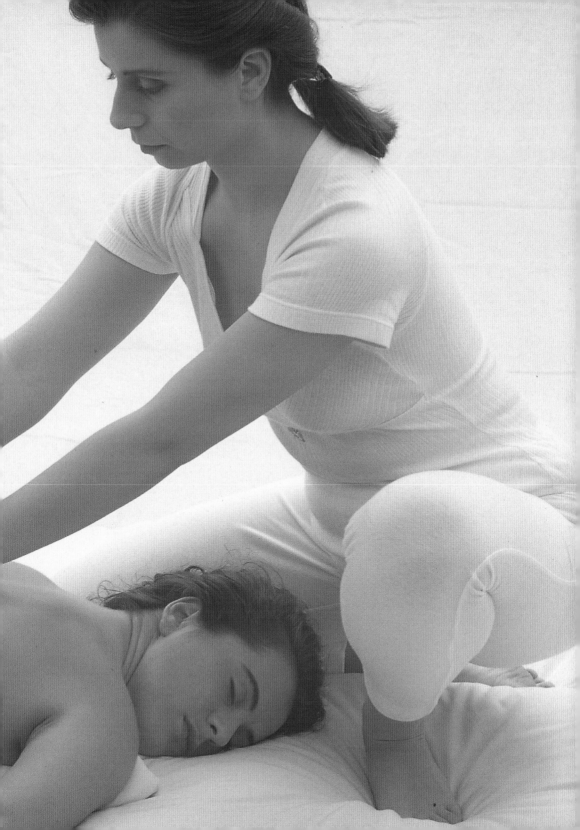

Massaging the back

There are several good reasons for beginning a body massage on the back. Some people need time to relax sufficiently to allow the process of massage to work properly, and the back presents a broad surface that does not feel as immediately intimate or as vulnerable to touch as, for example, the chest or stomach. At the same time, the muscles of the back are especially prone to tension resulting from stress, uncomfortable posture, and injury.

A thorough back massage can take the strain out of the whole body. Combine your strokes to prepare, soothe, warm and relax the back, while working therapeutically on all the main areas of tension, such as the spine, the lower back and the shoulders.

relaxing the spine

The first stage of the back massage focuses on relaxing the spine and the muscles that support it. Begin from a position behind your partner's head so that you can carry out a series of soothing effleurage strokes over the whole back, followed by some deeper pressure strokes to release tension from alongside the spine.

caution

During a back massage you should never apply pressure directly on the spine. The focus should be on releasing tension from the muscles alongside the spine.

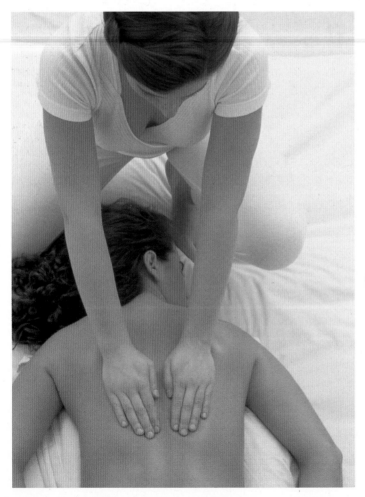

the initial integration stroke

This initial main effleurage movement embraces the whole shape of the back, warming the muscles and tissues. It can be applied up to five times as the preparatory stroke in a continuous sequence of motions.

◁ **1** To start, place your hands flat on each side of the spine, fingers pointing towards the lower back. Lean your weight into your hands and slide them steadily downwards to stretch the long muscles beside the spine.

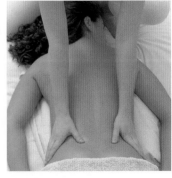

△ **2** As your hands reach the lower back, swing them out and around the hips to enfold the sides of the body. Your fingers should slip slightly under the front of the body.

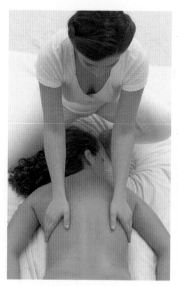

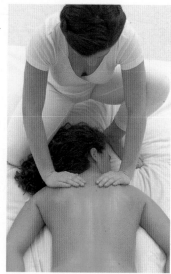

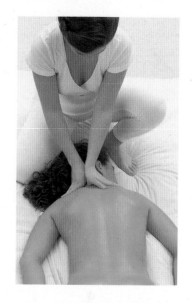

△ **3** Draw your hands gently but firmly up along the sides of the waist and ribcage until they reach the shoulder blades. Turn your wrists so that your hands glide in and around the edges of the shoulder blades.

△ **4** As your hands draw out across the top of the shoulders, shift the pressure into their heels to give a good stretch to tense shoulder muscles.

△ **5** Slip your hands softly around the shoulder joints and swivel your wrists to glide them lightly back in across the top of the shoulders. Take the stroke up the back of the neck and out through the head and hair.

rocking the body

Some variation can be added to the above stroke to bring extra vitality and movement to the body. Complete both rocking sequences with a sweep around the shoulders, drawing your hands towards the neck and up over the head.

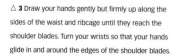

◁ **1** After your hands have curved around the sides of the lower back, draw them in towards the base of the spine. Slip your left hand on top of your right hand to add support. Slightly cup your right hand to create a suction effect and rock gently and rhythmically up over the length of the spine.

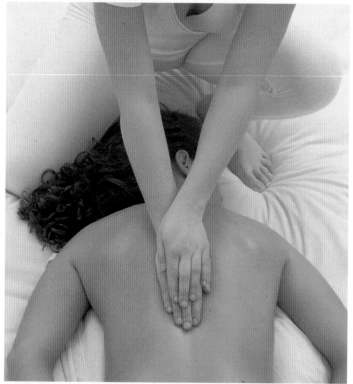

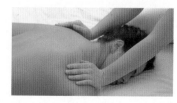

△ **2** Separate your hands at the top of the spine. Put pressure into the heel of each hand to create an alternating press-and-release movement, which works out towards the shoulders. This rocking motion is similar to the way in which a cat kneads a soft surface with its paws.

fanning

To enhance the overall relaxation of the back, perform three sequences of fanning strokes. Massage towards the lower back, and then return your hands by sweeping them out and up along the sides of the body in the same manner as the initial effleurage stroke.

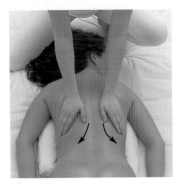

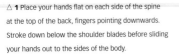

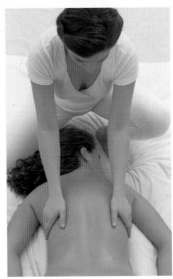

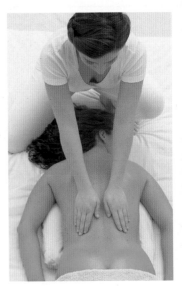

△ **1** Place your hands flat on each side of the spine at the top of the back, fingers pointing downwards. Stroke down below the shoulder blades before sliding your hands out to the sides of the body.

△ **2** Mould your hands to the sides of the body, gliding them up the ribcage for a short distance before flexing your wrists to draw them very lightly towards the centre of the back.

△ **3** Turn your hands so they are once again lying flat against each side of the spine, fingers pointing to the lower back. Stroke down another hand's length to repeat the fanning motion.

double stretch stroke

This stroke focuses on the long muscles, or erector spinae, which give support to the spine and help it extend and rotate the trunk of the body. Its stretching and rubbing effect releases tension and brings heat to the muscles, creating greater flexibility and movement in the back.

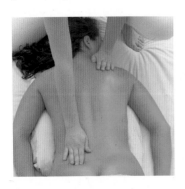

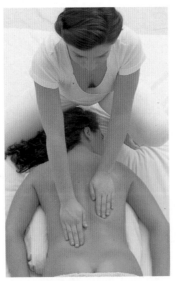

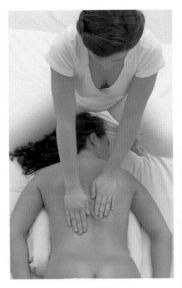

△ **1** Place both hands over the top of the shoulders and close to the spine, fingers pointing down the back. Using a firm and steady pressure, slide the right hand down over the long muscles while keeping the left hand in its original position.

△ **2** When the right hand reaches the small of the back, curve it around the hip and back to the base of the spine, before drawing it back up the long muscle on the left side of the spinal column. At the same time, slide your left hand down to repeat the motion on the right side of the spine.

△ **3** Continue to move both hands back and forth over the long muscles for up to five sequences. Increase the speed and pressure to create a heat-producing friction and rippling effect in the tissue as the hands pass each other. Complete the stroke with both hands resting by the shoulders.

pressure strokes along the spine

Now is the time to increase the pressure of your strokes along the spine in order to ease tight spots and bring relief. Sink the weight slowly into the muscle tissue at the top of the shoulders before starting the stroke, remaining sensitive to your partner's response to the pressure. Keep the strokes close to the spine, but avoid pressing directly on the bone. Once your stroke has reached the base of the spine, open out your hands to sweep them around and up the sides of the body so that each sequence can be repeated.

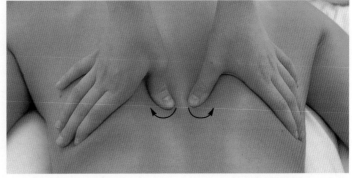

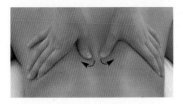

◁ **1** Starting at the top of the back, place your thumb pads on either side of the spine. It is important to remember not to apply pressure directly to the spine. Shift the weight into your thumbs while your fingers rest on the body. Massage in small circular motions close to the edge of the bone.

△ **2** Deepen the pressure as your thumbs rotate towards and away from the spine in the first half of the circle, and release the pressure to glide softly back and around. Work down the length of the spine in a spiralling motion. Repeat the stroke, increasing the pressure.

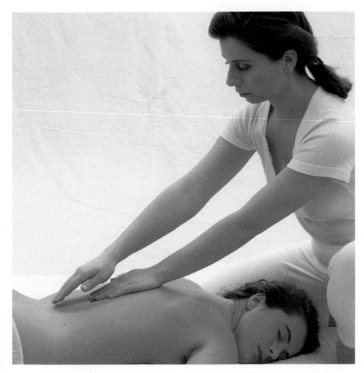

knuckle stretch

To complete this stage of the back massage, carry out an invigorating knuckle stretch.

▽ Starting at the lower back, use loose knuckles, crossing your thumbs over each other for support, to work up either side of the spine. Wait until your knuckles have settled comfortably into a deeper level of tissue, and slide them slowly and steadily down the spine again to give a good stretch. Repeat this twice, remaining aware of your partner's breathing. To integrate the different strokes and to complete the spine massage, make several large effleurage strokes to encompass the back, and finish by placing your hands softly over the spine for several moments.

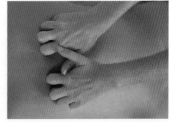

overlapping strokes

Following the double stretch and pressure strokes on the long muscles, soothe the areas with soft, gentle movements.

△ Carry out a series of strokes up over the spine, with one hand following the other in short, overlapping motions, with the fingers relaxed and spread apart.

focus on the lumbar region

Change your position so that you are kneeling beside the hip and facing towards the head. Spread a little more oil on the skin if necessary. Your focus is now on relaxing the lower half of the back, known as the lumbar region. This area is particularly prone to aches and pains which are the result of compression and strain caused by uncomfortable posture, awkward movement or prolonged sitting. Many of the following strokes also benefit those muscles that cross over the sides of the body from the abdomen to the back. These muscles, known as abdominus obliques, support abdominal organs and flex the spine.

soothing with effleurage

Start with a series of relaxing effleurage movements over the whole back before working specifically on the muscles between the pelvic girdle and the shoulder blades. To avoid twisting in your own posture, you can straddle your partner's body while doing these strokes. Keep one foot on the mattress, and use your leg muscles to lever yourself back and forth, and to support your own weight. Ensure that you remain at some physical distance from your partner.

fanning upwards

A firm fanning motion towards the heart can give a boost to the blood circulation. Massage with smaller fanning motions, moving up the back until your hands reach the shoulder blades, and then adapt the stroke to encompass the broad surface of the upper back before gliding back down the sides of the body.

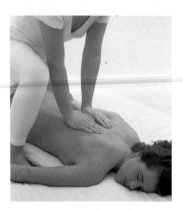

△ **1** Begin a large effleurage stroke from the lower back. Place both hands flat beside the spine, fingers towards the head. Lean into your hands, stroking up the back towards the head with a steady pressure.

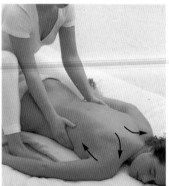

△ **3** Moulding your hands to the body, glide them over the shoulders, down the sides of the ribcage and waist as far as the lower back.

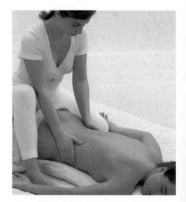

△ **1** Place your hands on each side of the spine, fingers pointing to the head. Stroke upwards with a steady pressure before fanning your hands outwards.

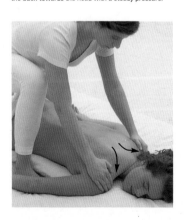

△ **2** As your hands reach the top of the back, fan them out towards the shoulders in a continuous flow of motion.

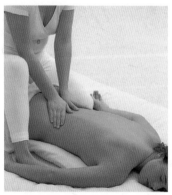

△ **4** Swivel your wrists and softly stroke towards the centre of the back in order to repeat the stroke two more times.

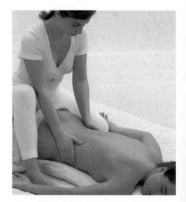

△ **2** Sculpting the sides of the body, pull softly but firmly downwards. Flex your wrists to stroke very lightly back into the body.

pressure circles on the lower back

Pressure circles are excellent strokes for removing tension from a tight lumbar region. Start the stroke softly, and as the tissue warms, increase the pressure into the heels of your hands. Build up speed to massage vigorously on the small of the back. Use firm pressure on the upward and outward half of the circle, flexing your wrists to glide your hands very lightly around to the start of the stroke. Complete the sequence with a full and soothing effleurage stroke over the back.

soft circle strokes

To accomplish the next series of strokes, turn to face into the back. Once you have finished the sequence, change position to repeat the whole sequence from the opposite side of the body. Flow from stroke to stroke without breaking the movement of your hands.

Soft circle strokes feel wonderful on the skin, with their overlapping and fluid motion easing and stretching tension out of the body's soft tissue. They are a perfect stroke for the broad yet rounded dimensions of the back. Begin circle stroking up the side of the body opposite to you, spiralling from the hip to the edge of the shoulder blade. Without breaking the flow, swing the stroke out to cover the spine and massage down towards the sacrum. Repeat three times.

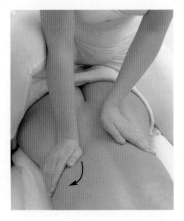

△ **1** Place both hands flat on each side of the base of the spine, with the fingers slightly tilted towards the sides of the body. Stroke your right hand up a short distance, fanning it outwards into a circular motion.

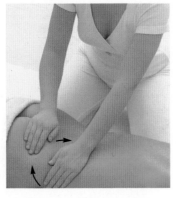

△ **1** Lay your hands over the opposite side to you, keeping the hands about 10cm/4in apart. Circle both hands in a clockwise motion.

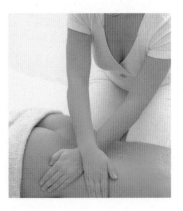

△ **3** As the left hand continues to circle over the side of the body, cross the right hand over it, dropping it lightly back on to the skin.

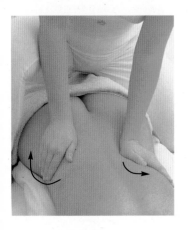

△ **2** At this point the left hand begins to stroke upwards. As the right hand decreases pressure and glides lightly back in a circular motion towards the start of the stroke, the left hand fans up and downwards.

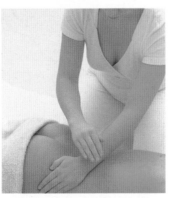

△ **2** Lift up the right hand as it completes the first half-circle to allow the left hand to pass underneath it in an unbroken motion.

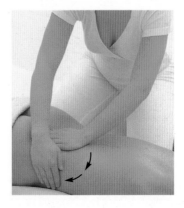

△ **4** Let the right hand form another half-circle stroke before lifting off as the left hand completes the full circle, spiralling upwards.

wringing the back

The wringing action on the lower back is done by crossing your hands from side to side, creating a warm friction on the muscle fibres. Work the stroke across the back, from the hips to the shoulder blades, and down again three times, always making sure that your hands fully encompass both sides of the body. Increase the speed and pressure of the wringing for an invigorating effect, and then slow it down for a soothing finish.

▽ **1** Place your right hand over the hip opposite to you, with your fingers wrapped slightly under the belly, the left hand cupped over the hip closest to you. Slide your hands towards each other with enough pressure to lift and roll the flesh on the sides of the body.

▽ **2** Decrease the pressure as you stroke across the back, hands passing each other to the opposite sides of the body. Without stopping, immediately begin to slide them back. Continuously stroke your hands back and forth while you wring up and down the lumbar region.

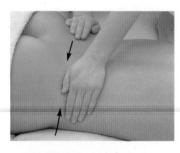

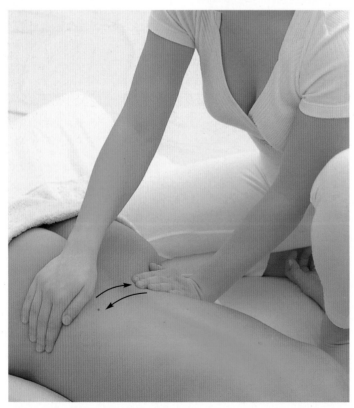

kneading

Invigorating kneading on the buttocks, hips, and along the flank of the body will help to release weight and tension from the back, bringing relief to the whole area. Scoop, squeeze, and roll the flesh with your right hand and then roll it towards the left hand. Without breaking the motion, repeat the action with the left hand so that it passes the flesh back. Keep the stroke moving back and forth in a rhythmic and circular manner. Take care to relax your own shoulders, wrists and hands. Knead thoroughly from the hip to just below the arm and back down again. Repeat once more.

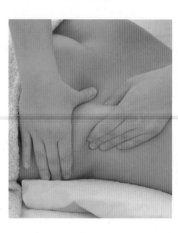

△ **1** Knead over the top of the buttock and beside the hip on the side of the body opposite to you. Work the kneading stroke up alongside the waist and rib cage. The amount of flesh on this area varies considerably from person to person.

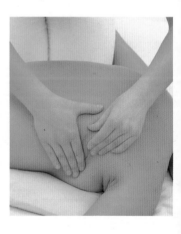

△ **2** Thorough kneading beside the shoulder blade will help the upper back to relax and the shoulder to drop.

hip, shoulder and spine stretch

This stretch stroke brings a pleasing sense of integration to the body as the hands move diagonally from the hip to the opposite shoulder, fan around and over the shoulder blade several times and then finish with a soft stretch over the length of the spine.

▷ **1** Place your hands close together, fingers pointing towards the opposite shoulder, over the hip nearest to you. Stroke across the body to make a sweeping diagonal stretch.

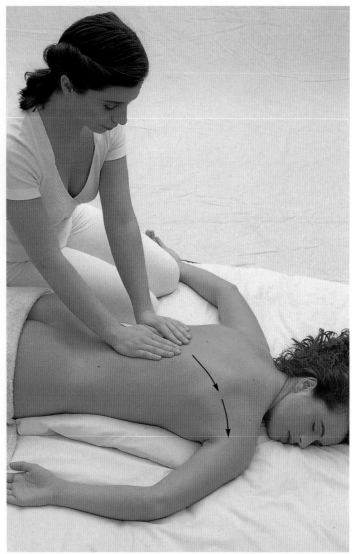

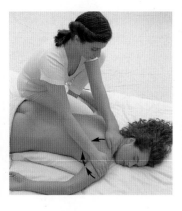

△ **2** When your fingers reach the tip of the opposite shoulder joint, mould them to curve into the shape of the shoulder blade. Draw your hands outwards to surround its circumference until the fingers of both hands meet at the centre of its inner ridge.

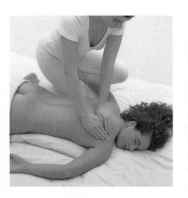

◁ **3** Sweep your hands several times over and around the bone, keeping your hands supple and wrists loose in order to fully enfold its flat triangular shape. Feel the muscles warm up beneath your touch.

▷ **4** Now pull both hands back towards the spine and draw your hands in opposite directions over the vertebrae, one towards the neck and the other towards the lower back. Stop briefly to rest your hands in a calm, still hold over each end of the spine. Move to the other side of your partner and repeat these strokes, following up with harmonious effleurage strokes to cover the whole surface of the back.

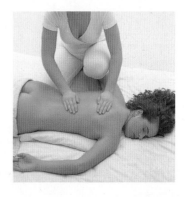

focus on the upper back

The upper back tightens under stress, and most people welcome the therapeutic touch in this region. The following strokes will help to disperse the tension, allowing a greater sense of freedom and vitality.

criss-cross and squeeze

This criss-cross stroke requires coordinated movement. It combines effleurage with a squeezing action and follows the line of the diamond-shaped trapezius muscle that lifts and lowers the shoulder girdle and helps to raise the head.

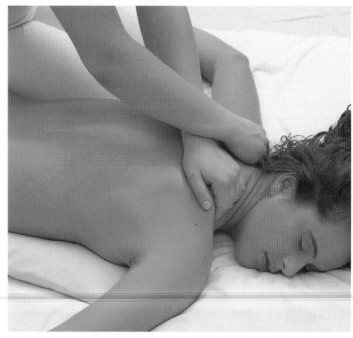

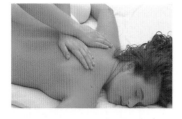

△ **1** Place your hands over the spine at the mid-point of the back. Both hands should be slightly angled towards each other, with the fingers of your right hand resting lightly over the fingers of the left hand. Stroke both hands directly out towards the opposite shoulders in a cross-over action.

△ **2** Without breaking the motion, wrap your fingers slightly over the front of the shoulders, then, adding pressure to both your fingers and the heels of the hands, lift, roll and squeeze the flesh. Release the pressure and pull your hands back towards the mid-point so that your arms are no longer crossed.

▽ **3** Now glide your hands out again to the shoulders, so that the hands form a V-shape. Again let your fingers wrap over the top of the shoulder, but this time slide your hands back without squeezing the muscles. Repeat at least two more times.

kneading the shoulders

Use a kneading action to roll and squeeze the muscles between the thumbs and fingers in order to ease tight spots at the base of the neck and over the shoulder.

▽ Work on the shoulder opposite you and ask your partner to turn her head to you so that the shoulder's surface is fully exposed.

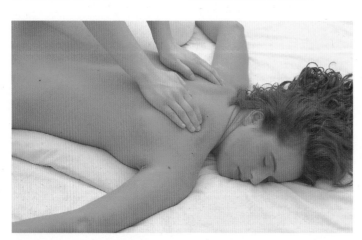

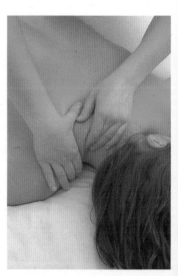

friction strokes

Friction strokes act to release tension from the upper back by pushing the tissue down towards the bone, then stretching it. Apply these strokes after kneading in fleshy areas, or after effleurage in areas where the bone is close to the skin.

easing the vertebrae

The thumbs and fingers are the perfect massage tools with which to penetrate deeper tissue around the shoulder blades and spine. The following friction strokes will bring help to bring relief to sore, constricted muscles.

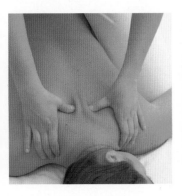

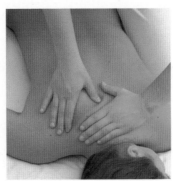

△ **1** Anchor your fingers gently but securely in front of the shoulders, placing your palms on either side of the spine. Apply pressure into your thumbs and sink them into the tissue alongside the vertebrae. Begin to slide firmly up towards the top of the shoulders.

▽ **2** Without releasing your fingers, circle your hands lightly back to their original position. Repeat the thumb slide several times.

△ **3** A further deep friction stroke can be achieved by using the thumb pad to press tissue against the bone, helping to dispel toxic build-up in muscle fibres. Using one hand to push the muscle towards the stroke, make a sequence of short slides with the other hand, using the thumb pad to stretch and relieve tense areas. Always remember to sink into and release pressure slowly and gently from a friction stroke.

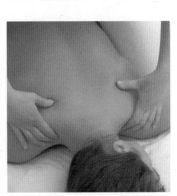

calming holds

Mark the end of each of the body massages with soothing strokes and a calming hold.

Bring a restful sense of completion to this section of the back massage by doing three full integration strokes. Then place your hands on the neck and the base of the spine before moving on to the next sequence.

a soothing finish

The deeper tissue work of kneading and friction strokes should now be followed by a series of soft and soothing effleurage strokes to bring a sense of overall relaxation and integration to the upper back.

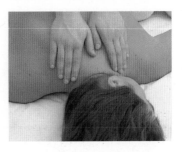

△ **1** Place your hands on the mid-back, flat against each side of the spine with the fingers pointing towards the head. Sweep your hands up towards the top of the shoulders.

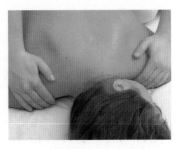

△ **2** Using your hands to mould perfectly to the curve of the body, spread them out to the edge of the shoulders, and in a flowing movement glide them soothingly around the joints.

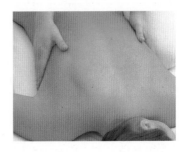

△ **3** Draw your hands down the sides of the ribcage until they are once again on the mid-back. Turn your hands so they can slide lightly to the centre of the back and repeat the effleurage stroke two more times.

Massaging the backs of the legs

The following sequence of massage strokes focuses on the lower half of the body – the legs and buttocks. This is an area of primary importance to the body's posture, weight and locomotion. By combining the techniques of effleurage, kneading, friction, percussion and passive movements, this programme of massage will help to warm and stretch the muscles, improve the circulation of blood and lymph, ease tension from the large strong muscles, and free contracted joints. Begin the massage on the left leg before repeating all the strokes on the right side of the body.

preliminary strokes

These opening strokes are important because they prepare the leg's soft tissues and warm the muscles for all deeper massage movements.

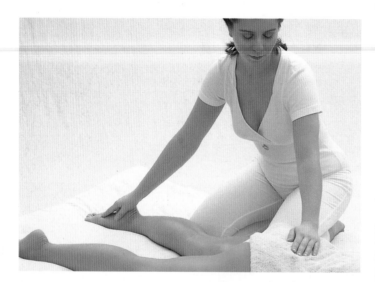

△ **1** Connecting the leg and back: Bring your partner's awareness to the leg with a connecting hold on the sacrum and foot. The gentle pressure of your hands begins the process of relaxation.

▷ **2** Integration stroke on the leg: Spread the oil smoothly down the whole leg, from the buttocks to the foot, then begin with the initial integration stroke. Repeat the stroke three times, increasing the pressure with each upward movement. Be sure to mould your hands to the shape of the leg and to adopt a posture that enables you to stroke upwards and pull back with ease. Place one foot on the mattress ahead of your body to lever your position back and forth.

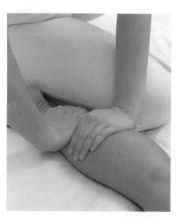

gentle leg stretch

For this stroke, start on the left leg. Wrap both hands over the back of the ankle, little fingers leading, with your left hand in the top position.

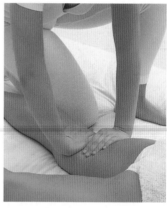

△ **1** Slide with a steady pressure up over the calf. Continue to stroke both hands towards the thigh, sliding lightly over the back of the knee. Then use enough pressure to create a ripple in the strong thigh muscles.

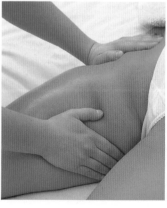

△ **2** As your hands approach the top of the leg, glide the lower one on to the inside of the thigh to rest for some moments while stroking the upper hand over the buttock and out around the hip joint.

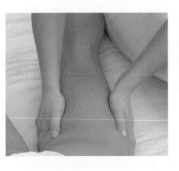

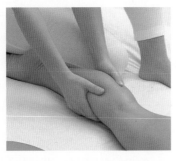

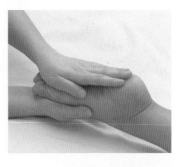

△ **3** When the moving hand descends to the outer thigh and is parallel with the waiting hand, slip your fingers slightly under the front of the leg so that you are holding it securely.

△ **4** Moulding both hands to the leg, lean the weight of your body backwards, returning the stroke steadily towards the ankle in an unbroken motion. This gentle stretch brings a feeling of length and release.

△ **5** As your hands reach the ankle, slip the hand on the outside of the leg over the back of the heel of the foot and, lifting the foot slightly, pass the other hand over the instep. Stroke out over both sides of the foot.

focus on the calf

The function of the calf muscles is to flex the knee and ankle joints, while the Achilles tendon flexes the foot and provides leverage for body movement. Keeping this area supple is important for general health. Muscle stiffness causes a sluggish blood circulation and poor lymphatic drainage, which results in low energy levels. The purpose of this sequence of strokes is to bring relief and relaxation to sore calf muscles.

Begin the sequence with some integrating effleurage strokes, which cover the lower leg from the ankle to just below the back of the knee.

fanning to the knee

Perform a series of fanning motions on the lower leg, moving up from the ankle to just behind the knee. Then glide your hands back down the sides of the leg and repeat the sequence.

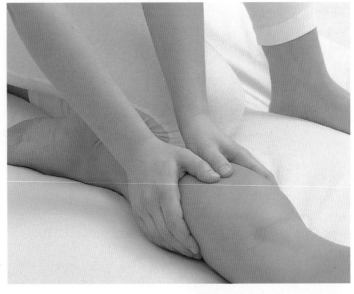

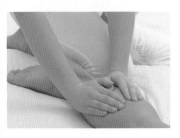

△ **1** Softening your hands to the shape of the leg, place them side by side so that the fingers tilt towards each other but point to the back of the knee. Stroke a hand's length up over the calf muscles.

△ **2** Fan both hands out to wrap around the sides and front of the leg, before sliding down and back towards the original position. Stroke further up over the calf to repeat the motion.

relaxing the achilles tendon

Cup your fingers under the front of the ankle, with the heels of both hands snugly on each side of the heel, and your thumbs on the lower calf.

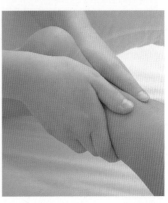

▷ Flex your wrists to rotate your hands in steady circular motions, soothing away strain from the heel and the Achilles tendon.

draining the lower leg

This stroke drains blood and lymph from the extremity of the body. It also creates a long, firm stretch on the lower leg muscles.

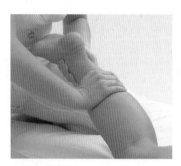

△ **1** Raise the foot and lower leg off the mattress by lifting and supporting the front of the ankle with your left hand. Wrap your right hand over the back of the ankle so that the palm and heel of the hand folds over the inner half of the leg.

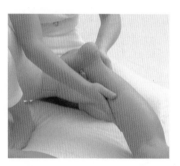

△ **2** Stroke with a firm and steady pressure up the leg towards the back of the knee. Swing the hand to glide down the front of the leg to the ankle.

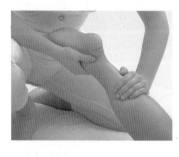

△ **3** Pass the leg to the right hand and repeat the motion with the left hand up over the outer half of the leg; return the stroke to the ankle. Repeat the sequence two more times.

kneading the calf

Kneading strokes will revive fatigued or aching calf muscles resulting from poor circulation, prolonged standing, or excessive exertion. Position yourself to face the calf and knead thoroughly from the ankle to just below the back of the knee and down again. Follow up with effleurage strokes.

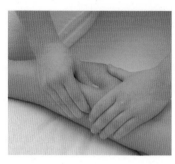

△ **1** Keeping both hands slightly apart, place them over the leg with the thumbs angled away from the fingers. Scoop, lift, and squeeze the muscle by applying pressure between the thumb, heel, and fingers and push it towards the left hand.

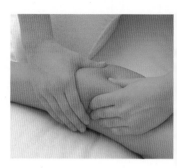

△ **2** Pick up and squeeze the flesh with the left hand and push it back to the right hand. Keeping both hands on the leg, pass the muscle back and forth in a rhythmic and circular movement.

deep friction

These deep friction strokes use the thumbs to penetrate and stretch a deeper level of muscle tissue, freeing it from underlying tension. Sink into the muscle slowly, always remaining aware of your partner's response to the pressure. Both strokes are achieved by rotating the thumbs from their base joints. Once your hands have reached to just below the knee, glide them back down the sides of the leg and repeat the sequence.

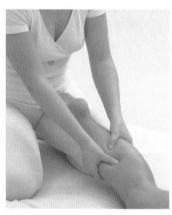

△ **1** Clasp the front of the leg with your fingers and stroke one thumb after the other up over the calf. Using short sliding movements, press firmly into the upward movement and then swing each thumb out and glide lightly back to perform the next upward stroke. At the same time gently roll the leg from hand to hand, squeezing the sides of the calf muscles with the heels of your hands.

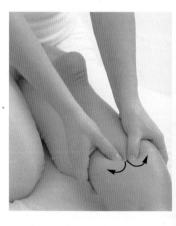

△ **2** Focus the pressure into your thumb pads, and rotate them in alternate and tiny outward flowing circles. Soften the stroke on the last half of the circle. Move up over the calf in three separate lines from above the back of the ankle to just below the knee. Follow up with several flowing integration strokes to cover the whole leg from the ankle to the top of the thigh.

focus on the thigh

A thorough massage of the thighs brings relief to this ample area of powerful body muscle, which provides essential support to the body's posture and mobility.

fanning and soft circle strokes

These flowing, relaxing strokes warm and soothe the leg, from the back of the knee to just below the buttock.

▷ **1** Glide your hands down the sides of the leg, swivelling around on to the back of the knee. Repeat the fanning sequence two more times.

▽ **2** Turn your body so that you face into the thigh and cover the top of the leg with continuous circle strokes to relax and soften the tissue. Pay special attention to the inner thigh muscles, which draw the leg towards the centre of the body.

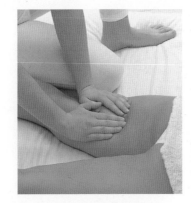

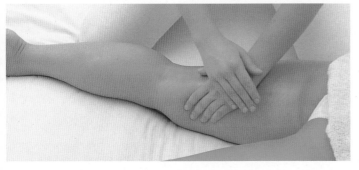

wringing the thigh

This wringing action massages across the bulk of muscle fibres and connective tissue that surrounds them on the thigh.

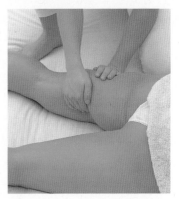

△ **1** Wrap your right hand over the inner edge of the thigh so that your fingers slip slightly under the leg. Place your left hand over the outer side of the leg so that the fingers rest on the thigh. Pull firmly to scoop up the flesh before crossing your hands over the top of the thigh to the opposite sides.

draining and kneading the thigh

These strokes help to break down excess fat deposits and boost the exchange of tissue fluids. With the soothing effleurage strokes, this boosts the lymph drainage and blood circulation in the thigh.

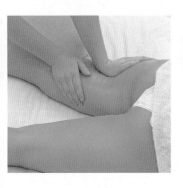

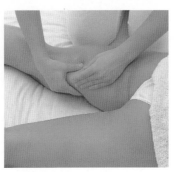

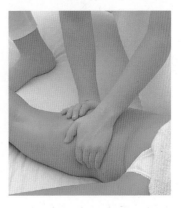

△ **1** Lean your weight into the heels of both hands for a series of firm, alternating pressure circles, one hand following the other. Lessen the pressure of the stroke as each hand fans out to the sides of the leg and glides back and around.

△ **2** Vigorous kneading of the thigh muscles will enliven the upper leg. Lift, squeeze and roll the flesh from hand to hand, working first up along the inner thigh and over the bulk of the muscles. Follow up with soothing fanning motions and other effleurage strokes.

△ **2** Continue to pass your hands rhythmically back and forth over the thigh, creating a slight twist in the movement to produce a wringing effect in the muscles. Stroke from above the knee to the top of the leg and back down again. Repeat once.

final strokes for massaging the backs of the legs

The powerful buttock muscles help to elevate the body and move the thighs. Massage aids a relaxed posture so the body's weight is supported by the lower half of the body, taking strain off the lower back. After massaging the thigh, focus on the buttock on the same side.

focus on the buttocks

Begin with some flowing integration strokes that cover and connect the thigh and buttock and mould into its contours. The strokes below are shown on the right side of the body for clearer instruction.

stimulating the whole leg

After applying the strokes on the leg and buttocks, return to a position by the ankle and repeat the initial integration stroke several times. Now begin a series of percussion strokes on the leg to enliven the skin and tone the muscles.

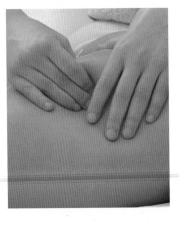

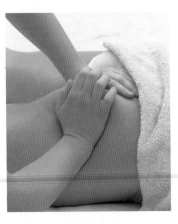

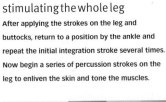

△ **1** Release tension from the buttocks by thoroughly kneading this fleshy area. You may find it easier to knead from a position on the opposite side of the body; stretching your arms will enhance the squeezing and rolling action of the stroke.

△ **3** To press deeper into the muscle, sink the heel of your hand into the buttock and rotate. Lean your weight into the first half of the circular motion and release the pressure on the return. Place your other hand close to the stroke and push the muscle towards the action. Apply these heel-pressure rotations over the whole area.

△ **1** Turn to face into the leg and briskly cup it, working from the calf up to the thigh, one hand following the other in rapid succession. Form a vacuum in the palms of your hands by bending the base knuckles and holding the fingers straight and close together while pulling the thumb in tight to the palm. As the hands cup the leg, flick them off the skin at the moment of contact. This creates a suction of air, drawing the blood supply up to the surface of the skin and leaving it with a healthy glow.

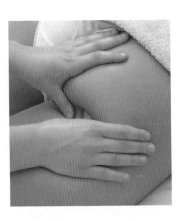

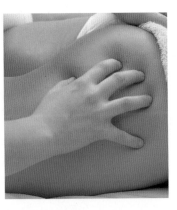

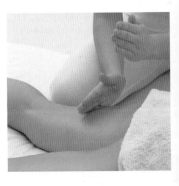

△ **2** Continue the massage from the left side of the body, and use your thumbs to work around and under the bones at the base of the pelvic girdle. Placing both hands over the buttocks for support, roll one thumb after another in short firm slides into the crease at the juncture of the buttocks and thigh.

△ **4** Shaking the buttocks can loosen any remaining stiffness and tension in the muscles. Place one hand softly over the sacrum to add support. Sink the fingers of the other hand into the muscle and vibrate rhythmically.

△ **2** Now use the hacking stroke, moving up the leg from the calf to the thigh, but taking care not to strike the delicate area on the back of the knee. Keeping your shoulders and wrists relaxed, hold your hands straight with the palms facing. Briskly strike the flesh with the sides of your hands, one hand following the other in quick, rhythmic succession so that they bounce off the skin immediately.

passive movements on the leg

Once the leg muscles are relaxed, you can introduce passive movements to gently stretch and ease tension from the joints, ligaments, and tendons. The most important thing to remember while making passive movements is never to move a part of the body beyond its point of resistance, and always to work within its natural range of movement. Your hands should impart sufficient confidence to encourage your partner to relax completely and allow you to lift, move, and stretch that part of the body.

enlivening the skin

Complete the percussion strokes by stimulating the skin with soft feather touches.

gentle hip and knee stretch

This passive movement helps to stretch the muscle attachments around the hip and knee joints by gently pushing the lower leg towards the thigh.

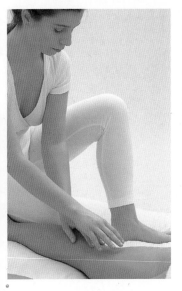

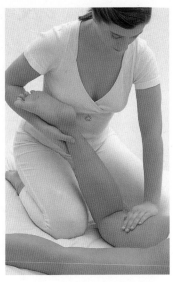

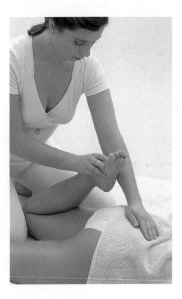

△ Starting at the top of the thigh, use your fingertips to brush down the leg in short strokes with one hand at a time. Lift each hand off the leg to cross above the other in a stream of downward overlapping motions.

△ **1** Kneel alongside the foot and slip your right hand under the ankle so that you will be able to support the leg. As you are sliding your right hand under the ankle, place your left hand just above the back of the knee. Slowly begin to raise the lower leg off the mattress so that the knee is flexed.

△ **2** Move your left hand to rest securely on the sacrum and lean forward to ease the raised part of the leg down towards the top of the thigh. Bounce the lower leg in tiny movements, gently against the point of resistance, and then lower it slowly back down to the mattress, keeping it in a straight line with the thigh.

lifting the leg

Take care of your own posture while doing this passive movement. Ensure that your back is straight, and elevate your own body from the muscles in your haunches during the upward lift. Do not attempt this movement if you have a weak back or the leg is too heavy.

▷ Raise the lower leg so the knee is flexed and then clasp the ankle firmly with both hands. Lift the leg slowly upwards to take the thigh slightly off the mattress. Bob the leg up and down a little before lowering the thigh.

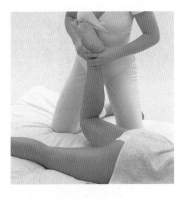

completing the first stage of the body massage

Once all the sequences of strokes have been carried out on the left and the right legs, lay your hands in a firm, but soothing hold on the back of the calves. This brief hold will bring a sense of balance and will also indicate to your partner that this initial stage of the body massage is now complete.

Massaging the front of the body

When your partner has turned over and you are ready to apply your strokes to the front of the body, take a few moments to compose yourself and relax your own body, so that you can focus your full attention on the massage. You will be touching the more vulnerable areas of the body, such as the face, chest and belly, so you need to bring sensitivity, confidence and care into your hands. Give your partner a few moments to settle into her new position, and reassure her with a calm and tender hold.

focus on the front of the leg

You will now begin working on the front of the body and continue the leg massage. Most strokes are similar to those used on the back of the legs. Specific strokes are required for the shin and knee as the bones are closer to the surface of the skin.

balance and joint release

These opening holds and stretches prepare the front of the legs for massage.

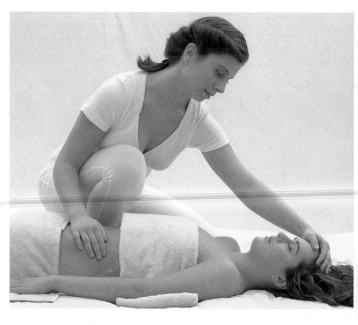

△ A calm and tender hold signals the beginning of the next stage of the body massage.

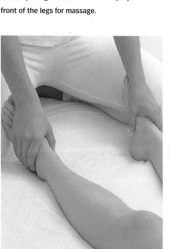

△ **1** Hold the feet for several moments to bring a sense of balance to both sides of the body. Then begin your massage on the left leg.

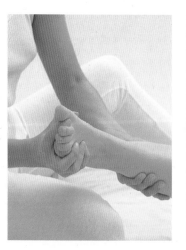

△ **2** Create space in the ankle joints with passive movements. Support the back of the lower leg with one hand, and place your other hand over the sole with your thumb and fingers lightly clasping the foot.

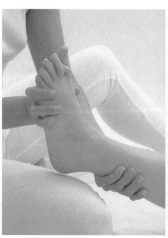

△ **3** Slip the index finger between the first and second toes to maintain a secure grip. Circle the ankle three times to the right and then three times to the left to rotate its joints.

a long stretch

This friction stroke stretches and eases the tissue between the two long bones that form the shin.

▷ Secure the back of the leg with your left hand and pull gently on the leg to create a slight traction. Wrapping your right hand over the inside of the lower leg, sink the right thumb sensitively between the two bones at the point where they join the front of the ankle. Slide the thumb slowly and steadily along the edge of the large bone until your hand reaches the knee. Lighten the pressure and glide your hand around the kneecap and back down the side of the leg. Follow this deep stretch with some effleurage.

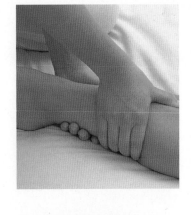

the main integration stroke

Begin by using the same flowing effleurage motion that you applied to the back of the leg.

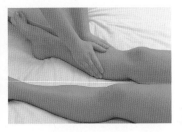

△ **1** Spread your essential oil on the front of the leg, stroking it down the length of the leg from the hip to the foot. Glide gently over the knee before taking the stroke up to the thigh.

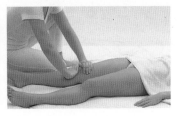

△ **2** Warm and stretch the muscles that cover the shin with a series of fanning strokes, moving up from the ankle to just below the knee before gliding your hands back down to the lower leg.

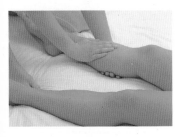

△ **3** Glide one hand after the other over the shin in a series of alternating fanning motions, slipping your fingers under the leg on the return movement to stroke back down over the calf.

relaxing the knee

The knee, like the ankle, plays an important part in the support and mobility of the body's weight and structure. The kneecap itself is bound by tendons and ligaments, which attach to the muscles and long bones in the thigh and lower leg. Strain and injury in the knee are common complaints, and it is important to include this area in your massage strokes to help keep it flexible. When working on and around the kneecap, settle your fingers beneath the knee to give it support.

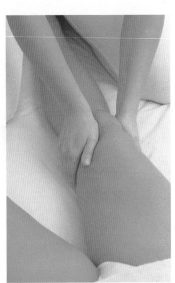

△ **1** Using the heels of both hands at the same time, rotate them firmly around the sides and above the top of the kneecap.

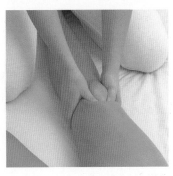

△ **2** Place both thumbs, one above the other, across the base of the knee. Slide them over the bone and then draw them out in opposite directions to encircle the edge of the kneecap until they return to their first position. Repeat the stroke several times as a continuous motion.

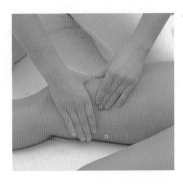

△ **3** Face towards the leg and knead thoroughly just above the knee. This will increase suppleness and circulation to the ligaments, tendons, and the muscles that attach to the joint.

the front of the thigh

The fanning, wringing and kneading strokes applied to the back of the thigh can now be used on the front of the leg.

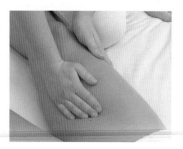

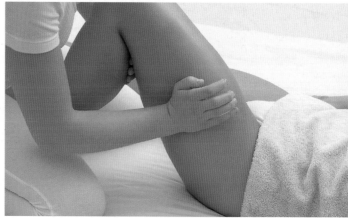

△ **1** Use a firm pressure to fan each hand alternately up over the thigh muscles.

▽ **2** Ask your partner to bend her knee so that the foot supports the weight of her leg. While the thigh is in a raised position, add some strokes to drain the blood flow towards the heart, followed by some deep tissue stretches on both sides of the leg. Wrap your hands around the leg so that your thumbs rest on the centre of the thigh. Firmly slide the heels of your hands and the thumbs a short distance up the thigh before drawing them out to the sides of the leg. Glide your hands down and around to their original position before taking the stroke further up the thigh.

△ **3** Hold the lower leg with one hand, using the heel pressure of the other hand to make a steady stretch up along the band of connective tissue that runs from the knee to the hip.

▽ **4** Continue the stretching stroke by sliding the heel of your hand around the hip socket before gliding your hand back down the leg.

▽ **5** Lean the leg outwards into the support of one hand, using the heel of the other hand to make a similar long, deep stretch down the inner thigh muscles stopping just below the groin. Then slide your hand around and back to the knee. Lower the leg gently on to the mattress and follow up with a sequence of stimulating percussion strokes to the thigh.

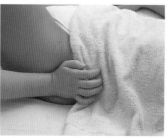

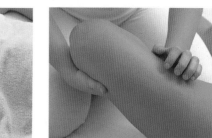

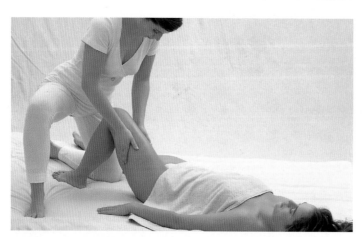

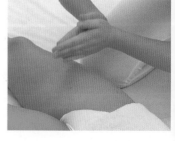

△ **6** Hack briskly to tone the muscles. Bring both palms together and strike the skin rapidly with the sides of the hands. End the leg massage with several full-length effleurage strokes, and repeat the whole sequence of massage strokes on the other leg.

focus on the abdomen

Massage on the abdomen can relieve symptoms of stress, deepen breathing, and help dissolve tensions formed when strong emotional feelings are retained. The abdomen is an extremely sensitive area containing many vital organs that are unprotected by skeletal structure. Before applying your strokes, take a few moments to allow the abdomen to relax under the caring touch of your hands.

the integration stroke

Rub a little essential oil into the palms to warm them, and spread the oil gently over the abdomen. Kneel on the right side of your partner, and begin with an integration stroke that flows over the abdomen from the pubic bone to the ribcage. Continue the stroke by gliding under the back to the spine and then out above the hips. Repeat three times in a continuous movement.

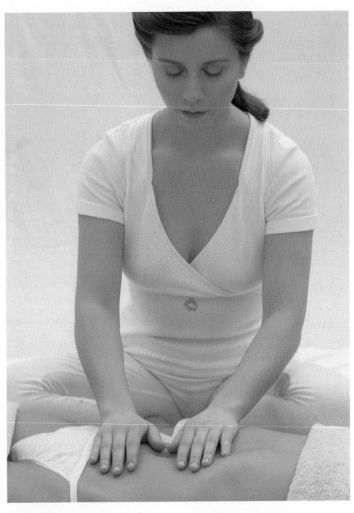

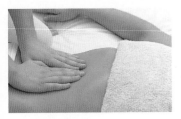

△ **1** Place both hands flat over the centre of the lower abdomen, fingers pointing towards the head. Stroke softly up to the base of the breast bone.

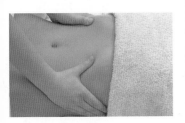

△ **2** Continue the stroke by fanning both hands out to either side of the ribcage and gliding under the back of the body.

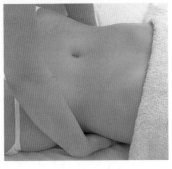

△ **3** Let the fingers of both hands slide under the back to meet at the spine. Lift the body slightly to arch the back before pulling your hands out towards the hips.

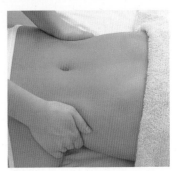

△ **4** Firmly draw your hands over the waist and then glide them back to their original position to repeat the stroke.

circling the abdomen

These circle strokes act to soothe and relax the abdomen. They flow over the area and fit perfectly to its shape.

▷ **1** Repeat continuous circles with the whole surfaces of your hands, moving in a clockwise direction until you feel the abdomen becoming soft and warm.

▽ **2** As the abdominal muscles relax, sensitively shift the pressure into your fingertips as you make the circular strokes. Decrease the circle so that you are stroking around the navel, then widen the circular movement outwards to cover the abdomen, shifting the weight back into the full surface of your hands.

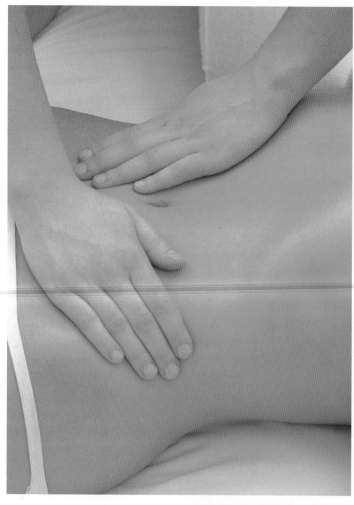

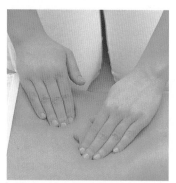

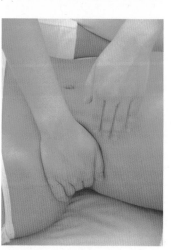

relaxing the sides of the abdomen

The muscles that cross from the back of the body to the front of the abdomen help to support the vital organs and rotate the spine. Make the following milking and kneading strokes on both sides of the body to increase suppleness.

◁ **1** Using one hand after the other in a milking action, pull firmly over the sides of the abdomen from just under the back. Glide lightly to the centre of the abdomen before lifting the hand off to repeat the stroke. Stroke in this way from the hip to the ribcage.

▷ **2** Lift, squeeze and roll the flesh from hand to hand in a kneading stroke along the sides of the abdomen from the hip to the base of the ribcage.

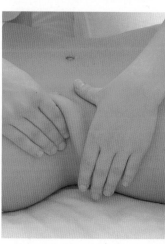

deeper strokes for the abdomen

If your partner is responding well to this massage and the area is relaxing, you can begin to apply the deeper abdominal strokes. Be very sensitive and alert to your partner's responses, applying and releasing pressure slowly, ensuring that any deeper strokes are appropriate.

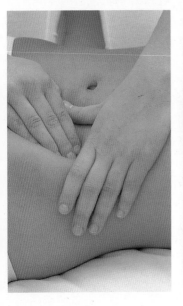

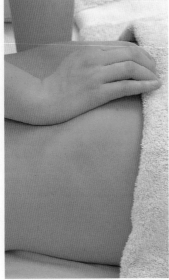

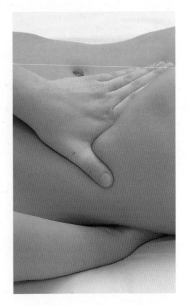

△ **1** Sink the first three fingertips of one hand slowly into the abdominal muscles. Place the other hand close to your fingers, with the thumb at an angle in order to anchor the muscle and push it slightly towards the stroke. Rotate the fingertips in tiny circles on one spot at a time, moving in a clockwise motion. Pay specific attention to the areas close to the wings of the pelvic bone.

△ **2** The upper abdomen can be tense in times of stress, as the diaphragm muscle between the chest and abdomen tightens, and the solar plexus, a nerve centre, becomes hyperactive. Once the area has been relaxed by softer strokes, and the breath deepens, slip your left hand under the body to rest below the spine. This creates a sense of support as you use the heel of your right hand to massage gently, but with increased pressure, in circles around the base of the ribcage.

△ **3** Ease constriction from under the ribcage with a firm, steady slide of one hand, while the other hand rests parallel and just beneath the body for support. Keeping your fingers close together and your thumb at an angle, sink the side of the index finger and hand gently under the edge of the lower rib. Slowly slide your hand down to the side of the body, lightening the pressure towards the end of the stroke. Repeat this stroke on the other side of the body.

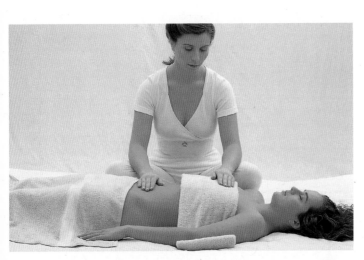

harmonious finish and hold

To bring a harmonious finish to the deeper sequences of strokes, repeat the flowing, soft, circular motions on the abdomen.

◁ To complete this part of the massage place one hand over the abdomen and the other on the chest so that it rests over the heart. Maintain this hold for a few moments to bring a calming sense of equilibrium and unity to the body.

Focus on the arms

Muscular tension forms in the arms and hands for a number of reasons. Poor posture can cause the shoulder girdle to stiffen and inhibit the flexibility of the upper limbs. Repetitive movements at work put strain, wear and tear on the muscles, tendons and ligaments. On an emotional level, the arms and hands represent the ability to reach out and contact the outside world, or the means of expressing creativity. Arm and hand massage feels wonderfully relaxing, bringing relief and ease to the upper body and renewing vitality. Using the following strokes, work first on one arm and hand, and then on the other.

opening out

This first movement helps the upper chest and shoulders to open out to create freedom from contraction in the shoulder joint and a feeling of length in the arm. The oil remaining on your hands from the previous strokes should be sufficient for this opening stretch but, if necessary, add just a little more to your hands as you work.

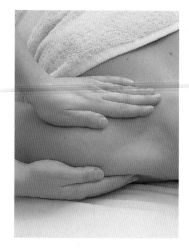

▷ **1** Face in towards the shoulder to lift it, and slip the hand furthest from the body under the top of the back so that the fingers point towards the spine. Place the other hand across the top of the chest, fingers pointing towards the breast bone. As you feel the shoulder relaxing between your hands, pull firmly and steadily out towards its edge.

▽ **2** Keeping one foot on the mattress, manoeuvre your position so you are able to sandwich the top of the arm between both hands, and then pull steadily down its entire length to give a gentle stretch to the shoulder joint.

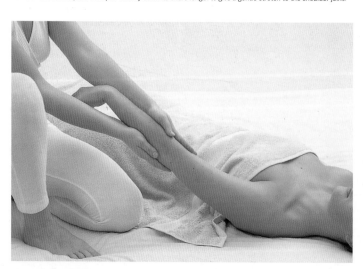

the integration stroke

Use oiled hands to mould the shape of the arm in overlapping strokes.

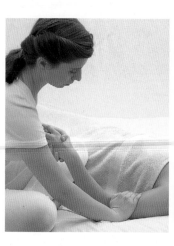

△ **1** Hold your partner's hand with the hand closest to the body. Wrap your other hand across the wrist, to lead the stroke with your little finger. Glide your hand firmly up the arm towards the shoulder.

▽ **2** Forming your hand to the curve over the shoulder, glide it around the joint.

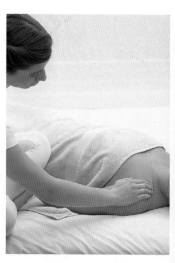

relaxing the forearm

Continue to relax the forearm with a series of alternating fanning motions. Fanning can be used to stretch and manipulate tension away from the muscles.

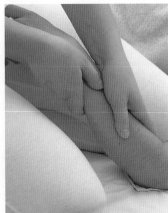

◁ **1** One hand following the other, move the fanning strokes up from the wrist to the elbow. Squeeze the muscles gently between the heel and fingers as the hand curves outwards, stroking firmly with your fingers on the underside of the arm as your hand glides back round. Slide your hands from the elbow back to the wrist to repeat the sequence again twice.

▽ **2** Secure the wrist with the hand closest to the body, and pull the arm gently to create a slight traction. Wrap the other hand around the outer forearm, sinking the thumb slowly into the groove where the long bones of the forearm join the wrist. Stroke firmly and slowly up the arm, between the bones, releasing the pressure at the elbow. Slip your hand around the joint and glide it back down to the wrist.

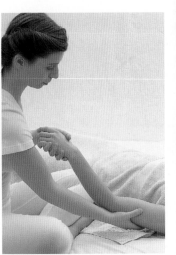

△ **3** Lifting the arm slightly off the mattress, stroke lightly down the back of the arm to the wrist.

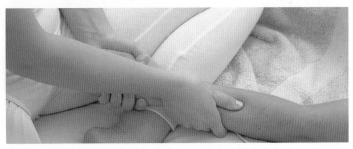

▽ **4** Pass your partner's arm to your other hand and clasp it by the wrist. Stroke up along the inside of the arm with the hand closest to the body, the little finger leading. Swivel your hand around just below the armpit and glide it back down the arm. Repeat the sequence two more times.

draining strokes

These strokes boost the circulation towards the heart and help to drain the lower arm.

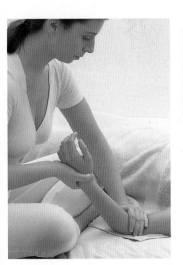

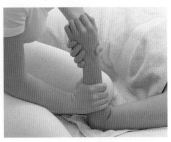

△ **1** Raise the forearm vertically so that it rests on the elbow. Clasp your partner's hand with your left hand and wrap your other hand around the top of the wrist, the little finger leading the stroke. Slide firmly down the arm as if to drain it. Open your hand to glide softly around the elbow joint and lightly back up the forearm.

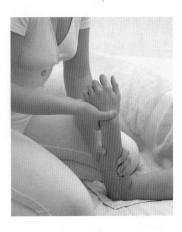

△ **2** Repeat the same draining motion on the inside of the arm, changing the position of your hands.

loosening the upper arm

The position and narrow structure of the arm can make the application of strokes more difficult than usual, so be sure that the limb is supported comfortably before massaging the upper half of the arm.

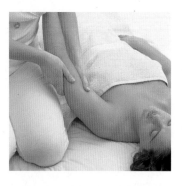

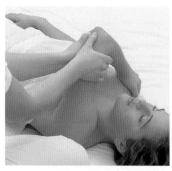

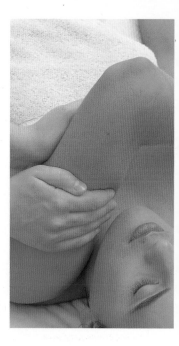

△ **1** Start with a series of alternating fanning motions, one hand following the other, from just above the elbow to the shoulder. Squeeze the muscles gently between your fingers and the heels of the hands as each hand fans outwards. When your hands reach the top of the arm, sweep them around and back down towards the elbow. Repeat once. To keep the arm in a raised position, secure its lower half between your own body and arm.

△ **3** Keeping the elbow flexed, lift the arm and place it across the body, asking your partner to clasp her other shoulder so that the upper arm remains steady and vertical. From this position, it is easy to apply your strokes. Holding the inside of the arm with your fingers, work around the back of the elbow joint with tiny alternating thumb circles.

△ **5** Wrapping your fingers around the inside of the arm, squeeze and knead down the upper arm muscles with circular fanning motions, applying pressure from the heels of the hands as they move outwards, and then gliding them back around more lightly.

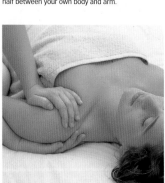

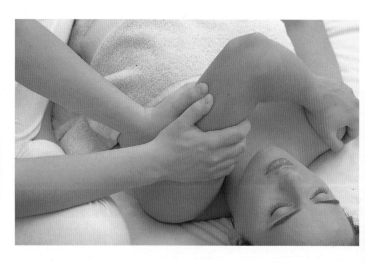

△ **2** Cradle the shoulder joint between both hands, placing the hand furthest from the body beneath the shoulder, and the hand closest to the body on top. Slide both hands back and forth over the top of the shoulder several times, making a see-saw motion for a warming effect.

△ **4** Clasping the upper arm firmly with the thumbs placed centrally next to each other, slide both hands steadily downwards in a draining action. Complete by gliding the right hand softly around the back of the shoulder and then repeating the stroke.

passive movements on the arm

These passive arm movements create a sense of length and space in the upper body and shoulder girdle by gently stretching the joints. Carry out these passive movements slowly and sensitively, working with the natural movement of the shoulder joint. Never force the arm or shoulder beyond its point of resistance or tension.

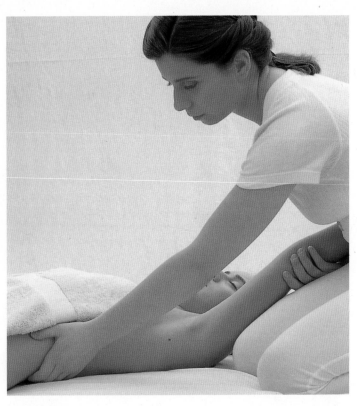

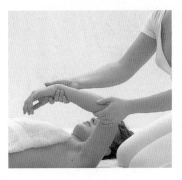

△ **1** Kneel behind the shoulder to remove the arm from its previous position. Support this movement by wrapping your right hand around the wrist and the left hand under the elbow. Begin to circle the arm slowly in a low arc-shaped motion, compatible with the movement of the shoulder joint, until it is stretched out behind your partner's head.

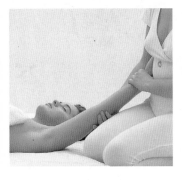

△ **2** Tuck the arm into the side of your body and change the position of your hands to support the elbow with your right hand. Pull very gently on the arm to create a slight traction.

△ **3** Lean forward to mould your left hand to the waist, and then slide it firmly up along the side of the body and softly under the shoulder joint in a steady stretching motion, bringing the feeling of length to the upper body.

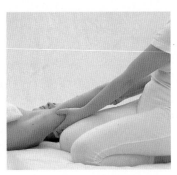

△ **4** Continue sliding your left hand up the back of the arm towards the elbow to increase the stretch in the shoulder joint. Now relax the shoulder and move yourself slowly back to the side of the body, taking the arm with you in a fluid arc-shaped movement. Ensure the arm is properly supported by your hands and the elbow stays flexed until the whole limb has relaxed back on to the mattress.

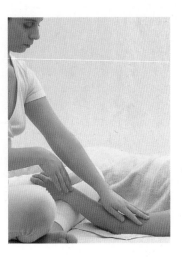

△ **5** Complete the passive arm movement with soft feathering touches, letting your fingertips sweep over the whole limb, one hand following the other in overlapping strokes.

Focus on the hands

Once the arm is relaxed, turn your attention to the hand. Your strokes will ease away tension from the tendons, muscles and bones to increase suppleness and dexterity. They will also stimulate the hand's many sensory nerve endings. A hand massage soothes away the stress of a day's activity: it is an essential part of a whole body massage, or can be done as a session in itself.

hand massage sequence

Kneel or sit below your partner's hand so that it can rest comfortably on your lap with the forearm slightly elevated. Change hands when necessary to complete the strokes on both sides of the hand. Use only a small amount of oil in order to secure a firm slide with your strokes.

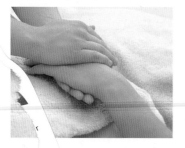

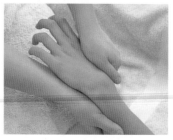

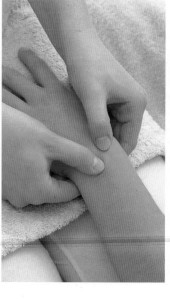

△ **1** Cradle_____ nd gently for several moments to allow the warm___ diating from your palms to melt away tensions. The ___llness of this calming hand-to-hand hold will enhance the deep sense of connection between you.

△ **3** Support your partner's palm and wrist with one hand, and use the heel of your other hand to make firm circular motions over the near-side of the top of the hand. Apply pressure in the heel on the outward fan of the circle, while stroking the palm firmly with your fingertips on the return slide. Perform the same stroke over the other half of the hand.

△ **5** Place your fingers under the wrist and make small, alternating thumb circles to ease the strain away from the tiny bones and surrounding ligaments on the top of the wrist joint.

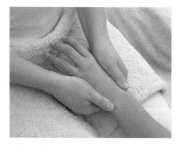

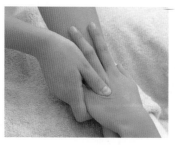

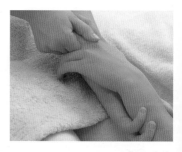

△ **2** Support the palm with your fingers and place your thumbs side-by-side over the centre of the top of the hand. Draw your heels and thumbs firmly out to the edges of the hand in a stretching motion, to create space between the bones and tendons. Repeat the stroke higher on the hand.

△ **4** Keep the hand supported and slide your thumb firmly in a straight line between each tendon and bone on the top of the hand, lightening the pressure as the stroke reaches close to the wrist.

△ **6** Relax the fingers and thumb, starting with the little finger and working across the hand. Begin by massaging the base knuckle with gentle circular motions using your thumb and index finger.

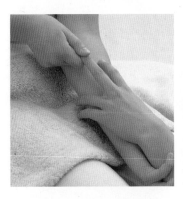

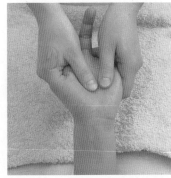

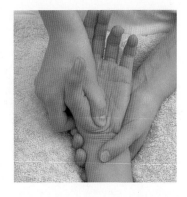

△ **7** Now pull firmly but gently along the top and bottom of each digit and out of its tip as if you are releasing tension away from the extremities of the body. Use smooth actions as the joints in the fingers are relatively delicate.

△ **9** Use both thumbs to make short, alternate sliding strokes over the surface of the palm to stretch and release tension from the muscles. Be sensitive to your partner's reactions.

△ **11** To massage more vigorously on the palm, support the back of your partner's hand with your hand, and use your other thumb to apply stronger pressure circle strokes, working on one spot at a time. Focus particularly on the area at the base of the thumb.

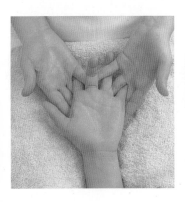

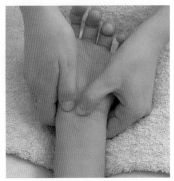

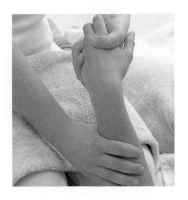

△ **8** Turn the hand so the palm is facing upwards. Interlock your fingers between those of your partner's hand, as shown, so that they rest against the back of the hand. Push them gently upwards, using enough pressure to open up and spread out the palm.

△ **10** Once the palm is relaxed, unlock your fingers and place them behind the back of the wrist. Massage over the inside of the wrist with small, alternating thumb circles.

△ **12** Apply some passive movements to loosen the wrist joints. Raise the forearm by flexing the elbow and supporting it with one hand. Firmly clasp your partner's hand with your other hand. Rotate the wrist several times, first in one direction, and then in the other.

how to finish a body massage

To complete your body massage apply a restful and calming hold. Bring your full attention to your touch, allowing both of you time to assimilate the beneficial effects of the session and to bring it to a gentle close.

Once you have withdrawn your hands from your partner's body, stand silently for several minutes. Make sure the whole body is covered with a sheet or blanket, and allow time for a few moments of complete relaxation, while you go to wash your hands. When you are ready, offer assistance to get up from the mattress or couch and have a warm towel ready to wrap around the shoulders if necessary. Encourage stretching and moving around a little to allow for adjustment to the standing position.

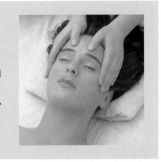

Instant neck and shoulder massage

Sometimes the idea of having tension in your shoulders and neck massaged away on the spot, without having to find a special place to do it and the time to undress, is a particularly tempting one. There is increasing interest in learning how to do a shoulder massage with the minimum of disruption, especially in offices. Even at home, there are times when nothing is better than someone giving you a ten-minute shoulder and neck massage, in the comfort of an upright chair. There is no need to use oil if you prefer not to, and you can work through light clothing if it is simpler.

neck and shoulder sequence

This instant massage can be carried out on any upright chair, using a pillow for support.

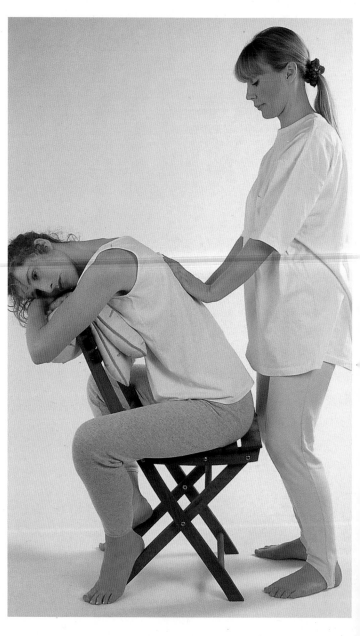

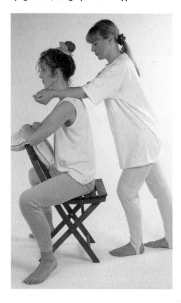

△ **1** Ask your partner to sit astride a chair, facing the back. You can offer a folded towel or cushion for comfort. Standing behind your partner, begin by leaning on your forearms so that your weight presses down gently on to the fleshy part of the shoulders.

△ **2** With your partner leaning forward, use effleurage strokes from the bottom of the shoulder blades, up the back and out over the top of the shoulders to finish at the top of the arms. Repeat four times.

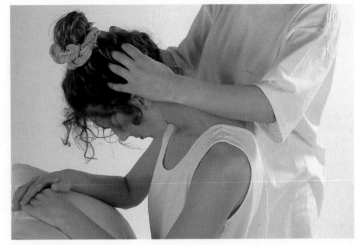

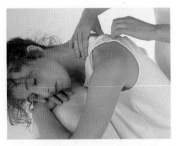

△ **3** With a firm petrissage, use both hands to knead out along the shoulders from the sides of the neck to the upper arms.

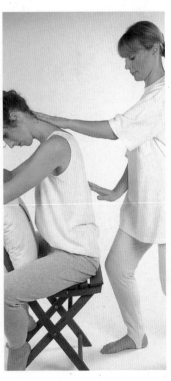

△ **6** Working from behind your partner again, massage the back of the head with both hands coming over the forehead and down to the temples with small circular pressures, moving the scalp against the skull. Lighten your touch at the temples.

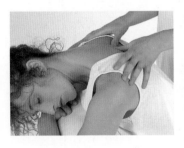

△ **4** Starting as far down the lower back as you can, work up the spine with the thumb, making small circular frictions. Continue up the sides of the neck to the base of the skull, then glide back down and work up again, this time moving out over the shoulders as you reach the top.

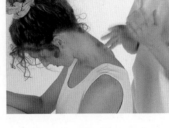

△ **7** First on one side and then on the other, do some hacking across the fleshy parts of the shoulders and upper back, using the outer side of your hands to make short, brisk movements. Keep the wrists and hands very relaxed. This movement helps to free up tension in the large shoulder muscles.

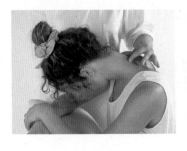

△ **5** Moving round to the side of the chair, tilt your partner's head forward and support it with one hand. With the thumb and finger of the other hand, grasp the neck firmly and massage with circular movements, working up the neck and into the base of the skull.

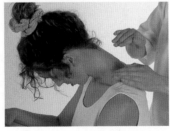

△ **8** Continue with a brisk cupping action across each shoulder, working on one side at a time.

△ **9** Finish the sequence by gently stroking down the entire back with one hand following the other. Repeat five times with each stroke getting lighter.

Self body massage

A simple, effective self-massage can do wonders to ease away tension and restore energy after a stressful, tiring day. After a shower or bath, massaging the body with lotions and oils is very relaxing and helps keep the skin in glowing condition. You can use self-massage to target particular aches and pains or areas of tension, for relief just where you need it. The beauty of self-massage is that you can do it to suit your needs and moods at any time – to unwind in the evening or to energize yourself in the morning.

working on the shoulders

Tense, knotted muscles in the shoulders are very common, making them an obvious starting point for a self massage.

▷ **1** Sitting upright, start from the base of the neck and press down with your fingers along the top of the shoulders. As you reach the bony part of the shoulder, slide your hand back to the base of the neck, and repeat the pressing at least three times. Finish by stroking firmly from neck to shoulder and then repeat on the other side of the neck.

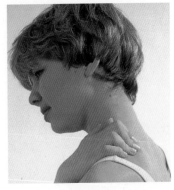

△ **3** Knead each shoulder with a firm squeezing action, rolling the flesh between your fingers and the ball of the hand. Repeat several times on each side.

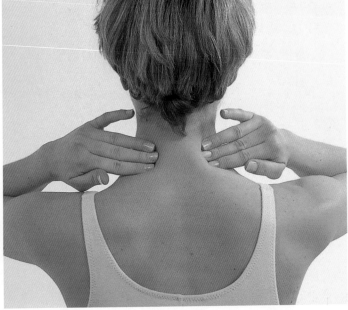

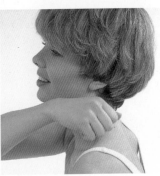

△ **2** Use the fingertips of both hands to make small circular movements, working up the back of the neck. Gentle circular movements, where you can feel yourself easing muscular tightness, are better than direct, static pressures on this area. Continue up and round the base of the skull towards the ears. Repeat the sequence a few times, paying particular attention to any knotty areas.

△ **4** With your hand in a loose fist, pummel your shoulder lightly, keeping the wrist and elbow relaxed. Use light, springy movements to stimulate the area. Repeat on the other shoulder.

Take care of yourself

Being massaged by someone else is of course the ideal, and many of the beneficial effects of massage result from the touch, care and attention of another person. However, self-massage does have an important part to play, particularly when regular massage by a professional therapist is not possible for reasons of time or personal finances.

It is becoming increasingly recognized that people in the busy modern world need to take time out to care for themselves. The great advantage of self massage is that you can do it when you need it most and adapt the strokes and pressure to your needs at the time. As part of a regular self-care routine, massage can be combined with meditation, yoga or other relaxation practices. It will help alleviate stress and induce a sense of well-being.

Most massage strokes can be used as they are, or adapted for the purposes of self-massage. And many of the benefits of a full body massage can be achieved, such as the relief of muscle tension, stimulating the circulation, improving skin condition, and lymphatic drainage.

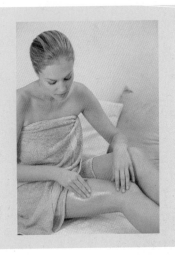

working on the arms

An arm massage is lovely and relaxing, and you can do some deep work on the triceps and biceps in the upper arm.

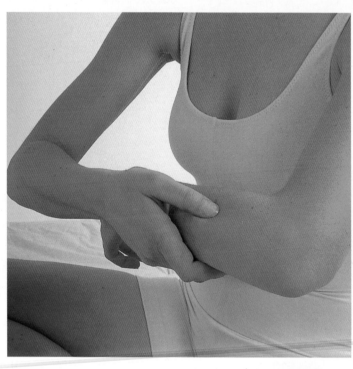

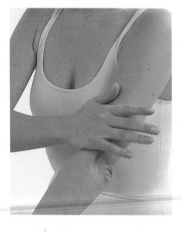

△ **1** Stroke firmly up the arm from the wrist to the shoulder, returning with a lighter touch. Repeat the stroke several times on different parts of the arm until the whole arm begins to tingle.

△ **3** Starting from the wrist, knead up the forearm toward the elbow, using your thumb to make circular movements. Follow a straight line up the forearm, then move your thumb across a little and follow another straight line up to the elbow until all the forearm has been worked.

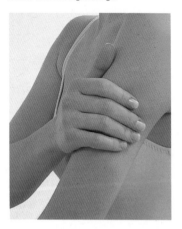

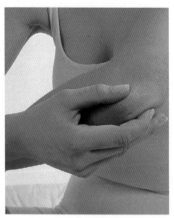

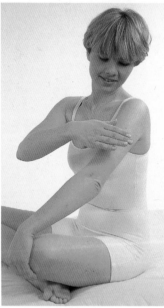

△ **2** Pressing your fingers toward the palm of your hand, knead up the arm from the elbow to the shoulder. Cover the area thoroughly, working right round the arm.

△ **4** With thumb and fingers, make circular pressures round the elbow. First, work round the far side of the elbow with your working arm coming over the top of the arm you're massaging, then bend that arm up and work from the inside of your elbow.

△ **5** Gently but briskly pat your upper arm, or use some gentle cupping. Follow with some effleurage stroking up and down the whole arm again to finish. Work on the hand (see opposite) before massaging the other arm.

working on the hands

The hands benefit from firm pressure, particularly on the palms, which can store tension from too much driving, continued computer use or any other repetitive hand work.

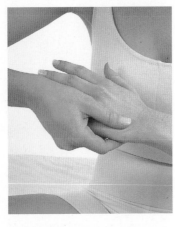

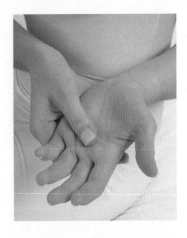

△ **3** With circular thumb pressures, work up each of the furrows between the bones in the hand, from the knuckle to the wrist. When you have covered each furrow, smooth the hand by stroking it gently with long strokes from the knuckle to the wrist.

△ **4** Turn the hand over to work on the palm. Cover the area with circular thumb pressures, paying particular attention to the heel of the hand and the wrist. Follow this with some deeper, static pressures all over the palm.

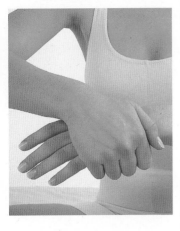

△ **1** Squeeze the hand firmly, spreading the palm laterally. Cover the whole of the hand from the fingers to the wrist.

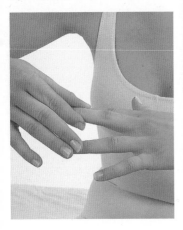

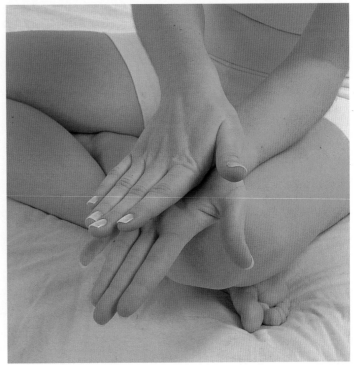

△ **2** Using circular pressure, squeeze each finger joint between your finger and thumb. Then hold the base of each finger and pull the finger gently to stretch it, sliding your grip up to the top of the finger in a continuous movement.

△ **5** Finish by stroking the palm of one hand with the other. This can be quite a firm stroke, working from the tips of the fingers to the wrist, leading with the pressure from the heel of the hand. Stroke back to the fingers and repeat twice more, each time using slightly less pressure. Finally, stroke the inside of the wrist. Repeat the whole of the arm and hand massage sequences on the other side.

working on the back and abdomen

The back is particularly difficult to massage for yourself using standard massage techniques. Rocking gently on a firm surface provides an manageable yet effective alternative.

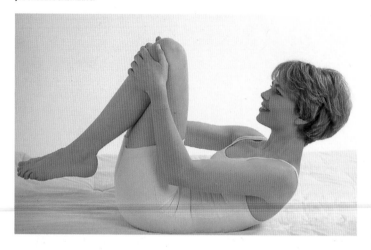

△ **1** Lie on your back, clasp your knees and gently rock backward and forward to massage the lower back, buttocks and hip joints and gently stretch out the vertebrae.

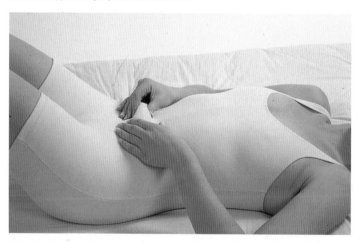

△ **2** Bend your knees up and use some gentle petrissage to knead the whole of the abdominal area. When you have finished kneading, place both hands flat on the centre of the abdomen, fingers pointing slightly together, and pause for a few moments. Then smooth your hands outward over the hips and thighs in a long, slow, moulding movement.

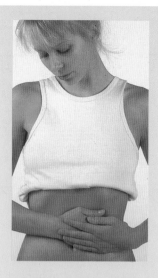

Abdomen and lower back care

Self-massage provides an opportunity to experiment with the varying pressures needed when massaging different regions of the body. The abdomen requires much lighter strokes than most other areas, as there is no bone protecting the underlying organs.

Thinking about the area you are working on and how you might be affecting the internal processes can help you give a more sensitive and effective massage.

Some common causes of lower back problems include:

- Lack of exercise
- Poor posture when standing and sitting
- Tense, hunched shoulders when driving or using a computer
- Sitting cross-legged
- Wearing high-heeled shoes
- Lifting heavy weights incorrectly.

Forms of exercise that are particularly beneficial for correcting postural imbalances and strengthening the muscles of the lower back and abdomen are pilates and yoga. Swimming and walking are also helpful.

working on the buttocks, hips and thighs

The big muscles of this area will benefit from a vigorous massage. Regular firm massage with deep kneading can help to disperse cellulite.

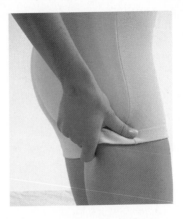

△ **2** With the thumb and fingers, squeeze and release the muscles firmly and slowly, working from the top of the thigh over the buttock. Repeat on the left side.

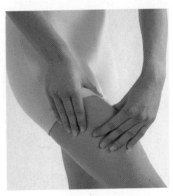

△ **3** Use both hands to squeeze and release the muscles on the front and side of the thigh, kneading the entire upper leg. Repeat on the other side.

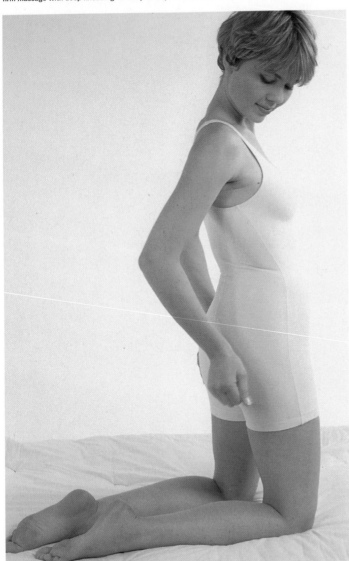

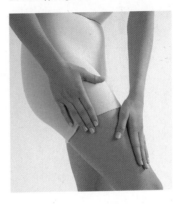

△ **1** Kneel up and pummel your hips and buttocks, using a clenched fist and keeping your wrists flexible. You can afford to use quite a bit of pressure here.

△ **4** Starting at the knee, stroke up the thigh with both hands to soothe the leg.

working on the legs

Stroking up the legs aids the return of blood to the heart, helping to boost the circulation and eliminate toxins. It can also revive tired legs. Massage will also help release tension in the calf muscle, which tends to build up.

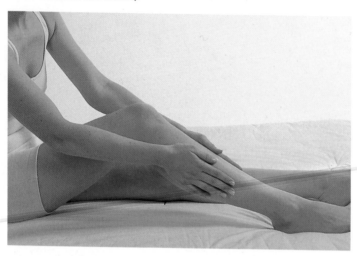

△ **1** Sitting down, with one leg raised slightly, stroke the leg with both hands from ankle to thigh. Begin the stroke as close to the ankle as you can reach. Repeat several times, moving round the leg slightly each time to stroke a different part.

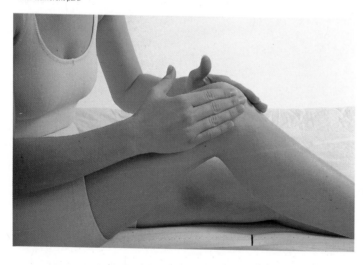

△ **2** Massage the knee, stroking round the outside of the kneecap to begin with, then using circular pressure with the fingertips to work round the kneecap more firmly.

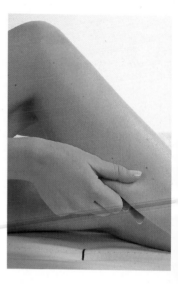

△ **3** Knead the calf muscle with both hands, using a firm petrissage to loosen any tension in the muscle.

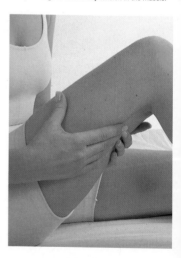

△ **4** Continue the kneading on the thigh, working over the top and outside areas with alternate hands. Whilst the leg is still raised, do some soothing effleurage strokes up the back of the leg from ankle to hip. Continue with the foot massage (opposite) before repeating all the steps on the other leg.

working on the feet

This is one of the hardest-working and most neglected parts of the body, so it's not surprising that a foot massage is particularly pleasurable. Use plenty of cream or oil on the feet as the skin can be dehydrated and hard.

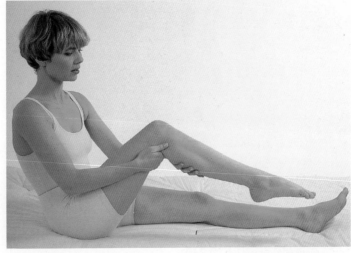

▷ **1** Sitting down and leaning back, raise a leg, supporting the weight with your hands. Rotate the ankle five times in each direction.

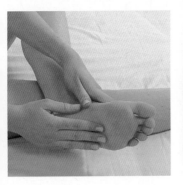

△ **2** Gently bring your foot over the other leg. With one hand on top of the foot and the other one underneath, stroke up the foot from toes to ankle. Repeat three times.

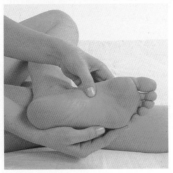

△ **4** Supporting the foot with one hand, continue the circular pressures over the raised instep, working from the inner to the outer edge. Repeat this part of the sequence three times.

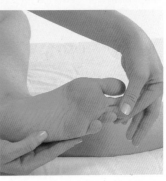

△ **6** Beginning with the small toe, massage each toe. Slowly stretch the toe between the thumb and finger, pull gently, moving your fingers up the toe each time, until you reach the tip.

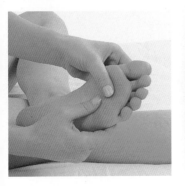

△ **3** With the thumbs, apply circular pressure over the ball of the foot. Work in lines from the inside of the foot to the outer edge. Repeat three times.

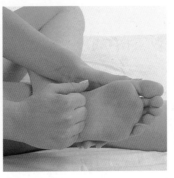

△ **5** Still holding the foot with one hand, make a loose fist with the other and firmly rotate your fist over the instep. Work thoroughly into the arch.

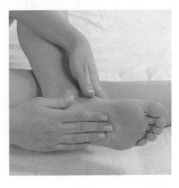

△ **7** Repeat the effleurage strokes of the foot, with one hand over and one under the foot, working from toes to ankle, several times. Repeat the leg and foot massage sequence on the other side.

Raising energy self-massage

Tone up your body and give yourself an energy lift with a self-massage programme that uses a variety of strokes to relax tense muscles and stimulate the circulation. Self-massage is not only beneficial to your physical system; it also gives you a psychological boost when you are tired or under stress. It increases your awareness of your body, an essential part of learning how to help others become more conscious of their bodies through massage. Another benefit is that it helps you to practise the techniques and gain the confidence to apply them to a partner when you are carrying out a body massage.

wake-up programme

This self-massage programme is guaranteed to invigorate you when you wake up in the morning and need a energizing boost, or whenever you are feeling generally run-down. It is also an excellent programme to use prior to giving a massage, so that you can begin the session with a fresh mind and body. Both you and your massage partner will feel the benefit.

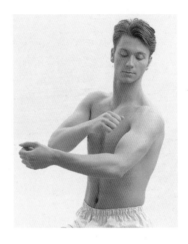

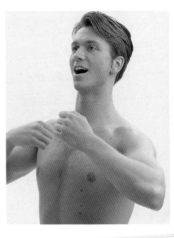

△▽ **2** Use your fist to pummel from the shoulder down the outside of the arm and hand. Feel how the skin begins to tingle. Turn the arm and, with the other fist, steadily pummel the inside of the hand and up the arm to the shoulder. Shake the whole arm to loosen up the joints. Then repeat steps 1 and 2 for the opposite side of the body.

△ **3** Use both hands to vigorously pummel your ribcage and pectoral muscles. Open your mouth and let out a roar to clear your throat and chest.

▽ **4** Warm up your abdominal muscles and boost your digestive processes with a brisk abdomen rub. Place one hand flat over the other and massage in a clockwise direction several times.

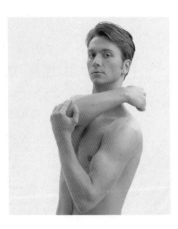

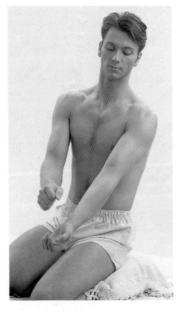

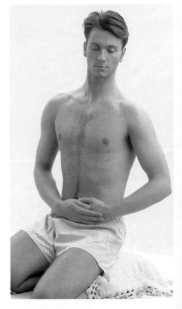

△ **1** To relax a stiff neck and shoulders, support your elbow with one hand and make a loose fist with the other hand. Use the flat edge of your knuckles to pummel the muscles on the opposite side of the body. Pound gently but firmly down the back of the neck towards the edge of the shoulder.

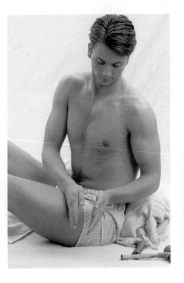

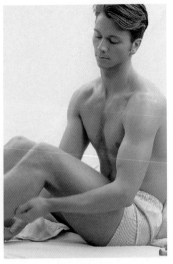

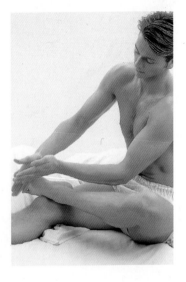

△ **5** Tone the muscles and stimulate the circulation in your legs using hacking strokes, repeatedly striking the skin with the sides of both hands.

△ **6** Tight calf muscles can slow blood circulation. Use one hand after the other to pummel the lower leg to relieve tension and revitalize the system.

△ **7** Hack briskly, but gently, over the top and bottom of the foot to relieve stiffness in the muscles, joints and tendons.

Repeat steps 5–7 for the opposite side of the body. When you have completed the Wake-up Programme, stand up and shake your whole body to release any remaining tension and loosen the joints. Then stand completely still so that you can appreciate the sensation of vitality it gives.

massage instruments

Nothing feels better than the touch of hands on the body, but massage instruments can be used successfully in self-massage to reach awkward areas. A two-ball roller, for example, is ideal for working on sore points on the back.

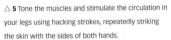

self-massage for the hands

Keeping your hands supple and relaxed is an important part of massage. While practising the strokes, you may find yourself using certain hand movements for the first time, so it is a good idea to exercise the hand joints frequently to increase their flexibility. Use one hand to gently squeeze all over the other. Repeat for the other hand. Rub the palms together briskly to increase warmth and vitality.

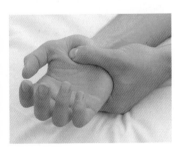

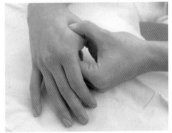

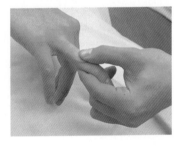

△ **1** Release tension in the muscular pad at the base of the thumb by pressing into it with the thumb of the other hand and then rotating it on one spot at a time. Support the back of the hand with the fingers. Work over the entire palm in a similar way.

△ **2** Sink and rotate your thumb into the web between the thumb and index finger of the other hand. You will find a tender spot that can bring relief from toothache, headaches and digestive problems.

△ **3** Pinch the base of a finger on one hand between the thumb and index finger of the other hand, then pull the thumb and index finger in alternate short, firm slides along the length of the finger to its tip to stretch it. Repeat this movement on all the digits. Repeat the whole hand massage sequence for the other hand.

Sensual body massage

Research has shown that the art of massage and touch has therapeutic effects, both physically and emotionally. The skin is the largest organ in the body, feeding the brain with information on our external environment, and if it is caressed gently and lovingly, then the brain will also relax and unwind. After a stressful day, massaging your partner allows you some time to wind down and enjoy each other's company.

Being massaged in a brightly lit room with blaring rock music may appeal to some, but for true sensuality it is better to create a relaxing and inviting atmosphere. Dim the lights or even use candles, prepare some aromatic oils and put on some relaxing background music.

Have a warm, not hot, shower beforehand and make sure the room is warm enough. Both you and your partner must be really comfortable, so the bed or the floor are usually the best places for a massage. Massaging in front of – but not too close to – an open fire is also extremely sensual, as the warmth and flickering light from the flames, combined with the soft crackle of burning wood, will help create a tender and loving atmosphere.

basic technique

The secret to a really good massage is to maintain a constant confident touch, using flowing, unbroken strokes. Experiment with different pressures and speeds, exploring a range of different techniques and communicating with each other as to what feels most delightful.

To lubricate the areas that you intend to massage, pour some blended oil into your hands, rubbing them together to warm them up. Apply enough oil that your hands glide smoothly over the surface of your partner's body, but remember that a little goes a long way.

circle strokes

These stretch out the muscles, releasing tension from the soft tissues. They are best applied to broad surfaces, such as the back, thighs, chest and belly. Place both hands flat on the body, side by side. Lead with your right hand and move both hands in a clockwise direction, using a constant, fairly gentle pressure.

fanning strokes

These strokes also release tension from the soft tissue and are ideal on the back, as it is a large broad surface. To fan upwards, place both hands flat at the base of the spine on each side of the vertebrae. Glide them both up, concentrating pressure in your palm before fanning out to the sides of the body.

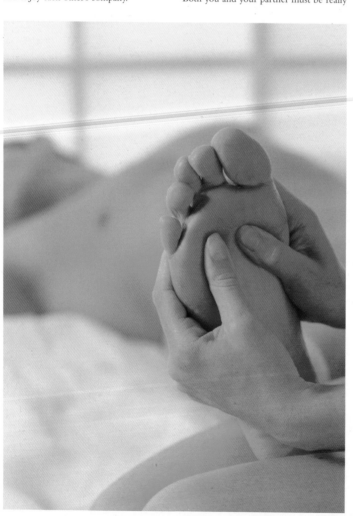

◁ A foot massage can be very sensual but it is important to use a firm touch to avoid tickling a sensitive partner.

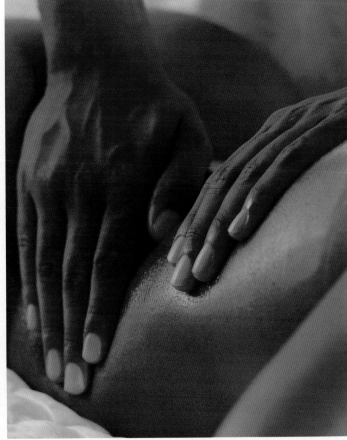

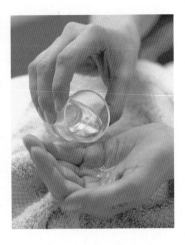

△ Warm some oil in your hands to avoid the shock of a cold touch.

◁ With circle strokes, keep both hands next to each other, so your right hand will have to pass over the left.

▽ Percussion strokes can be fun, but be gentle.

From here, mould your hands around the sides of your partner's body and drag them down to the base again.

kneading strokes

These are ideal for fleshy areas, such as the buttocks and thighs, and release tension from the larger muscles. Imagine that you are kneading dough by squeezing a portion of flesh in your fingers and then rolling it from one hand to the other and back again.

percussion strokes

Rapid strokes that create a vibrating sensation help to improve skin tone and circulation to nerve endings. Hacking involves a series of chopping movements, with alternate hands concentrating on the same area. The wrists must remain relaxed, so the action is bouncy rather than stiff. Take care not to use too much pressure.

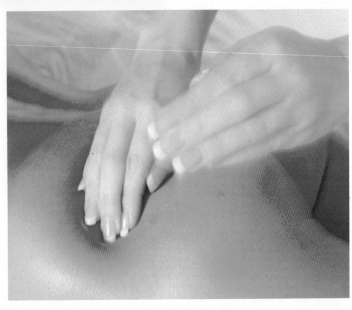

A loving massage

There are few more lovingly intimate ways of spending time with your partner than giving each other a massage. As a powerful form of nonverbal communication, massage can strengthen an already loving relationship and build bridges where there are problems.

head

A head massage is one of the nicest gifts you can give your partner, especially if they have had a hard day, as it releases all tension.

Ask your partner to sit comfortably, while you sit or stand behind them. Take off jewellery that might catch on their skin, then place your fingertips on the scalp. Run your open fingers softly through the hair. With quite a firm circular motion, rotate your fingers around the scalp, changing the size of the circles and gradually increasing the pressure. Concentrate on areas such as behind the ears, along the hairline and the base of the skull.

Now concentrate on the forehead, gliding your thumbs from the top of the nose in an arch to the sides of the head and back. Repeat, following the line of the eyebrow, and adapt it by using small circular strokes with the balls of your thumbs. Next, sweep your thumbs gently down the sides of the nose and across the sinuses, then out towards the cheekbones before repeating.

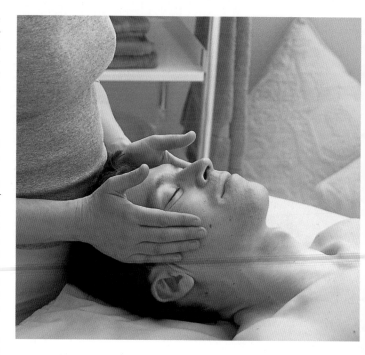

△ **Massaging the delicate skin of the face feels wonderfully intimate.**

Cup your hands into a loose fist and support the back of the ears with the side of your first finger, using your thumbs to make small circular motions all around the rims. Then move down to grasp the lobe between the tips of your thumb and index finger and gently pull it down, allowing it to slip through your fingers before repeating.

shoulders

A good place to start a full body massage is the shoulders and back, as these areas often contain the most knots and tight muscles. By easing the tension there, you pave the

way for a totally relaxing and sensual full body massage – truly a great act of love.

Ask your partner to lie on their front. Put a small amount of massage oil on your hands and rub them together to warm it.

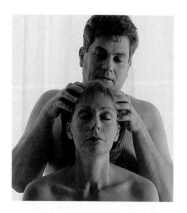

◁ **A head massage is superbly relaxing, helping to release all the day's stress and tension.**

▷ **The ears are a powerful erogenous zone – massaging them can be erotic.**

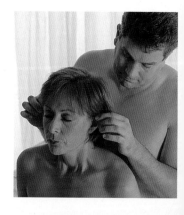

Start at the top of the shoulders with both hands flat on the skin with the neck between them. Run your hands up the back of the neck, then down and along the tops of the shoulders in long sweeping strokes. Repeat with a firmer pressure using your thumbs. Begin to focus on specific areas, gradually increasing the pressure, pressing your thumbs into the muscular areas using small circular strokes until you can feel the muscles loosening up. Punctuate the more intense circular strokes with the sweeping strokes to add variety and encourage relaxation.

Extend your massage down your partner's back. Place your hands flat on either side of the top of the spine and sweep down to the base. On the upward sweep, apply more pressure by using your bodyweight. Vary this stroke by sweeping your hands out to the sides using fanning strokes or a harder circular pressure with the heels of your hands. Avoid directly massaging the spine.

breasts

Massaging a woman's breasts is a sensual experience for both parties. It is best done with the woman lying on her back. You may find it easier to straddle your partner, but do not sit on her. Begin by placing your hands palms down under each breast with your thumbs out to form an "L" shape and the breast cupped in the crook of the "L". Using quite firm pressure, circle your hands upwards and inwards and as they rotate inwards, bring the thumb and index finger together so that they end up lightly pinching the nipples before beginning again. If you want, you can concentrate on one breast, using a similar technique but this time with one hand following the other to complete the circle.

Another technique is to use your fingers and thumbs to pinch the nipple area gently before slowly fanning your fingers out across the breast. Use a light pressure around the nipple and increase the pressure as your fingers span out.

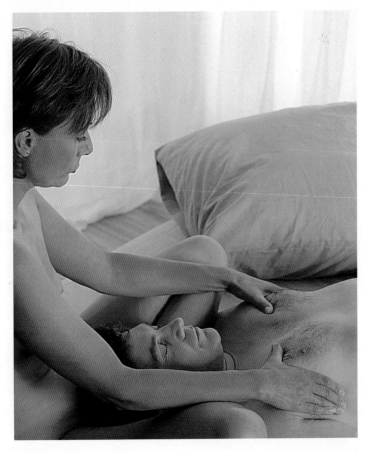

thighs

It is easier to massage the thighs with your partner lying on their back, as they can bend their knees. Cup one hand on the underside of the thigh and the other on the top, just above the knee. Increase the pressure in the tips of your thumbs and fingers as you glide your hands up the length of the thigh and down again. Vary your strokes from feather-light to harder fanning, using the heel of your hand to give pressure in a constant sweeping motion.

buttocks

Sit at your prone partner's side and softly knead the buttocks with both hands, gradually increasing the pressure. Next, hold your hands above one buttock, keeping them taut, flat, straight and parallel, and use a sharp chopping motion to strike it. Use alternate hands and move up and down the length of the buttock.

△ Men also enjoy having their chests massaged. As the pectorals are less sensitive, you can use a firmer pressure. Use the balls of your fingers to do small circles on the whole area, but especially the sides and the groove of the armpit.

▽ Buttocks are usually the fleshiest part of the body but need different treatments.

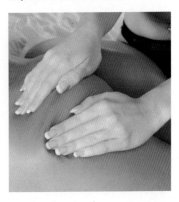

A sensual massage

In the right circumstances, with a softly lit room, relaxing music, and using some of the more aphrodisiac essential oils such as rose, patchouli, neroli or sandalwood, a massage can be a highly pleasurable and sensual experience, relaxing the body and arousing the senses. Intuition will play a larger part in a sensual massage, as you discover which areas have the strongest impact on your partner's senses. It certainly isn't just the most obvious erogenous zones that bring pleasure – the back of the neck, scalp, solar plexus, inside of the elbows, hands and feet are just a few others.

a sensual body massage

The back can be extremely sensitive to touch and starting here will help your partner to relax into the massage.

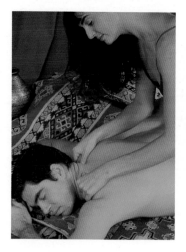

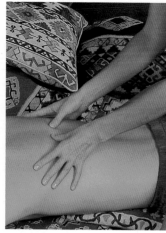

△ **2** Knead firmly along the top of the shoulders, squeezing and releasing the muscles each side of the neck and shoulders where a lot of tension builds up. As the shoulders start to relax, work more deeply into the muscles.

△ **3** Beginning at the nape of the neck, let your thumbs stroke down each side of the spine. Return up each side of the spine with slightly more pressure and rotating the thumbs to release muscular tension. Work up and down two or three times.

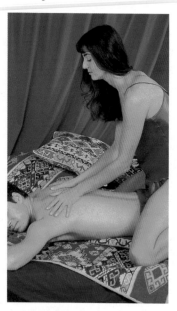

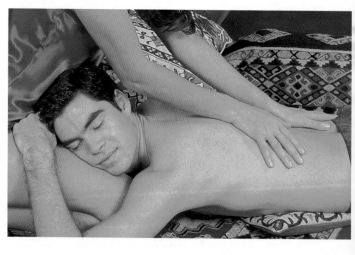

△ **1** With your partner lying on their front, start by resting your hands gently on the back of their shoulder blades. Fan the palms out across the back, sweeping your hands out and around over the shoulders and top of the back.

△ **4** Move round so your partner can rest their head on your thighs, and with long, effleurage strokes, slowly massage the length of the back, from the neck right down to the buttocks and back up the sides of the trunk. Repeat this three times.

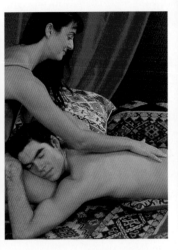

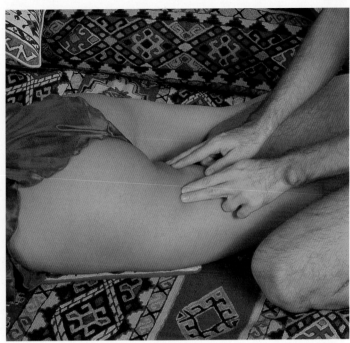

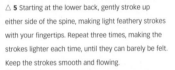

△ **5** Starting at the lower back, gently stroke up either side of the spine, making light feathery strokes with your fingertips. Repeat three times, making the strokes lighter each time, until they can barely be felt. Keep the strokes smooth and flowing.

△ **7** Curling your third and fourth fingers under, place your hands toward the top of the left upper leg and circle your first and second fingers outward, one hand alternating with the other. This should be a slow, leisurely stroke with varying pressure. Slowly move down the leg towards the knee, working from the inner thigh outward each time. Once you have reached the knee, repeat the entire sequence on the right leg. Only apply light pressure to the back of the knee joint.

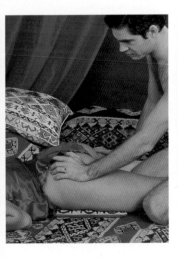

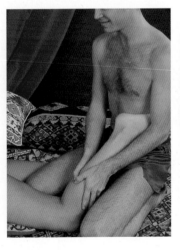

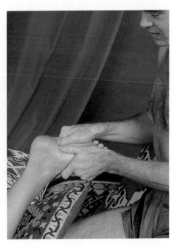

△ **6** Massage the lower back with some kneading. Using the flat and, in particular, the heel of the hand, knead the buttocks, then come back to the start and work over a different area.

△ **8** Move back to the left leg. Support your partner's leg across your thigh and circle your thumbs over the whole calf muscle, alternating the thumbs and applying firm pressure. Repeat on the right leg.

△ **9** Raise your partner's foot, supporting its weight in your hands. Knead the instep firmly, using the thumbs to apply the pressure. Work all over the ball of the foot up toward the big toe.

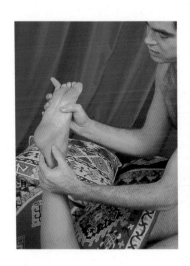

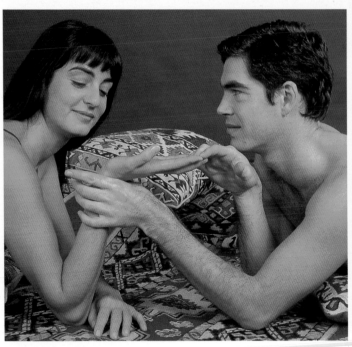

△ **10** Support your partner's foot in one hand, placing the thumb of that hand firmly over the centre of the instep. With the thumb and first finger of the other hand, stroke round the ankle with circular movements. Repeat the foot sequence on the right foot.

△ **12** Gently stretch and release your partner's wrists, by flexing the hand backward and forwards. Softly stroke the inside of the palm with your fingers. Repeat on the other hand.

▽ **13** Gently massage each finger, beginning with the thumb or little finger and working from the base joint to the tip. Try squeezing, rubbing and circular movements, and gentle pulling.

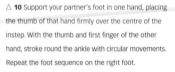

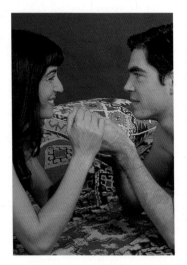

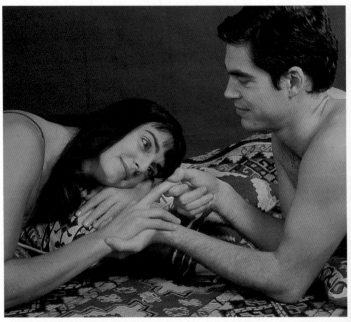

△ **11** At this stage, lie down facing each other, making sure you are both comfortable and well supported with plenty of cushions. Gently caress your partner's hands.

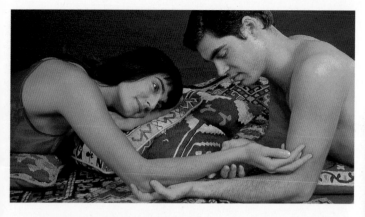

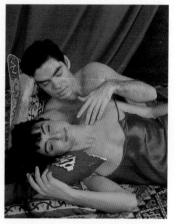

△ **14** Supporting your partner's elbow in one hand, use the other to caress and stroke the inside of the wrist just below the thumb, which is a particularly sensitive area. Continue working over the whole of the wrist area, using gentle circular thumb movements. Repeat on the other wrist.

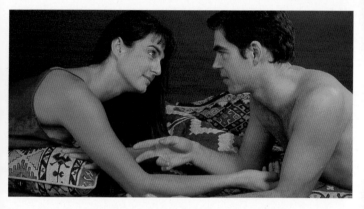

△ **17** With a feathery touch, stroke across the shoulders and up the neck, covering the sides, front and back. You can run your fingers up through the hair as well. Spend more time caressing the base of the neck, which is extremely pleasurable.

△ **15** With feather strokes, use your fingers to stroke up the soft inner arm. This is a highly sensitive area when lightly touched and the effect is both stimulating and relaxing. Repeat on the other arm.

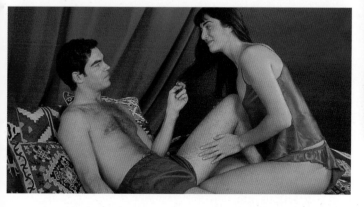

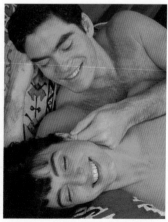

△ **18** Finally, trace round the ear with your fingers, starting at the outside and circling toward the centre. Continue with soft pinching movements round the outside edge and on the lobe, which is another highly sensitive area.

△ **16** Use long effleurage strokes up and down the inner thigh. Slow, gentle movements will be the most effective in a sensual massage.

Therapeutic Body Treatments

Once you have mastered the basic massage skills you will want to broaden your knowledge and technique. The beauty of this healing art is the process of discovering how the body functions, and the way it responds to treatment. This section shows how oil blends can be combined with strokes to treat a whole range of conditions. Your enhanced skills will enable you to bring greater relief, relaxation, invigoration and comfort.

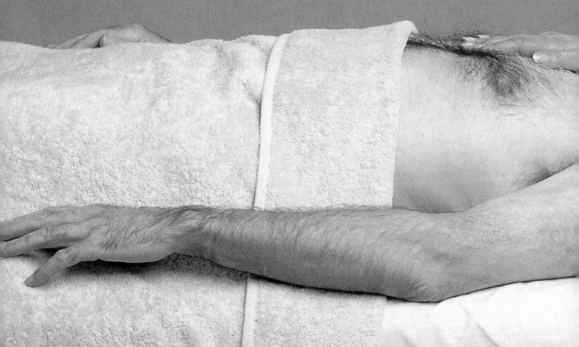

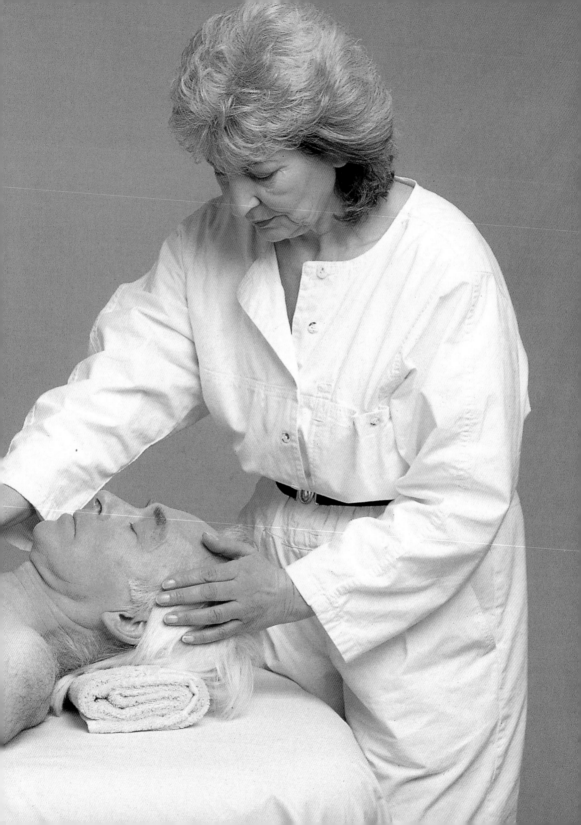

Aromatherapy and massage

When essential oils are used for aromatherapy massage, different oils are combined to increase their therapeutic effect. As you become more practised in the art of blending you will begin to develop a nose for compatibility, in much the same way as a perfumer blends scents, and you will be able to judge the best blend for your requirement by its aroma. Once you have mixed your oils, use them immediately, as they are perishable.

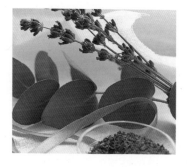

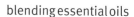

blending essential oils

Blending oils for massage enables you to alleviate various physical and emotional symptoms in a single treatment, and while the combination of therapeutic properties is of prime importance, the value of fragrance should also be taken into account – nobody enjoys taking unpleasant medicine, so don't underestimate the beneficial effects of a pleasing and sweet-smelling odour when mixing your oils.

The ratio of essential oil to carrier oil may vary, but as a general rule, 5 drops of essential oil in 10ml (2 tsp) carrier oil is enough for a body massage. This gives a standard 2.5 per cent dilution, the recommended dilution for most purposes.

However, if you are using oils for purely emotional problems, half the number of drops can be equally effective, while physical symptoms often respond better to a slightly higher percentage of essential oil. If your massage partner has a lot of body hair you will need to use more carrier oil, but keep the amount of essential oil the same. If you are using bottles or jars bought from the chemist they will usually have their capacity marked on them. To work out how many drops of essential oil you will need in a container, simply divide its capacity by two. For example, if you have a 30ml (1fl oz) bottle of carrier oil you will need to add 15 drops of essential oil, or for a 50g (2oz) jar, 25 drops of oil.

◁ **Lavender is one of the most useful essential oils, and it combines well with peppermint and eucalyptus for a relaxing, yet stimulating, blend.**

useful conversion guide		
1ml	=	20 drops of essential oil
5ml	=	1 teaspoon
30ml	=	2 tablespoons
600ml	=	1 pint

synergy

When essential oils are blended, a chemical reaction occurs and the oils combine as a new compound. For example, when lavender is added to bergamot the sedative qualities of bergamot are increased; but if lemon is added to bergamot, then its uplifting, refreshing aspect is enhanced. This process is known as synergy. Using this principle, oils can be blended so that they treat a person's emotional and physical needs at the same time. The blend can also be modified from treatment to treatment, depending on the time of day or the person's mood (for example, changing the balance of the blend, or substituting a different oil to the basic blend, can raise someone's spirits if they are low).

top, middle and base notes

Essential oils are categorized by what are known as top, middle and base "notes", which is how perfumers categorize scents, using different combinations of notes to create a new perfume. A good blend combines an oil from each category, and each oil is classified according to its dominant characteristic. It is not always

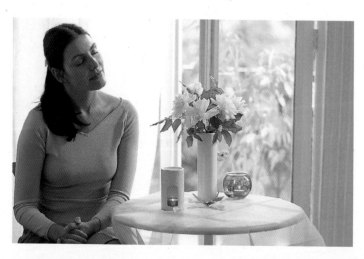

◁ **You will develop a nose for top, middle and base scents, but generally fresh, herbaceous oils such as lemon, eucalyptus or tea tree are good top notes. Floral oils and some herb oils make up the majority of the middle notes, while woody, resinous oils are base notes.**

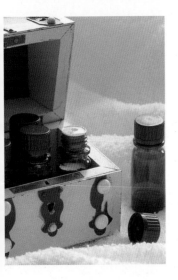

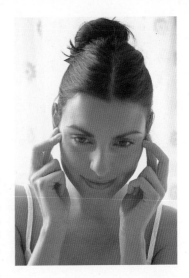

◁ Essential oils should be stored away from direct light and heat. Specially made boxes are ideal and must be kept out of reach of children.

▷ A soothing blend of essential oils and an appropriate carrier oil can make all the difference to a massage to relieve a headache.

It is useful to know the Latin or scientific name of each oil because most reputable suppliers put this name on the label of the bottle. If you are in any doubt about where to buy oils, seek the advice of a qualified practitioner, who will recommend a reputable retail supplier.

Essential oils last for a relatively long time if a few simple precautions are taken. They should be bought and then stored in dark-coloured glass bottles with a stopper that dispenses them a drop at a time. Keep the lid firmly closed to prevent evaporation, and store them in a cool place out of direct sunlight. Citrus oils tend to go off more quickly than other oils, so it is a good idea to buy them in small quantities as you need them. It is easy to tell if an oil has deteriorated because it will become cloudy and give off a distinctly unpleasant odour.

simple to classify oils by note. For example, rose and jasmine are heady fragrances, and are floral oils but are usually considered to be base notes. Because they evaporate quickly, most blends should contain a higher number of top-note oil drops to middle-note and base-note oil drops. For example, a well-balanced blend would be made up from three drops of orange (top note), two drops each of clary sage and geranium (both middle notes), and two drops of cedarwood (base note).

buying and storing essential oils

Make sure the oils you buy are pure, undiluted essential oils. In general, price is an excellent guide, and it is wise to compare various suppliers' prices so that you can recognize an expensive oil and a very cheap one. Be aware that essential oils are easily adulterated, and that there is no such thing as cheap rose oil, for example; cheap rose oil is probably a similar-smelling product to which geranium or palmarosa oil has been added. If you buy from a reputable source you will also avoid buying oils from a second or third distillation. These contain only a few active ingredients as the majority are removed during the first processing.

▷ Vegetable carrier oils are ideal for massage. Essential oils readily dissolve in the carrier oil, and the blend allows the hands to move over the skin without dragging or slipping.

carrier oils

Massage is a wonderful way to use essential oils, suitably diluted and blended with an appropriate carrier oil. Suitable carrier oils for massage include sweet almond oil (probably the most versatile and useful), grapeseed, safflower, soy (a bit thicker and stickier), coconut and even sunflower. For very dry skin, a small amount of jojoba, avocado or wheatgerm (except in cases of wheat allergy) may be added.

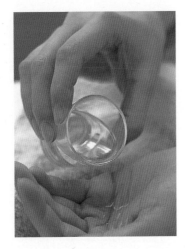

cautions
• Never take essential oils internally, unless professionally prescribed.
• Always use essential oils diluted.
• Do not use the same essential oils for more than one or two weeks at any one time.
• In pregnancy, some oils can be dangerous. Do not use without professional advice.
• For problem or sensitive skin, dilute the oils further, and if any irritation occurs, stop using them.
• Some oils, such as bergamot, make the skin more sensitive to sunlight, so use with caution in sunny weather.
• Anyone with a specific complaint such as epilepsy or asthma must be treated with extra care. If in any doubt, seek professional advice.

More detailed information on the range of essential and carrier oils is provided on pages 318–339.

Massage for sports

Professional sports people value massage very highly, not least because it works on several levels. Used before exercise it can prepare the body for the increase in activity not only by warming and loosening the muscles and joints, but also by stimulating the system, both physically and mentally. This is the key to improved performance. After an exercise session, massage speeds up the elimination of waste products (in particular lactic acid) by stimulating the lymphatic system. The accumulation of these waste products during exercise is the cause of much of the stiffness and pain experienced afterwards.

strains and sprains

A burning sensation under the skin is likely to indicate that muscles, fibres or ligaments have been strained – stretched beyond their natural limits. This is often the result of exercising without an adequate warm-up routine, or over-exertion. A routine of pre-exercise massage and limbering will help to prevent strains. Try not to exercise beyond your level of fitness. Gently massaging the affected area will help to speed recovery.

Sprains are more serious and are caused by violent wrenching of a joint, most commonly the ankle, wrist or knee. The surrounding muscles, ligaments and tendons may also be damaged and the affected area may be extremely painful and swollen. Apply an ice-pack or cold compress for 15–20 minutes to reduce the swelling. When it is removed you can start to massage the area gently (as shown opposite), taking care not to work directly on the swelling. Rest the ankle as much as possible and use a support bandage.

A serious sprain should always be checked by a doctor in case a bone has been fractured, and a sprained knee always requires medical attention.

cramp

You don't have to be a fitness fanatic to suffer from cramp. On the contrary, it is usually underused or ill-prepared muscles which go into cramp. It doesn't even take movement to set it off: the searing pain of cramp can occur in the middle of the night, when the reduced circulation has caused muscles to contract. Frequent cramps may indicate generally poor circulation or a deficiency of calcium or salt. Massage will increase the blood circulation to alleviate the pain. You should also try to stretch out the affected muscle.

backache

Back strain is the most common source of debilitating pain. Most sports put increased strain on the legs, buttocks and back. Previous injuries can make the back prone to recurrent pain. Awkward, inappropriate or excessive exercise can also cause trouble. With regular and thorough back massage (particularly before exercise), the likelihood of injury is reduced. If, however, you want a quick warm-up for the back, or an after-exercise sequence, follow the instant back and shoulder massage. Always consult a doctor, osteopath or chiropractor if in any doubt about the seriousness of a back problem.

with or without oils

You don't always have oil at hand, and it certainly isn't crucial for massaging unexpected strains, sprains and cramps. If you do have some light vegetable oil nearby, all the better, but don't worry if you don't.

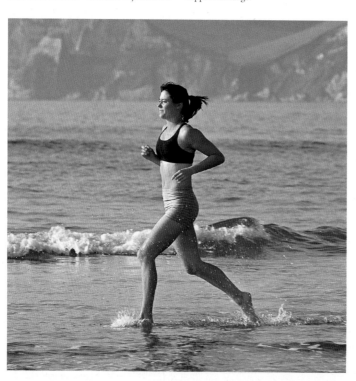

◁ **Warming up before exercising helps reduce the risk of injury – gentle jogging is one way of achieving this.**

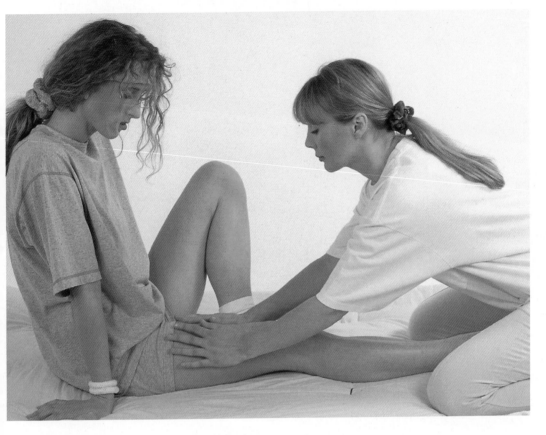

ankle strain or sprain

One of the most commonly injured areas is the ankle. Gentle massage can help.

△ **1** Avoid working directly on the swollen area. Start with gentle effleurage strokes working from the knee toward the thigh. Massaging in the direction of the lymph nodes in the groin will help drain away the fluids that have accumulated round the joint. Lightly stroke back to the knee. Repeat several times.

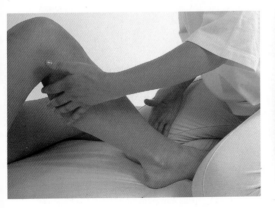

△ **2** Help your partner to bend the affected leg. Continue the effleurage strokes on the lower leg, this time working from the ankle to the knee, alternating your hands. Repeat several times, then gently squeeze the calves with one hand, while the other supports the foot.

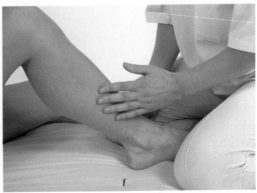

△ **3** Concentrating on the ankle area, stroke extremely gently all round the ankle with short upward movements. Check with your massage partner that this is not causing them any discomfort.

calf cramp

Cramp occurs when a muscle contracts and won't relax. Massage can provide instant relief.

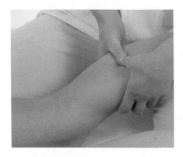

△ **1** With your partner lying face down and the foot supported across your leg or a small pillow, gradually apply direct thumb pressure into the belly of the cramped calf muscle for eight to ten seconds.

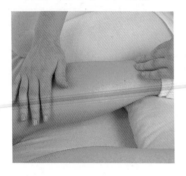

△ **2** Do some effleurage strokes, working from ankle to thigh and back down again.

self-help stretch

Cramp could be caused by lack of stretching before exercising. Stretching the affected muscles will help ease the cramp.

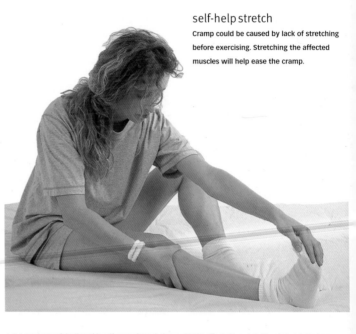

△ **1** A good way of dealing with calf cramp is to sit down with the affected leg straight and stretch the toes toward you. Hold this position for eight seconds and then release. Repeat a few times, until the spasm seems to be lessening. Then knead your calf muscle using firm pressure. When the muscle feels more relaxed switch to effleurage strokes, working up the leg.

hamstring cramp

The hamstring is a very active muscle that can become very tight if not sufficiently stretched after use. Hamstring and calf cramp are two of the most commonly occurring kinds of cramp and can be treated in similar ways.

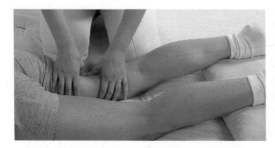

△ **1** With your partner lying face down and the ankles raised on a small pillow or cushion, begin massaging up the back of the thigh using alternate hands in slow, rhythmical stroking movements. Then apply static pressure to the middle of the thigh with the thumbs, holding for eight to ten seconds.

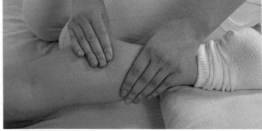

△ **2** Firmly knead the calf muscle. Squeeze, press and release the muscle using one hand after the other. Finally, do some soothing effleurage strokes up from ankle to thigh and back down again.

hamstring self-help stretch

**To prevent muscle cramp avoid over-extending
yourself and always warm up properly.**

▷ **1** Lie down flat, with the affected leg raised and
the other knee bent. Stretch the muscle by pulling
the thigh gently toward the chest. Then firmly stroke
up the back of your thigh for eight to ten seconds.
Start to knead the back of the thigh until you feel
the muscles begin to relax. Finally stroke over the
area to soothe it.

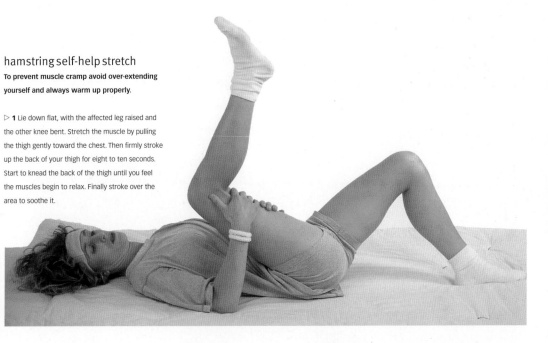

tennis or golfer's elbow

**Inflammation and damage to the tendon cause
the pain associated with these conditions.
Massage can help relieve the pain.**

▷ **1** Support your partner's wrist in one hand and use
soothing effleurage strokes along both sides of the
arm, stroking from the wrist to the elbow and back
again. Repeat several times.

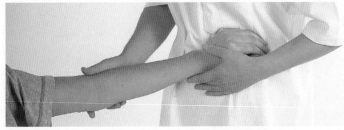

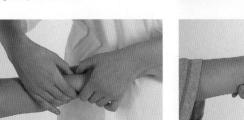

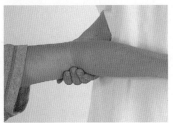

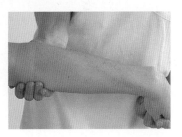

△ **2** Rest your partner's hand against your side.
Continue working up from the wrist to the elbow and
back, making small circular movements with both
thumbs, paying particular attention to the muscles in
the forearm.

△ **3** Secure your partner's hand in yours, and with
the other hand supporting the elbow, flex the elbow
gently forward.

△ **4** Bring the hand back to give the tendons that
attach to the bones a good stretch, taking care not to
cause your partner any pain.

Convalescence and recuperation

After an illness or injury the body is left in a vulnerable condition, and a period of convalescence is vital to give the immune system time to rebuild its defences. Massage helps to promote this important transition.

healing holds

Gentle, hands-on holds are ideal for the first fragile stages of convalescence. The power of touch can be very useful because it can comfort the body, stimulating the nerves

▽ If recovery from illness or injury involves being confined to bed for some time, massage can be invaluable. Initially it is helpful to soothe and calm the body, and later more gently invigorating treatments will speed the recuperation process.

that replenish the vital organs, and return the body to a normal resting stage. As your partner recuperates, whole body massage will tone up the muscles, boosting circulation and increasing the body's overall vitality and sense of well-being.

Soothing holds help to balance the nervous system and increase the body's energy levels. Start at the head, gently placing your hands over the forehead, temples and cheeks, then work slowly and methodically down both sides of the body to the feet.

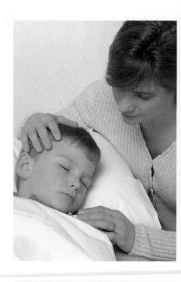

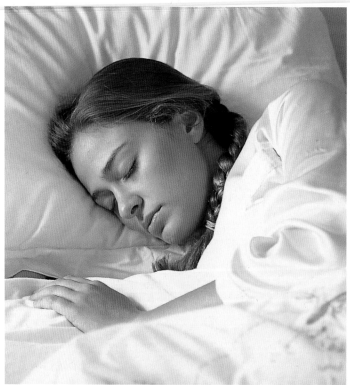

useful essential oils

The period of convalescence is often a time of physical and emotional change. The patient may experience bursts of energy, followed by fatigue when the spirits fall. The oils that are useful for convalescence include ginger and orange to stimulate the appetite, which may still be lacking at this time. The stimulating quality of eucalyptus and tea tree may help overcome lethargy. Orange and lavender both have an uplifting and comforting nature, and are more gentle, and these oils may be all that are needed to get over the last part of an illness. Also, during this recovery period the immune system needs boosting. The oils to choose for this are bergamot, frankincense, patchouli, lemon, rosewood and tea tree. Mandarin is a relaxing tonic oil, and clary sage is also very useful. Cypress and juniper are helpful for inducing sleep.

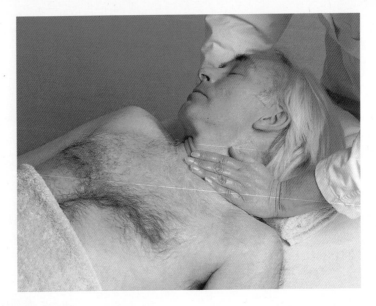

reducing tension and clearing the head

The prolonged periods of inactivity in convalescence can cause the shoulder and neck muscles to tense up. This tension restricts the circulation which, in turn, leads to discomfort and headaches.

▷ Gentle kneading of the shoulders can help to reduce tension in the shoulder and neck muscles. If appropriate follow this with a relaxing neck, head and face massage.

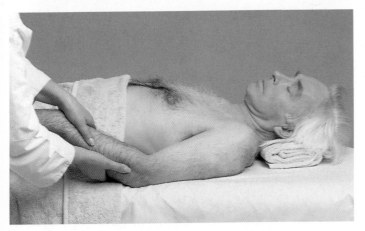

getting ready for action

As your partner recuperates and becomes stronger, the desire to resume normal activities grows. At this stage in convalescence, it is often useful to focus your massage on the feet and legs to boost a sluggish circulatory system, and massage the arms and hands to renew their strength and dexterity.

◁ **1** Begin the massage with a healing hold. Cup your left hand over your partner's temple and place your right hand over the heart area. This helps to encourage a sense of integration between mind and body.

▽ **2** Massage the hands and fingers to release tension and increase flexibility.

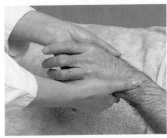

◁ **3** Now massage the forearms, using draining strokes to help the circulation flow back to the heart. To loosen and warm the muscles, use one hand after the other in a fanning motion, working from the wrist towards the elbow.

Massage for the elderly

Many elderly people live full and active lives, and aromatherapy massage provides a valuable contribution to the maintenance of their physical and emotional health. The contact of touch through the medium of massage is especially important for alleviating feelings of isolation, which may result from loneliness or bereavement. Whole body massage is beneficial to older people, but if they are uncomfortable about undressing, then massage on the hands, feet and face is equally helpful. Still, hands–on holds, to induce feelings of calm and peace, can be applied to the body while the person is fully clothed.

A condition commonly affecting the elderly is the onset of osteoarthritis, a degenerative disease of the joints caused by wear and tear. One or several joints of the body may be affected. Gentle massage with the recommended essential oils brings great relief. However, it is not advisable to massage over the joints if they are inflamed, swollen or disintegrated. In these circumstances, still holds will allow the warmth of your hands to subtly comfort the affected area.

recommended oils

Using essential oils for the elderly presents no particular difficulties, yet it is advisable to bear in mind two general points. First, as we age our metabolism slows down, so that any chemical introduced into the body will remain there slightly longer. Second, because of this slower metabolic rate and a less physically active life, the whole system can become more toxic. This is particularly true for those people who must necessarily live a more sedentary life, or are in residential homes or hospitals.

With these points in mind, it is best to avoid the highly stimulating oils and make use of the gentle essential oils that have similar uses. A more dilute blend of the essential oil should perhaps also be considered. Oils that are particularly appropriate are frankincense, geranium,

still hands-on holds

Lay your hands gently around an arthritic or painful joint to allow the warmth and presence of the hands to penetrate the tissues, helping to increase circulation and reduce stiffness.

▷ **1** Focus your attention and breath into your hands before gently cradling the shoulder. This supportive hold will help the shoulder relax.

▽ **2** Osteoarthritis commonly affects the knee joints in older people. Cup the knee between your hands to bring it warmth and comfort.

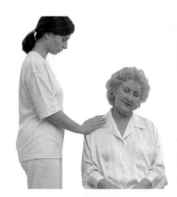

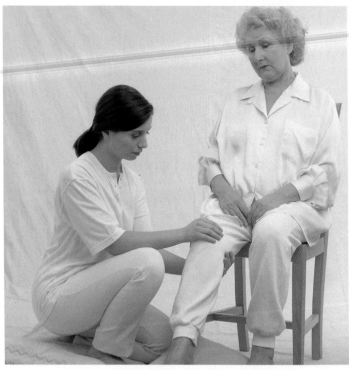

ginger, grapefruit, jasmine, juniper, lavender, marjoram, nutmeg, neroli, rosemary and sandalwood.
• For arthritis, try benzoin, black pepper, chamomile, cedarwood, eucalyptus, ginger, juniper, lemon, marjoram and nutmeg.

• For aches and pains, try ginger.
• For grief and loneliness, choose from marjoram, rose and nutmeg.
• For constipation, try fennel, ginger, marjoram or black pepper.
• For mature skin, try frankincense.

relaxing the spine

The vertebrae at the top of the spine are another potential trouble spot with the progression of age. As flexibility is lost, mobility in the neck and head is reduced. Gentle massage will boost the blood supply to the surrounding tissues, helping the whole area to remain supple.

staying supple

Regular hand and foot baths with essential oils are an excellent preventive measure against stiff and aching joints at the extremities of the body. Massaging the hands and feet will also help to keep the wrists, fingers, ankles and toes supple, giving the whole physical system an extra boost.

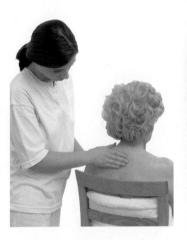

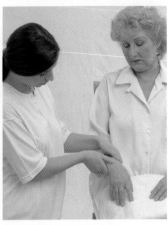

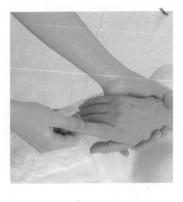

△ **2** Many older people wish to pursue their hobbies, which may require dextrous hands and fingers. If the joints are not inflamed or in a degenerated condition, regular hand massage with gentle passive movements and stretching of the fingers will assist this continued flexibility. (For other strokes suitable for the hands, see the whole body massage programme.)

△ **1** Soft, circular effleurage strokes over the top of the spine, at the base of the neck, and between the shoulder blades will ease away tension. While massaging with one hand, use the other hand to support the front of the body.

△ **1** Support the wrist with your fingers, and apply circular and sliding strokes with your thumbs to ease away tension from its tiny bones.

a soothing neck and face massage

Gentle and relaxing, this massage is an excellent means of easing away physical and emotional tensions in elderly people. The loving contact of your hands will be especially comforting in times of loneliness, distress and bereavement.

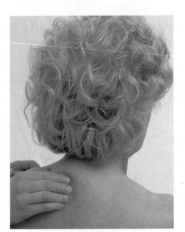

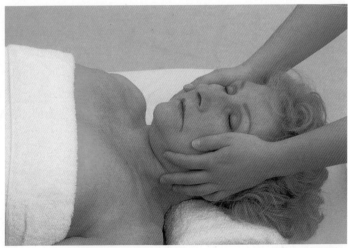

△ **2** Excess tissue frequently builds up over stiff, tense areas, further prohibiting flexibility. Once the muscles are warmed with effleurage, sink into a deeper level of tissue with friction strokes. Use small circular motions from your fingertips to loosen and stretch the areas surrounding the top of the spine.

Energy and auric massage

There is an electro-magnetic energy field known as the aura that surrounds all living things in both the animal and plant kingdom. The word "aura" derives from the Sanskrit for "air", and the same word in Latin means "breeze". Both words suggest that the aura is a subtle but constantly moving energy field.

The influence of the energy field on our health and well being is fascinating area to explore with massage and aromatherapy. The aromatherapy massage brings to the aura the benefits of healing and peace, thereby helping to prevent the physical body from manifesting symptoms of ill-health and emotional disturbance.

Knowledge of the body's auric and energy vibrations has always existed in spiritual and healing practices, but has been largely ignored by modern medicine and science. Today, healers, psychics, body workers, and massage therapists are again tuning into the subtle body energy when working on the health of the whole person.

the chakra energy levels

The centres of energy, known as "chakras", relate to the endocrine glands and so provide a bridge between the subtle and physical anatomy of the body. Their function is to transform energy from one level to another. The most important seven chakras form a line from the base of the spine to just above the head. In Eastern tradition, each chakra has a vibrating sound and a colour that relates to it. All seven chakras represent a different aspect of our physical, emotional and spiritual life, and have a positive and negative electrical charge. Although they operate independently of one another, they are also interrelated. Auric massage with essential oils can restore the balance between them. Knowledge of the chakras, their functions, and their positions is essential for anyone intending to do enery work. For an introduction to the chakras see the box on page 178.

preparation for energy and auric massage

Assemble the appropriate essential oils with some vegetable carrier oil or unscented moisturizer. Lay the person down comfortably, making certain they feel warm and safe. It is not necessary for them to undress. Take time to become still and attentive within yourself by bringing your whole attention to your own body and breathing. This will increase the sensitivity in your hands, helping them to tune in to subtle energy vibrations.

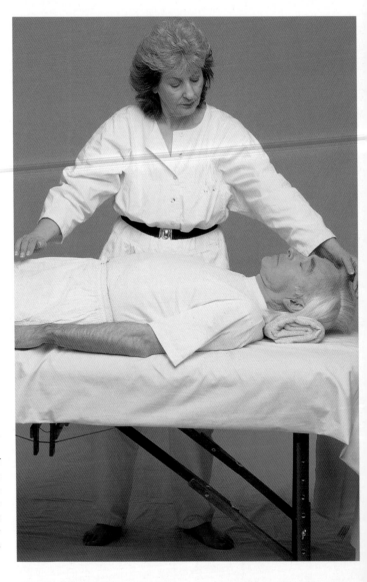

balancing body energy with healing holds

Begin the programme of auric massage with some healing holds to bring a sense of unity to the body, and equilibrium to the mind.

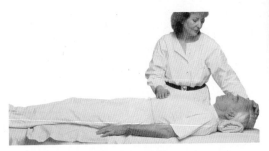

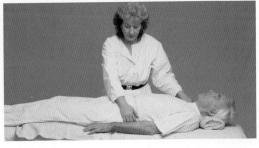

△ **1** If you are doing the healing holds for energy balancing in a session of their own, you can put the recommended oils in an aromatherapy burner to infuse the room with their healing fragrance.

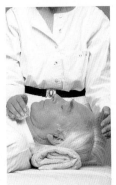

◁ **2** Raise your hands to shoulder level and let them drift down towards the body, with great sensitivity and awareness, to find the edge of the person's aura. This is felt as a tangible but subtle vibration. Softly enter this energy field, letting your hands come to rest, without weight, over the body. Tune in deeply through your hands to the person's essential energy, with the intention of restoring harmony to the whole being. Hold gently until your intuition tells you to move your hands to connect and balance other parts of the body.

△ **3** This polarity hold brings a sense of integration and balance to both sides of the body. When standing on the left side of the body, place your left hand over your partner's right shoulder, and the right hand over his left hip. Imagine a current of energy passing between your hands.

▽ **4** Healing holds on the legs and feet can help to earth the physical body, bringing an inner stability to the emotions. Start with a hip and foot hold to connect the whole leg. Then, when you are ready, place your right hand over the knee, keeping the left hand on the hip. Finally, place your left hand over the knee while cupping the right hand beneath the sole of the foot.

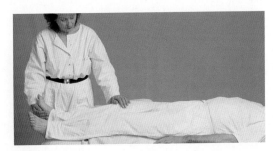

clearing the aura

When the person becomes calm through the loving touch of the healing holds, you can begin the auric massage.

▷ **1** Take the blended oils and spread a small amount into the palms of your hands. Alternatively, add one drop of the oil to a small quantity of moisturizer and rub it into your hands. Now stroke over the aura in smooth, slow, rhythmic strokes towards the feet, working down the body and then over the limbs, one at a time. Do this three times, working over the aura's spiritual, emotional, and physical levels. Start by clearing the spiritual plane (45–60cm (18–24in) above the body); then move lower down on to the emotional level (15–20cm (6–8in) above the body); and finally, on to the physical level (5–7.5cm (2–3in) above the body). Complete your session by letting your hands hover over the belly and heart, before settling softly on to the body.

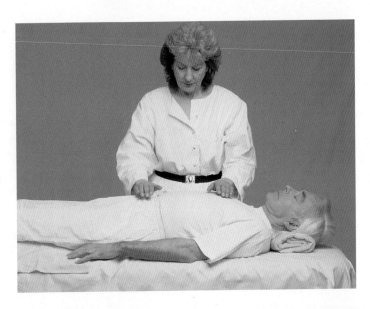

chakra balancing

By trusting your intuition, and moving your hands sensitively above the body in an auric massage, it is possible to detect subtle variations in the relationship of one chakra to another. Stress affecting a specific area of life may manifest in a related chakra, leaving that part vulnerable to disease. This can be felt as an overcharge of vibration or holes in the aura, which could represent potential ill-health. Harmony can be restored by using the essential oils related to the disturbed chakra, and applying auric healing holds to balance it with the other chakras.

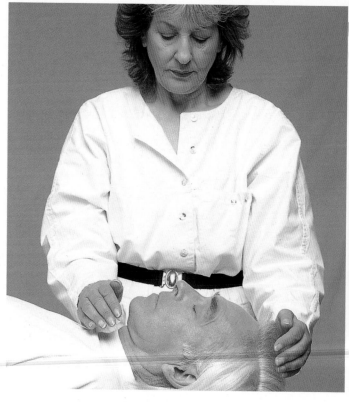

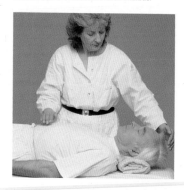

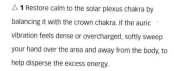

△ **1** Restore calm to the solar plexus chakra by balancing it with the crown chakra. If the auric vibration feels dense or overcharged, softly sweep your hand over the area and away from the body, to help disperse the excess energy.

△ **2** The throat chakra is the centre of communication. When someone is experiencing difficulties with self-expression, help to clear and recharge the energy on an auric level by gently undulating your hand above the throat. Visualizing a blue light around the throat can be helpful.

the seven chakras

- **The base chakra:** Associated with the colour red and the adrenal glands. Connection to basic life survival, stamina and physical drive, the basic constitution, and elimination. Essential oils: Frankincense, black pepper, clary sage
- **The belly chakra:** Associated with the colour orange and the reproductive gland. Sense of yourself, relationships with others, concrete activity, ability to put ideas into action, fertility. Essential oils: Chamomile, fennel, marjoram, orange, peppermint, rose, sandalwood
- **The solar plexus chakra:** Associated with the colour yellow and the pancreas and spleen. Decision making, activity in the world, intellect. Essential oils: Frankincense, fennel, juniper, lavender, peppermint, neroli, rosemary, rosewood
- **The heart chakra:** Associated with the colours green or pink, and the thymus gland. Vulnerability, hopes and dreams, self-esteem, empathy, spiritual purpose. Essential oils: Benzoin, bergamot, geranium, mandarin, peppermint, rose, sandalwood, ylang ylang
- **The throat chakra:** Associated with the colour sky-blue. Self-expression, inner growth, the place of synthesis between inner vision and outward expression in any form. Essential oils: Chamomile, clary sage, sandalwood
- **The brow chakra:** Associated with the colour indigo and the pituitary gland. Personal ethics, morality and spiritual law, perception of the arts, perception of inner vision. Essential oils: Benzoin, clary sage, jasmine, juniper, orange, rosemary
- **The crown chakra:** Associated with the colour violet and the pineal gland. Spiritual control of the physical plane, the point of connection between spiritual and physical life. Essential oils: Cedarwood, cypress, eucalyptus, frankincense, juniper, lavender, mandarin, neroli, rose, rosewood, sandalwood

Note: Some oils help re-balance the upper and lower chakras in a general way: try jasmine, lavender or sandalwood.

protecting the aura

You can use visualization techniques in conjunction with essential oils and auric massage to bring an energetic safety and protection to a friend at a time when he may feel particularly sensitive and vulnerable. Imagine that you are gently sealing the aura from harsh external forces with a layer of pink light. Rub the blended oils into your hands, and then send the intention of goodwill and protection into your hands as you draw them over the aura from the crown to the base of the body.

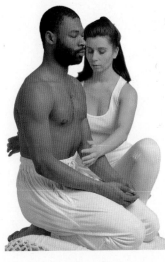

△ **2** Slowly draw your hands down over each side of the body to gently protect each chakra.

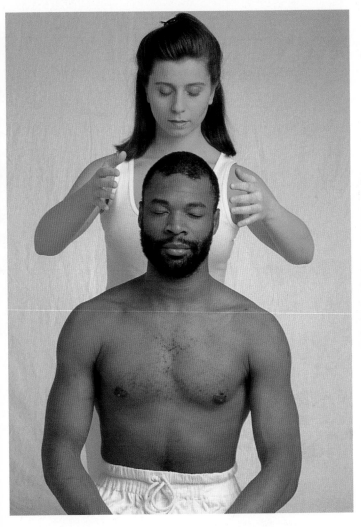

△ **1** Focusing your total attention into your hands, visualize spreading the seal of pink light over the aura, starting from the crown of the head.

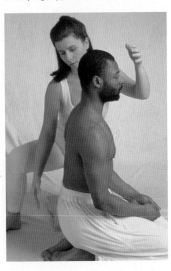

△ **3** Complete this aura protection massage with a balancing hold, letting your hands hover at a distance over the base of the spine and the head. When you feel ready, let your hands drift away from the body and sit silently with your friend for some moments.

completing auric work

When massaging the aura, your hands can feel overcharged and heavy with static energy. Release this down to the earth by shaking your hands gently towards the ground, or by placing them on wood. Consciously let go of the session when it is over and wash your hands in cold water.

Improving circulation

A healthy circulatory system is vital to the well-being of both mind and body. Massage, combined with a healthy diet and exercise, is an effective way to boost both blood and lymph circulation in order to promote health and vitality.

The circulatory system is divided into two parts: blood circulation that is pumped by the heart; and lymph fluid circulation that is moved by muscle action. The lymphatic system carries waste products to the lymph nodes, which act as filters to prevent harmful substances from entering the bloodstream, and is an important part of the body's immune defence system.

causes of poor circulation

Poor circulation may be caused by hereditary factors, but it can also be brought on by a sedentary lifestyle, smoking, an unhealthy diet, or emotional stress and tension. A sluggish circulation will cause a depletion of vital nutrients in the body leading to exhaustion, ill–health and even depression as toxins build up and the elimination process is impeded.

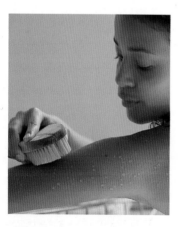

△ Use a natural bristle brush for a stimulating body massage while you are bathing. This stimulates lymph circulation, which helps the body rid itself of waste products.

boosting and draining

The signs of a sluggish circulation can be detected in pale, mottled or blue-tinged skin, which is usually cold to the touch. The most common areas of poor circulation are the extremities of the body. Lift the limb and apply flowing strokes to boost and drain the blood supply on its return to the heart.

▽ **1** Cold arms, hands and fingers indicate poor circulation. To assist the return of blood to the heart, raise your partner's forearm and clasp the hand with whichever of your hands is closest. Wrap the other hand over the back of the wrist and drain firmly down the arm towards the elbow with a long steady stroke. Glide lightly around the elbow and back up to the wrist. Swap hands to repeat the movement on the inner forearm.

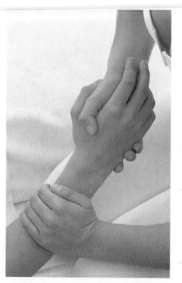

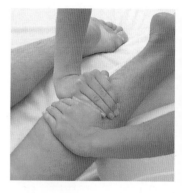

△ **2** Help to increase vitality in the legs and feet by first applying the basic effleurage stroke from the ankle to the back of the knee, with the lower leg in a raised position. Wrap both hands over the back of the ankle, little fingers leading, and firmly stroke up the calf. This position also helps to drain excess water from around puffy ankles.

▽ **3** Deeper drainage strokes can be achieved by using your thumbs to stroke, in alternating short slides, from the ankle to just below the back of the knee. Repeat several times.

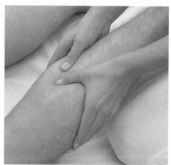

useful essential oils

The following essential oils aid circulation: cedarwood, cypress, eucalyptus, geranium, lemon, mandarin, neroli, rose, rosemary.

To address the problem more fully, create a blend that includes a detoxifying oil from the list of oils recommended for cellulite and one of the general tonic and stimulant oils.

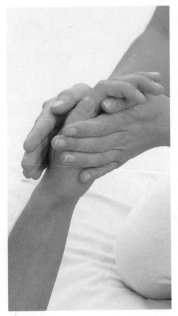

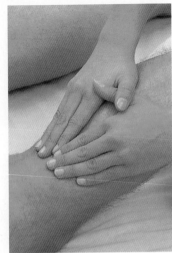

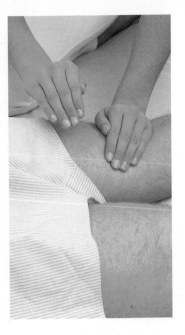

warming up

△ Hands and feet that are cold as a result of poor circulation can be warmed up by briskly rubbing them between both hands. The friction produces heat and stimulates the blood supply and the hands and feet very quickly begin to feel much warmer.

stroking towards lymph nodes

△ Lymphatic massage follows a specific procedure and requires the therapist to have a clear knowledge of the distribution of lymph vessels and nodes throughout the body. However, in a basic massage, gentle, upward effleurage strokes towards the major superficial lymph nodes – such as those in the back of the knee – can assist the lymphatic circulatory system to eliminate toxins from the body, particularly after kneading, friction and deep tissue strokes.

benefiting the skin

△ Pale, flaccid skin benefits from the stimulating effects of all percussion strokes. In particular, the suction effect of cupping draws the blood up towards the skin, bringing vital oxygen and nutrients to its peripheral nerve endings and underlying tissues.

---

self-massage for varicose veins

The return of de-oxygenated blood to the heart from the lower half of the body is against the pull of gravity, and so the veins have valves in them that open and close to prevent back-flow. When a valve is damaged the veins become dilated, causing the condition known as varicose veins. This condition can be exacerbated by pregnancy, obesity or prolonged standing. It is not advisable to massage directly above or below a varicose vein, but gentle upward-flowing effleurage over the sides of the leg, or away from the damaged vein, will ensure that the area is not neglected during a massage.

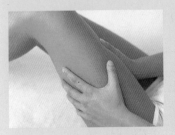

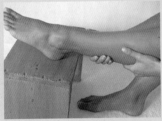

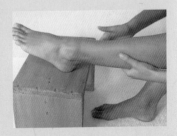

△ **1** Begin by smoothing the essential oil blend all over the leg. Then massage the upper half of the leg using upward movements. This helps to clear the valves so that blood passes more easily from the lower leg.

△ **2** Massage in an upward direction only, using the palms of both hands. Moving up the calf muscle, make long, firm strokes.

△ **3** Run the fingers of one hand up the calf muscle then repeat with the other hand. Finish by repeating step 2, then carry out the sequence on the other leg.

Anti-cellulite massage

Cellulite is detectable by the bumpy "orange peel" look of the skin on the fleshy areas of the body. It is caused by the accumulation of toxic deposits in the fatty tissues. Massage alone cannot rid the tissues of such deposits, but it can greatly assist the process.

Cellulite, which collects mostly on the hips, buttocks and upper arms, is not specifically related to body weight and affects people of all sizes, especially women. It usually results from a sluggish circulation and poor elimination of toxins from the body, and in order to improve the condition it is necessary to use a combination of approaches. This includes a change of diet to cut down on the intake of toxins such as refined carbohydrates, caffeine and alcohol. This should be combined with an increase in the daily intake of fresh vegetables and water. Regular exercise is also important, as it helps the lymphatic system rid the body of waste products.

The following massage programme, combined with the appropriate essential oils, should become part of a daily routine for six to eight weeks if you are to achieve a smooth and healthy skin. Mechanical massage instruments are also useful for this purpose.

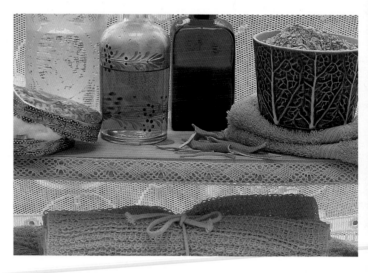

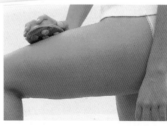

△ Brisk rubbing with a rough cloth, or a loofah, before applying essential oils in a carrier lotion or oil, can help to disperse cellulite.

◁ Hand-held massage instruments such as this wooden six-ball roller are ideal for making the circular pressure motions that help to smooth out cellulite spots on the thighs.

self-help

A quick self-massage programme to stimulate the circulation and elimination process from fleshy cellulite areas can be carried out several times a day, such as when dressing and undressing, or after taking a bath or shower. Squeeze and knead the thighs and buttocks, and follow up with percussion movements.

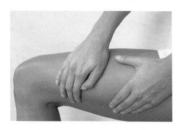

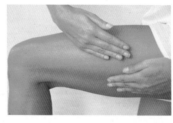

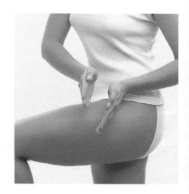

△ **1** After firmly rubbing in your prepared oil mix or lotion, move both hands alternately up the outside of the leg. Use a loofah or bristle brush if you prefer.

△ **2** Hack, cup, and pummel the thighs briskly to tone the area and revitalize the blood circulation. This stimulates the circulation and allows quicker penetration of the essential oils.

△ **3** Continue to work over the cellulite area using the heels of both hands alternately. Maintaining the firmness of the strokes, repeat step 1. Then repeat on the other leg.

cellulite reduction massage

If your partner is worried about cellulite, focus your attention on the problem areas of the thighs and buttocks during the massage. By using the correct sequence of basic massage strokes, you can soothe, tone and stimulate the whole area, boosting the blood supply to the tissues and helping to increase the lymphatic drainage of waste products.

useful essential oils

to stimulate and detoxify: juniper, eucalyptus, fennel
to stimulate circulation and prevent water retention: geranium, lemon, cypress, sandalwood

▽ A useful essential oil blend for treating cellulite would be three drops of lemon, two drops of geranium, two drops of fennel and one drop of cedarwood.

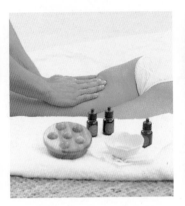

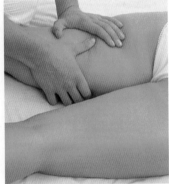

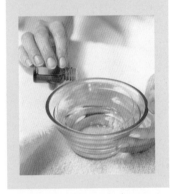

△ **1** Soothe, warm and relax the thigh muscles with upward-flowing effleurage strokes such as integration and fanning motions. Repeat several times, always returning the stroke to the back of the knee by gliding your hands around and down the sides of the leg.

△ **3** Deep friction strokes help to break up toxic deposits. Sink and rotate your thumb pad on one area at a time, using your other hand to push the tissue towards the stroke. Follow these strokes with fanning motions to aid the elimination process.

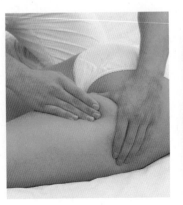

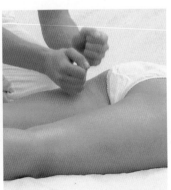

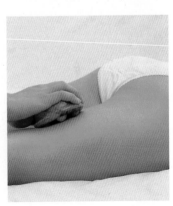

△ **2** The lifting, squeezing, and wringing action of kneading strokes enliven the thigh and buttock muscles and help the exchange of tissue fluids. Knead thoroughly over the whole area, following up with effleurage strokes to boost the circulation.

△ **4** Pummelling, hacking and cupping strokes are ideally suited to cellulite conditions. Briskly strike the thigh and buttocks, one hand following the other in rapid succession, flicking off the skin at the moment of contact.

△ **5** Soothe the thighs and buttocks with effleurage strokes. If you have a mechanical roller, use it to add to the benefits of your cellulite massage by moving it in circular motions over the flesh. This is particularly effective when the skin is oiled.

Strokes for insomnia

therapeutic body treatments

Soothing, hypnotic strokes and sedative essential oils help to separate the activities of the day from the vital period of sleep and rest at night, and enable the insomniac to break the cycle of sleeplessness.

In cases of insomnia or bad dreams that lead to broken nights, it is important to reduce the intake of stimulating drinks such as tea and coffee, and to avoid eating late at night. It is also helpful to create a relaxing ritual to prepare for falling asleep. The suggested massage treatments, given here and for the treatment of anxiety, combined with a recommended blend of aromatherapy oils, will prove invaluable for this bed-time preparation.

soft and soothing strokes

This sequence of strokes should wash over the body in outward flowing motions, creating a gentle stream of movement that draws tension and anxiety away from the central core of the body. The soft, downward pulling strokes have a hypnotic and sedative effect, which will calm the emotions and quiet an over-active mind, thereby helping to induce relaxation and sleep.

As you apply the strokes, be aware of your breathing, drawing your hands down on the inhalation and pausing briefly on exhalation. This slight pause in the motion will create a wave-like feeling, rather than a straight pulling effect. Rub a little oil into your hands and mould them to the body, imparting a steady softness, and always begin the sequence on any limb from above the major joint, such as the shoulder or hip, in order to draw tension away from the constricted area.

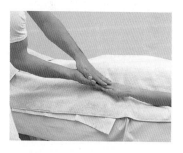

Take the stroke right out of the head, hands or feet, and beyond the actual physical body, as if you are emptying it of the stress and worries that may inhibit sleep. Each sequence should be performed up to five times on each part of the body. Begin by pulling your hands along the back of the neck to help to release tension.

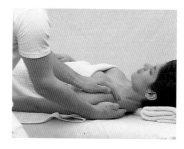

△ **1** Place one hand over the top of the chest, and the other over the muscles on the back of the shoulder, so that the fingers point towards the centre of the body. As you breathe in, pull your hands steadily outwards to the edge of the shoulder and down to just below the joint. Pause briefly as you exhale, letting your hands rest and lightly cradle the top of the arm.

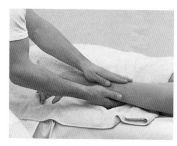

△ **2** Adjust your position so that you can continue the pulling motion down the arm. As you breathe in, pull both hands down to just below the elbow. Relax as you breathe out, and continue the slide down the forearm and below the wrist while inhaling.

◁ **3** Draw your hands over both sides of your partner's hand and fingers, taking your stroke out as the hand settles back on to the mattress. Repeat steps 1 to 3 on the other side of the body.

releasing neck tension
Place both hands, fingers pointing down, on each side of the spine. Ask your partner to breathe deeply and to relax the neck and head into your hands. Pull your hands gently but firmly, with the fingertips slightly indented into the tissue, up the back of the neck and then out from under the head.

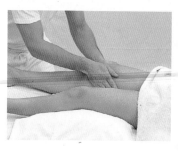

△ **4** Begin the hip, leg and foot sequence by laying both hands just above the pelvic girdle to cradle the side of the body. Pull both hands down over the hip socket as you inhale, separating them as they reach the thigh in order to hold each side of the leg: rest briefly as you exhale. With the next inhalation, draw your hands down the leg to just below the knee.

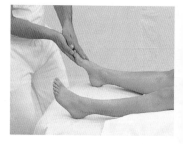

△ **5** Continue this wave-like motion down the lower leg to just below the ankle. Then slide one hand under the foot, with the other on top of the foot, pulling gently and steadily until your hands pass over the toes. Repeat the strokes on the other side of the body.

sedating strokes on the legs and feet

Soft, soothing, downward-flowing strokes over both legs will further enhance the calming and sedative effect of your massage.

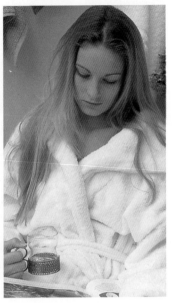

△ Sleeplessness is a very common response to stress. Learning to relax is vital, and massage can be extremely helpful. However, massage will need to be part of a daily routine that also includes a healthy diet and regular exercise.

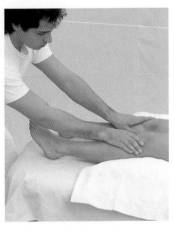

△ **1** Using the flat surface of both hands, softly stroke down the legs from the thighs until your hands pass over and off the feet. Repeat the movement as many times as you like to allow your partner to relax.

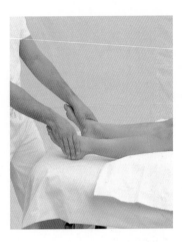

△ **2** To increase the sedative effect of your strokes, complete these sequences with a still, calm hold of your hands over the front of both feet. This will draw the energy down the body, bringing a sense of balance and peace.

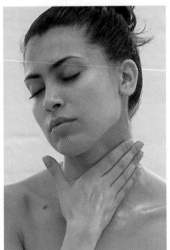

△ A soothing self-massage of the neck, shoulders and arms will relieve nervous tension and have a relaxing sedative effect. An ylang ylang oil massage blend can be particularly helpful for insomnia that has been caused by bad dreams.

useful essential oils

In cases of insomnia, all the relaxing, sedative oils are useful, these include: chamomile, clary sage, lavender, marjoram, mandarin, neroli, orange, rose, rosewood, and sandalwood. Use 2–3 drops of essential oil blended with 15ml (1 tbsp) of an appropriate carrier oil.

• frankincense or lemon blended with one of the oils listed above can help to calm and soothe.

• ylang ylang can be very helpful to relax and calm anxiety in cases of disturbed sleep following a bad dream.

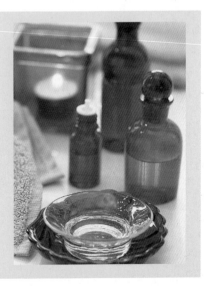

Massage for digestive disorders

When stress is manifested physically in the abdominal area, massage and touch can bring the sense of safety and comfort needed to relax and relieve mild digestive disorders and abdominal discomfort.

Emotional tension can cause us to tighten our abdominal muscles and reduce our breathing in order to avoid the experience of painful or uncomfortable feelings. If we are unable to assimilate those emotions, or express them appropriately, they can manifest themselves as physical disorders, particularly playing havoc with the digestive system. Massage helps to deepen breathing, allowing the muscles to soften and expand, and to restore harmony.

All the strokes shown on the abdomen in the Body Massage section are suitable when stress is felt in this area. Reflexology, shiatsu, hands-on breathing techniques, self-massage and passive movements can also bring relief to simple digestive disorders.

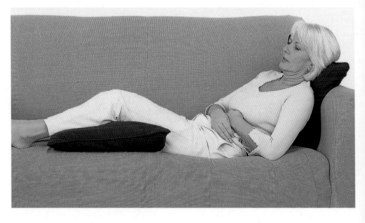

△ Abdominal pain can be a warning that there is disorder in the system, so always consult a doctor if it is persistent.

shiatsu elimination point

An important shiatsu point for the release of intestinal congestion is the one found on the web of skin between the thumb and index finger. The exact location is indicated by its tenderness to pressure. This point is known as Large Intestine 4, or in Chinese terms as "the Great Eliminator".

▽ Press gently on this point for up to five seconds, then release the pressure gradually.

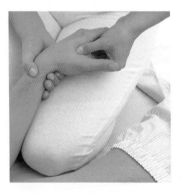

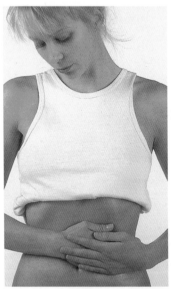

△ Peppermint essential oil is particularly useful for digestive disorders. For self-massage place your hands on your abdomen and move your hands in a clockwise direction to encourage digestive and bowel action.

holding and breathing

Still, calm holds over the abdominal area will encourage deeper breathing, allowing the release of pent-up emotions and stress. The following holds will all help to promote relaxation and eliminate tension, enabling the digestive tract to function properly.

▽ **1** If your partner is under extreme stress and is experiencing abdominal discomfort, the best position is to lie sideways with the knees drawn up slightly. Pillows under the head and between the knees will create a feeling of security. Place one hand over the lower back and the other on the belly, and encourage slow, deep breathing from the abdomen. When the abdominal muscles are relaxed, rub the abdomen with gentle clockwise strokes.

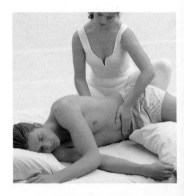

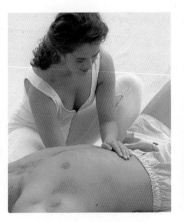

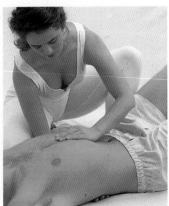

△ **2** With your partner lying down with knees raised, place one hand under the small of the back and ask that the weight of the pelvis be dropped towards your hand. Place your other hand over the abdomen so that its warmth helps to dissolve constriction in the muscles. Then ask your partner to direct breathing towards your hands and to imagine that each breath is helping the abdomen to expand and release tension. Keeping one hand under the pelvis, move your hand to hold different parts of the abdomen.

△ **3** Encourage deep but gentle breathing in the diaphragm and solar plexus region by placing one hand below the mid-back and the other over the top of the abdomen. This will encourage the release of tension that can lead to digestive problems. As the area relaxes, gently massage it with soft circular strokes of your palm.

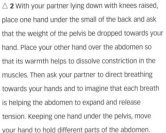

useful essential oils

For specific digestive complaints the following essential oils and blends may be useful:
- *constipation and pain:* three drops each of ginger, orange, bergamot and clary sage
- *sluggish digestion:* peppermint, juniper, rosemary
- *indigestion:* drop of peppermint, three drops each of ginger, lemon and bergamot
- *flatulence:* bergamot, fennel, ginger, lemon, marjoram, neroli, nutmeg, peppermint, rosemary
- *colicky pain:* bergamot, chamomile, clary sage, ginger, cypress, lemon, orange, peppermint, sandalwood
- *constipation:* fennel, ginger, marjoram, neroli, orange, peppermint, rose
- *diarrhoea:* cypress, chamomile, ginger, lemon, orange, peppermint

▽ **Rosemary has analgesic properties which will benefit headaches, painful digestion and muscular pain.**

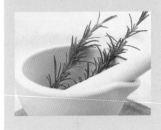

relieving abdominal cramp

Pushing the knees towards the abdomen can help to relieve tightness there. With your partner's knees bent so the feet are flat on the mattress, adjust your posture so that you can lean your weight forward as you perform this passive movement.

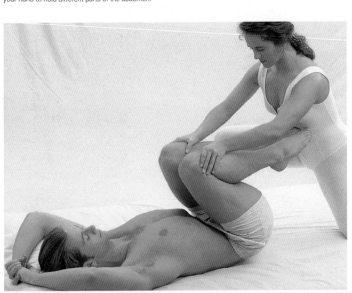

◁ Slowly push the knees towards the trunk of the body, taking care not to force them beyond their natural point of resistance. Help to lower your partner's feet to the mattress, then repeat the movement twice more.

Massage during pregnancy

Pregnancy is a time of great physical and emotional change for a woman, and it is important that, however busy, she finds the time to take good care of herself and her body. Massage is a soothing and beneficial therapy during this prenatal period, but because of complications and conditions that can occur, it is important to check first on its advisability with a family doctor or obstetrician.

Massage over the abdomen during the first three months of pregnancy should be avoided, and also in cases of toxemia, high blood pressure, severe water retention, and swelling of the hands, feet and face. However, when a pregnancy is going smoothly, massage with the appropriate essential oils can help reduce feelings of nausea, minimize stretch marks, combat fluid retention, and alleviate the stress and strain on muscles and joints that result from carrying the extra weight.

staying comfortable

As the abdomen swells during pregnancy, it becomes more difficult to lie down comfortably. Use pillows to support the body, so lying on the side is comfortable while you massage.

▽ Place one pillow under the head, one alongside the body, to lean into, and one between the knees. This position enables you to make a gentle and relaxing contact hold, placing one hand over the abdomen and the other on the nape of the neck, holding for several moments.

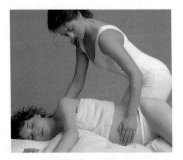

relaxing the shoulders

Loosening the shoulder joints takes the strain out of the upper back and chest, enabling the whole posture to carry the additional weight of the pregnancy.

▽ Encourage your partner to let go of the full weight of the arm and to allow you to control this passive movement. Place your right hand on the back of the shoulder to support it and, ensuring that the elbow remains flexed, begin to lift the arm by clasping the

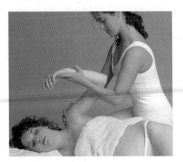

underside of the wrist and forearm with your left hand. Using your own forearm as a support, circle the arm forwards and back over the head. Do this three times with the movement coming from the shoulder joint. When you are ready to massage the other side of the body, rearrange the pillows and repeat this joint release movement on the right shoulder.

▽ Gently massaging the abdomen in the morning and evening with a suitable oil blend can help to prevent stretch marks.

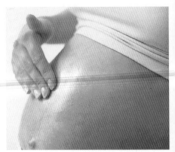

useful essential oils

The majority of essential oils are safe to use during pregnancy provided common sense is applied and the suggested guidelines given below are followed. Those to avoid are fennel, peppermint and rosemary. A number of other oils stimulate bleeding, although no evidence has been found to suggest they endanger the fetus. However, they should be avoided during the first three months of pregnancy and after that used only in moderation if no alternative is available. These oils, which should be used with care and awareness, are as follows: chamomile, clary sage, cypress, jasmine, juniper, lavender, marjoram, nutmeg, peppermint, rose and rosemary.

During the stages of pregnancy, some women can have a variety of uncomfortable symptoms, which may be eased by the following essential oils:
• for nausea: ginger, lemon, nutmeg, rosewood, sandalwood.
• to minimize stretch marks: mandarin and neroli or geranium and frankincense in a vegetable oil carrier enriched with carrot and wheatgerm oil.
• to combat fluid retention: choose from geranium, lemon, mandarin, neroli and orange.

In the last few weeks of pregnancy geranium can be used to tone the whole reproductive system and assist the body in preparing for labour. During labour a variety of oils can be used for massaging the lower back. They include geranium, lemon and neroli.

easing lower back strain

Pregnancy can put a great deal of strain on the curvature of the lower spine and the surrounding muscles, sometimes leading to chronic back pain. While your partner lies sideways, focus your strokes on the lower back and buttocks, enabling the area to release its tension.

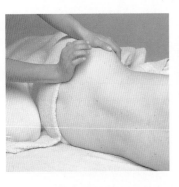

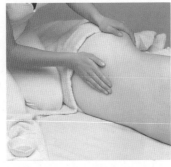

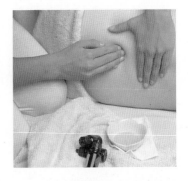

△ **1** Spread the oil over the lower back and buttocks, warming and soothing the muscles with soft effleurage strokes. Then begin to work deeper into the gluteal muscles of the buttocks, rotating the heel of your hand in one area at a time while supporting the hip with your other hand.

△ **2** It is common to see a pregnant woman instinctively placing a hand over the base of the spine to soothe away discomfort and pain. Bring relief to the muscles surrounding and covering the pelvic girdle and lower back with flowing, circular motions from the surface of your hand.

△ **3** Tiny, circular friction movements with your fingertips will deepen the remedial effects of your strokes on the lower back. Ease away tension in the muscle that covers the sacrum, the flat triangular bone at the base of the spine. Push the tissue towards the stroke with your other hand.

helping circulation

Smooth, flowing, and soft effleurage movements, stroking up over the feet, ankles and legs, will help to boost circulation and to reduce the likelihood of puffy ankles and varicose veins, both common conditions during pregnancy.

soft circles on the abdomen

After the first three months of a healthy pregnancy, you can gently massage the abdomen with the same soft circular motions that you would normally apply to the abdomen in a whole body massage.

spine and shoulders

The best position for this massage is leaning into the support of a pillow while sitting astride a chair. This will allow the shoulders to fall forward so that the upper back becomes more open and available to touch.

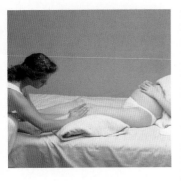

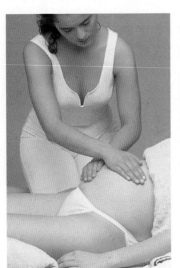

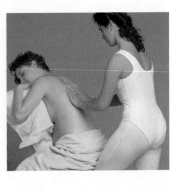

△ So that your partner can sit comfortably during a leg massage, the best position is usually to lean back on a mound of cushions or pillows, with a rolled-up towel to support the neck. It may also be helpful to place a pillow under the knees to take the strain off the thighs, buttocks, and lower back.

△ The warmth of your touch and the soporific motions will be very relaxing to both the mother and baby.

△ Begin with several effleurage integration strokes. Start at a point mid-back, and stroke your hands up each side of the spine before fanning out to encompass the shape of the upper back. When the muscles are relaxed, follow up with kneading on the shoulders and upper arms. Add some gentle friction with thumbs or fingers on tight spots beside the spine and shoulder blades. Complete with several more effleurage strokes.

Baby and child massage

It is never too soon to enjoy massage. In many parts of the world, it is customary for babies and children to be massaged by their mothers and carers. Touch is a natural expression of love, communicating warmth and security. In babies, massage helps strengthen the growing bond between mother and baby. Babies also enjoy it and usually sleep better afterwards. Children too are generally receptive to being massaged. The important thing to remember when working with babies or children is that their bodies are still developing, so they must be treated very gently.

massage for babies

When giving baby massage, focus on the chest and back, using light, smooth strokes. Do NOT massage the head, as this is too malleable. The best time to massage your baby is at the end of the day, before feeding and bathing. Although it may be the last thing you feel like doing, once you start you'll find it relaxes you both. If at any point you sense your baby is not enjoying the massage, then stop. The massage should only go on if you are both enjoying it.

preparation for massage

Make sure the room is warm, as babies feel the cold, and their body temperatures can drop quickly. Have a soft cloth or towel for your baby to lie on and, if you are using oil, warm it up before applying. In India, a blend of coconut and sesame oil is often used in baby massage, although almond, apricot or grapeseed oils are also suitable. Ideally the oil should be cold-pressed and organic.

▽ **All babies thrive on being cuddled and touched. Skin-to-skin contact is essential to the nurturing of an infant and an important part of the bonding process.**

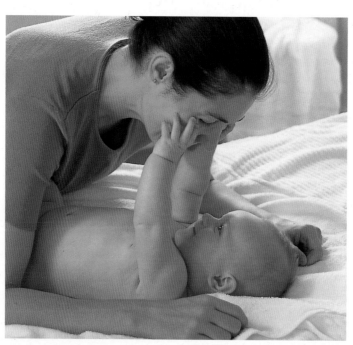

baby massage sequence

Begin the massage by playing and interacting with your baby. It is important to establish whether they are in the right mood.

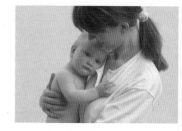

△ **1** Hold your baby close to you, so that the warmth of your body, the beat of your heart, and the rhythm of your breathing will comfort and soothe.

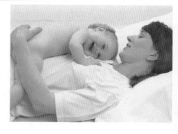

△ **2** Babies love to lie against the softness of your body. Place a soothing hand over the base of the spine, while gently stroking the head.

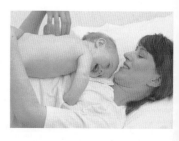

△ **3** Wriggling your fingertips softly up and down your baby's back will usually cause giggles of pleasure as the feather-like touches tickle and stimulate the soft skin.

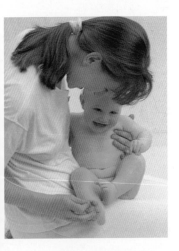

△ **4** Babies never seem to lose interest in their fingers and toes; use this fascination and wiggle and rotate the joints one by one.

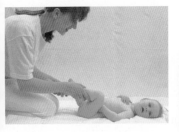

△ **5** Babies love a game of passive movements, where you move and gently flex the joints of the arms and legs. Bend one knee towards the body and then straighten out the leg. Carry out the same action on the other leg. Repeat several times.

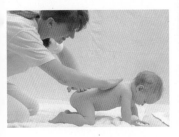

△ **6** If the baby can keep still for long enough, you can rub nourishing oil into the skin as you massage. Pour a little oil into your hands and rub it in gently, using circular movements on the baby's chest. Soft effleurage strokes on the back, such as a criss-cross motion and circles, will soothe and calm to complete the massage.

massage for children

When your massage partner is a younger child, you will probably need to find a higher chair, such as a kitchen stool, for them to sit on. You can also use cushions to raise the seat. Make sure the child's legs are not left dangling, by using cushions under their feet. Be flexible and creative in your approach, giving appropriate treatment when called for: you can offer a back or shoulder rub for instance if the child complains of a headache. A treatment that lasts between 5–10 minutes is usually sufficient. Be sensitive to how the child reacts, and don't try to persuade them to continue if they get restless or ill at ease.

When massaging teenagers, remember that they don't always welcome physical contact, and keep the massage as relaxed and informal as you can. Don't over-prepare the situation; take the opportunity when it comes to suggest a massage as part of your usual interaction with each other.

At the end of a massage with a young person, stand behind them and rest both your hands on their shoulders, with your fingers pointing forwards. Ask them to take a deep breath in and out. On the second out breath, gently press down with your hands and then let go. This helps to "ground" their energy and to release any remaining tension.

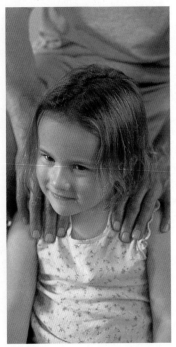

△ **You can do head massage on children from when they are aged about three years old. It is best to keep treatments light, short and sweet at this tender age.**

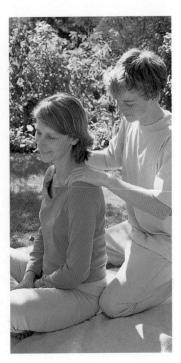

△ **Children learn by experience, and by receiving massage they can soon learn how to become proficient masseurs themselves, as happens in many parts of the world.**

A baby massage

A newborn baby instinctively responds to touch, and massage between mother and baby is a marvellous way of enhancing the natural bonding. All babies have this powerful sensitivity to being caressed and cuddled. Watch the reflex action of a baby tightly curling its fingers or toes as soon as something touches them.

There is no fixed sequence for massaging a baby. Keep the movements gentle and flowing. The simple action of gently stroking a baby will strengthen the natural bonding, and soothe and reassure the baby too. Massage has been shown to help calm difficult or colicky babies, and alleviate wind and other digestive problems. It may also build resistance to coughs and colds. Use a little light vegetable oil which is easily absorbed, such as sweet almond or sunflower, taking care to avoid the eyes. Vegetable oils are preferable to mineral oils, which are not absorbed by the skin.

A baby will benefit from many of the positive effects of massage, such as developing muscle tone. Effleurage towards the heart will help boost your baby's circulation, while some gentle clockwise abdominal strokes will stimulate the digestive system. From around six weeks old, you can begin using essential oils on your baby. Use only the safest oils, lavender or Roman chamomile, and no more than 1 drop in 15ml (3 tsp) of carrier oil.

getting comfortable

Lay the baby gently on its back on a warm, soft towel between your legs, or on your lap, whichever is most comfortable. Pour about 5ml (1 tsp) of sweet almond oil into a small dish. Make sure your hands are warm and that the room is quiet, very warm and there are no draughts. After a baby's bathtime is ideal.

working on baby's front

Make massaging your baby a pleasant game for both of you. Don't expect your baby to stay perfectly still for you, and keep the massage session quite short.

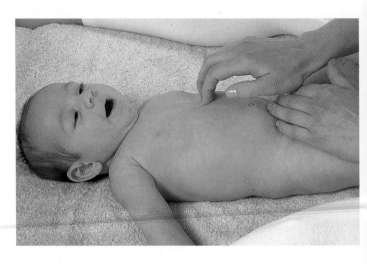

△ **1** Slowly and gently, smooth a little of the oil all over the front of the baby's body, shoulders to feet, avoiding the face. Lightly stroke down the chest and abdomen with the tips of your fingers. This is a delightful stroke which can be used to calm a baby at any time.

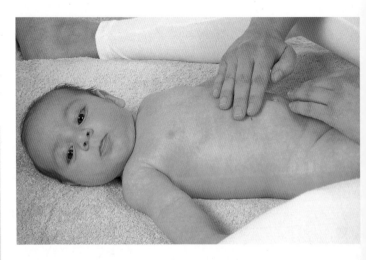

△ **2** Keeping the pressure very light, smooth both hands over the abdomen in continuous circular strokes, working up the baby's right side, across and down the baby's left side. Keep the movement continuous by lifting your left hand when your arms cross. Repeat these circular strokes several times.

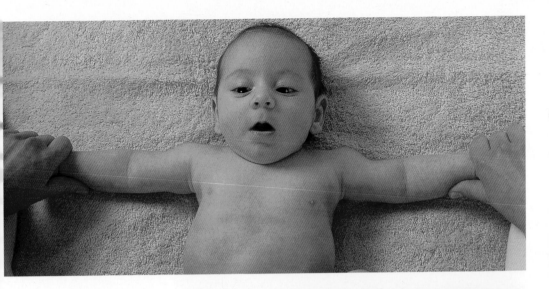

△ **3** Gently stretch out both arms to the side, spreading the hands and fingers if the baby will let you. Gently squeeze out along the arms, then massage the wrist and palms with light, circular thumb movements. Finish by stretching out each finger with a slight pull.

▷ **4** Move on to the legs and feet, working on one leg at a time. Support the leg with both hands and gently squeeze and release the fleshy part of the thigh. Then, supporting the leg with one hand, stroke the leg from the knee to the thigh and back down again.

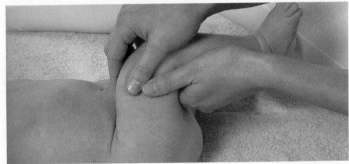

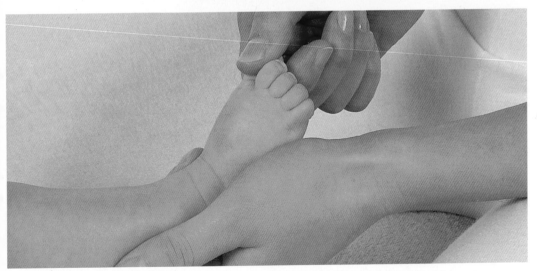

△ **5** Move your supporting hand down to behind the ankle. Gently smooth the palm of your other hand over the top of the foot from toe to ankle and back again. When you get to the toes, very gently stretch each one in turn. Repeat steps 4 and 5 on the baby's other leg.

working on baby's back

Respond sensitively to your baby's reactions during the massage – some strokes will feel more enjoyable than others and you can spend more time on these.

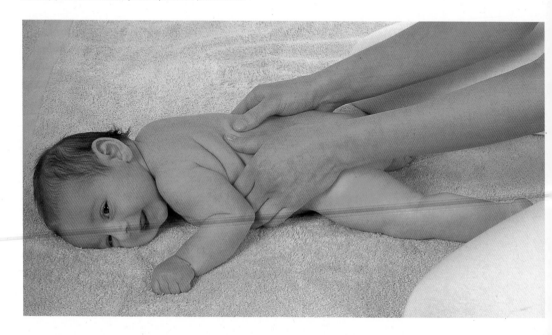

△ **1** Turn the baby over on to its front. Begin by stroking up the whole back to distribute a little oil. Take your strokes round the sides as well and then up the legs, back and out over the arms. Gentle massage on the back like this is particularly soothing because of its calming effect on the spinal nerves.

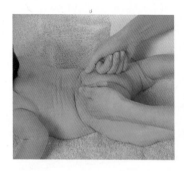

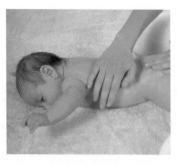

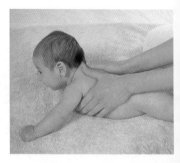

△ **2** Gently knead and squeeze the buttocks to stimulate the circulation. Make a loose fist and rotate over the buttocks, in circular movements.

△ **3** Alternating your hands, one over the other, gently stroke up one side of the back to the shoulders and down again. Repeat on the other side of the back.

△ **4** Bring both hands round the sides of the upper body, and use your thumbs to massage gently up the back to the base of the neck and down again. Include some gentle massage with the thumbs on the shoulders.

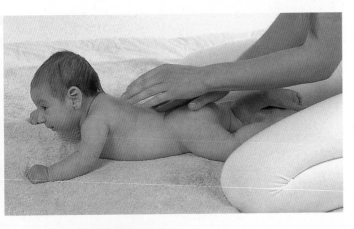

◁ **5** To finish, repeat the feather strokes used at the beginning of the massage, working all over the back from neck to buttocks.

▽ **The special connection between parent and baby is reinforced by the gentle and calming touch of massage. What better way to help your baby feel nurtured and cared for?**

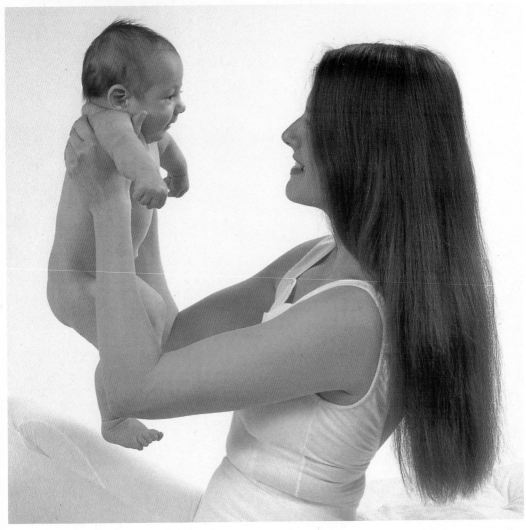

Massage for pets

Massage is the oldest and simplest physical therapy. Its most basic but profound form is when the mother "rubs it better" for her child. The fact that the skin and nervous system develop from the same cell layer when in embryo may have something to do with the fact that massage calms the mind as well as the body, and giving a sense of complete well-being.

Giving your pet a massage will induce a feeling of well-being in the pet, and can help to establish a valuable non-verbal communication that conveys an attitude of loving care. This strengthens the bond between pet and owner, and the sense of harmony that this generates will help to heal not only the pet's physical body but its mind and spirit as well. The act of giving a massage is therapeutic for the owner and has been found to reduce stress levels. In this sequence (opposite), a dog has been used, but the principle can be applied equally to cats and other domestic pets.

Physically, massage improves the pet's circulation, relaxes the muscles and helps to balance muscle function and joint action, and can help to disperse scar tissue. It also helps the lymphatic system to speed up the rate at which it detoxifies the body. It may also increase the production of the body's natural pain killers (endorphins) which help to increase the feeling of well-being.

Massage can be used as an aid to keeping a healthy pet fit. It should not be used to treat sick animals unless they have first been checked by a vet. It should definitely not be used in cases where there is severe pain or the skin is damaged or infected. Nor where there is muscle injury, or where there are severe joint pains. Massage is also contra-indicated where the pet has recently had a high temperature (in the case of an acute infection for example), and when the pet is known to have high blood pressure.

massage routine

A simple routine for an owner would be to begin with a few gentle strokes of even pressure along the body and limbs in the direction of the hair growth. These strokes should be slow and rhythmic and will help to relax the pet. They also allow the owner to locate any tender spots. Lubricants are not normally required, but if they are, baby powder is preferred to the oils used on humans; these make the fingers slide too quickly over the skin for the massage to be effective, and they can get very messy.

The pressure of the strokes should be gradually increased to a firmness that the pet will tolerate. Change the direction of these firmer strokes to work towards the heart so as to stimulate venous and lymphatic drainage. Ideally one would start at the feet and move upwards and forwards towards the head. If, however, the pet is footshy it may be better to start at the head and work back along the body.

The pet's feet should be massaged slowly and gently with the fingers, getting into the spaces between the toes if possible. Massage the legs upwards towards the body, starting just above the paw. Use your fingers for small pets and your palm where possible for larger pets.

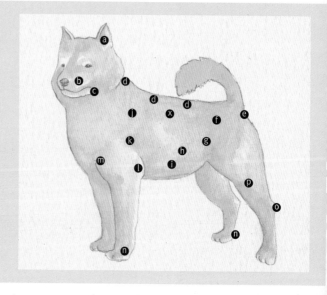

Diagnostic massage points in a dog
Pressure on these points can elicit a pain response to indicate potential problem areas:

a – ear
b – teeth and gums
c – throat and neck
d – back and spine
e – anal glands
f – hips
g – bladder
h – abdomen
i – lower abdomen and liver
j – ribs and lungs
k – ribs and lungs
l – elbow
m – shoulder
n – feet and toes
o – hock (ankle)
p – stifle (knee)
x – kidney and ovary

simple dog massage

Most dogs love the attention of a massage and are quite happy to stand still while you pummel them gently from head to toe. A regular massage will certainly improve your relationship with your dog. Add a simple massage at the end of your daily grooming routine, building up slowly until your dog is used to it.

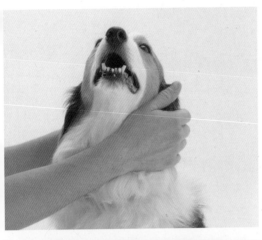

◁ **1** When first using massage on your dog, or if your dog is known to be footshy, start off with his head. Place your hands on his head and, with light pressure, start with slow strokes, moving down over the ears. Repeat several times until you feel your dog relax. Extend the strokes over the head, around the eyes, nose, mouth and ears.

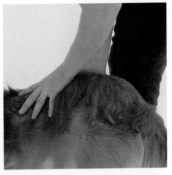

△ **2** Move slowly down the neck to the back area. Keep your hands on either side of the spine (never massage directly on the spine) and make long rhythmic strokes in the direction of the heart.

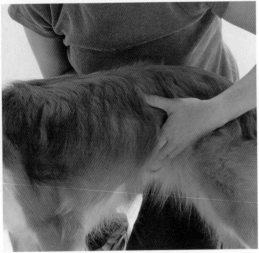

△ **3** Slide your hands round the dog's sides to the abdomen and make circular movements over the belly and groin area, using your fingers or the palms of your hands, depending on the size of the dog.

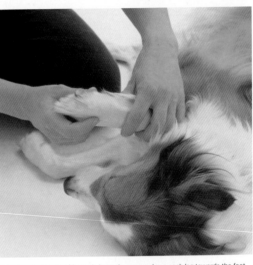

△ **4** Massage the shoulder and chest, then move down each leg towards the foot. The feet should be massaged very slowly and gently: try and rub between the toes if the dog will let you.

To tackle the abdomen, either keep the pet standing or get him to roll over. Massage with circular movements, again using either your palms or fingers depending on the size of the pet. The body and chest are best massaged first on one side and then the other. Start at the rear of the body and work towards the pet's head.

The spine should *never* be massaged. Instead, massage slightly to each side of the midline using your finger tips. It is here that you are most likely to find the tender trigger points. Do not massage these points at all vigorously. It will cause the surrounding muscles to go into spasm as a protective reflex. Light massage will help to reduce the reactivity of the point and to induce relaxation of the muscles. Finger pressure on a trigger point can deactivate it, whilst vigorous massage can increase the pain by stimulating further muscle contractions in an attempt to protect the damaged area.

Finally move to the head and neck. This stage of the massage is a favourite with most pets, and you may like to give a few minutes' extra attention here. Massage the head area gently, including around the eyes, nose, mouth and ears, remembering to stroke and not to poke. The neck should be treated as an elongation of the back, and massage applied to the side and not to the middle. End the session with a few light strokes along the body from head to tail.

Osteopathy for pets

Osteopathy is a form of treatment based on the manipulation of the body's bony skeleton. The basic premise is that imbalance and disharmony will result from the changes that occur in all parts of the body when one part of its structure is altered. Osteopathy is not a complete system of medicine. The idea of osteopathy for pets might seem strange, but most pets are surprisingly amenable to this therapy.

what is osteopathy?

Osteopathy was developed in the late 19th century by an American, Dr Andrew Taylor Still. He saw the skeleton as having a dual purpose. The commonly recognized function was that it provided the physical framework for the body. By the action of the muscles that were attached to it, it allowed the mechanical movement of the body. The other, equally important, function was to protect the body's vital organs. Dr Still theorized that if the skeleton were out of alignment, the body it supported and protected would not be able to maintain a state of good health. The basis of osteopathy is that structure governs function.

Osteopathy is used alongside orthodox Western medicine. Osteopaths are trained to treat each patient as a complete structure, paying close attention to the relationship between the musculoskeletal system and the function of the body. They look at a patient's history to decide if osteopathy is a suitable treatment. A thorough physical examination enables them to observe the ease and range of movement in the limbs and spine. By feeling the muscles and bones, the osteopath can locate painful areas and identify any misalignments of the skeleton. The osteopath is then able to make a diagnosis and develop a treatment plan.

how it works

Osteopathy on pets uses soft-tissue massage techniques and joint manipulations to make adjustments to the damaged neuro-musculoskeletal structure. The techniques used on pets and humans are very similar. Manipulation techniques make corrections which repair the damage and allow healing to occur. After the initial treatment, the osteopath will monitor improvements by sight and by feeling the changes that occur in the diseased area and in the body.

Osteopathic massage increases blood flow, which speeds up the elimination of toxic waste products that build up in the damaged areas. It increases the oxygenation of the tissues to relieve pain and stiffness.

The most common joint-manipulation technique used in osteopathy is the high-velocity thrust. Contrary to popular belief, although this causes popping noises, it does not realign bones and joints. It does, however, slightly separate the joint surfaces momentarily. This separation stretches the joint capsule and gives it greater freedom of movement. As the joint capsule is stretched, tiny bubbles of carbon dioxide come out of solution from the joint fluid and these are responsible for the popping sound.

The other techniques used are passive movement and articulation. These gently and painlessly stretch the soft tissues to result in greater joint and limb mobility. Passive movement involves the osteopath moving the pet's limbs while the pet relaxes and makes no physical effort. Articulation takes this a stage further, and uses the pet's limbs as levers to stretch the soft tissues. In all techniques, the osteopath monitors the pet's response and makes adjustments to its treatment plan accordingly.

availability

Osteopathy is now recognized as a valid treatment for animals, although there are as yet no recognized schools of veterinary osteopathy. If you wish to have your pet treated osteopathically, it must first be examined by a vet. If the vet also thinks that treatment would be beneficial, a qualified human osteopath will work on your pet under the vet's direction.

It is important that the vet and the osteopath co-operate with each other. The vet's notes, diagnosis and schedule should be made available to the osteopath, and the osteopath should discuss the treatment, benefits and outcome. Failure to liaise effectively can result in an inappropriate treatment being given. Osteopaths may use other therapies in their treatment of human patients, but by law they are not allowed to use techniques other than osteopathy on your pet without the permission of the vet.

when to use osteopathy

In the absence of scientific research it is difficult to evaluate the value of osteopathy in pets. However, where vets have referred pets for osteopathic treatment, the results have been encouraging. Osteopathy seems to be particularly useful to alleviate any joint pain arising as a result of road traffic accidents and degenerative diseases.

Although the theory of osteopathy is valid for all species, it is important to remember that cats, in particular, do not like being handled by strangers. Their reluctance to co-operate with osteopathic treatment is a great drawback to its use, except when the cat is trusting enough to relax and allow manipulation, in which case good results can be obtained. However, if the cat refuses to co-operate, do not force it, but postpone the treatment session to another date. Alternatively, you may wish to consider a different therapy after discussing the options with your vet.

General osteopathic treatment

The initial stage of any osteopathic treatment is a thorough examination of the animal's whole body. The osteopath will work through a sequence of movements, manipulating the pet's limbs in order to identify a suspected misalignment. This therapy is equally successful with dogs and other domestic pets.

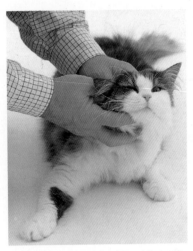

◁ **1** Examination and articulation of the cat's pelvic bones. Each hind leg is extended to stretch out the muscles.

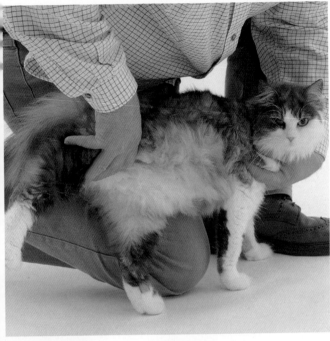

△ **2** Examination and articulation of the neck. The head is gently rotated clockwise to stretch the muscles in the neck and shoulder.

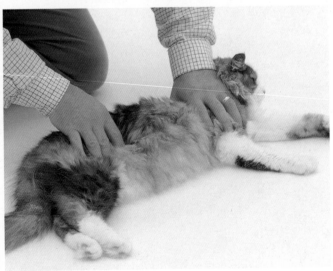

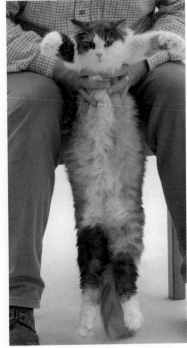

△**3** Examination of the front leg. The cat lies on its side with its muscles relaxed, while the positions of the skeletal structure are examined.

▷ **4** Examination and articulation of the hind legs. The cat is lifted clear of the ground to extend the hind leg muscles and bone structure.

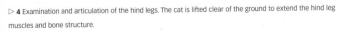

Using Shiatsu in Massage

A system of manipulating the body to restore balance, shiatsu draws strongly on the ancient Chinese practice of acupressure, and is based on the same theory of life-force energy flowing through the body in channels known as meridians. When performed with a relaxed body and an open and sensitive frame of mind, simple shiatsu movements can be used safely on oneself and others to help revitalize the body, mind and emotions.

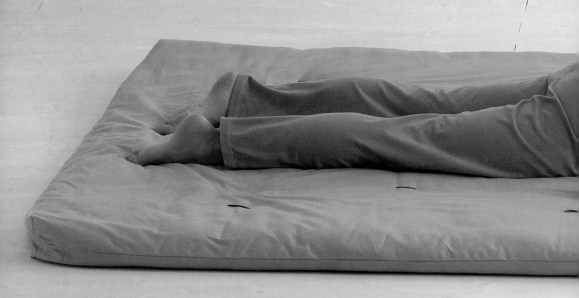

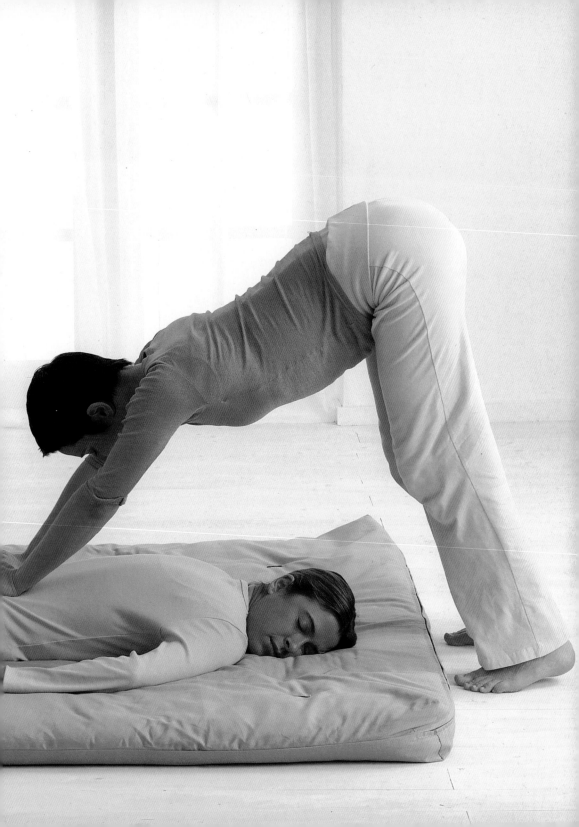

The principles of shiatsu

Shiatsu can be traced back over 5,000 years to its roots in ancient Chinese forms of medicine such as acupuncture and acupressure. However, it is a modern Japanese therapy, which fuses traditional Eastern practices with Western techniques of osteopathy. Literally translated, the name means finger pressure – *Shi* (finger) and *Atsu* (pressure) – although elbows, knees and feet are also used to press along the body's network of meridian lines and pressure points, releasing blocked channels of energy. It is a holistic method of alleviating pain and promoting health in the whole body.

giving a shiatsu session

If your partner closes their eyes, this can make the session a special time to relax and switch off from the world. There is no need to talk during a treatment as the communication of touch can say so much more. One of the fundamental principles of shiatsu is to have simultaneous touch from both hands. With a two-hand connection a

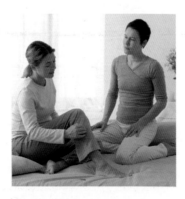

⊲ Spend a little time finding out about your partner's health concerns before you begin the shiatsu.

circuit is created, bonding the giver and receiver. To keep this link, one hand is stationary – the support hand – and plays the role of listening to and comforting your partner, while the other hand – the messenger hand – moves and does all the work. The amount of pressure from both hands will vary depending on the area of the body you are working on. The messenger and support hands change roles

many times throughout a shiatsu session. What you are trying to achieve is two points of contact merging and feeling like one to both therapist and partner.

Even as a beginner use your senses of looking, asking, listening and touching. Listen to your partner's needs and ask about symptoms before giving a treatment. Your motivation to help can be felt by your partner through the hands, transforming the simplest techniques into a caring bond. Before giving a shiatsu treatment, calm your own mind, as any tension will transmit itself to your partner.

the hara

The *Hara* is one of the most powerful energy centres of the body. In shiatsu terms it is known as the *Tanden*, and is located below the navel in the lower abdomen. It is the physical centre of the body and features prominently in all shiatsu treatments. The *Hara* incorporates the *Yin* (Earth) force flowing up the front of the body, and the *Yang* (Heaven) force flowing down the back merging into the lower abdomen. By focusing all movements from this centre, you can give harmonious and supportive treatments. Develop an open-posture principle in which your *Hara* is physically and energetically behind all your movements. This enables weight to be used instead of force. The simple rule is if you're not feeling comfortable and relaxed your partner will become aware of this.

It is very important to remember your own breathing when stretching and applying pressure. Breathe in deeply and exhale as you move into a stretch, encouraging your partner to do the same.

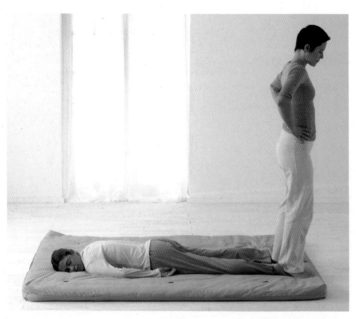

⊲ "Walking" on the feet stimulates reflex points and helps to ground an overactive partner.

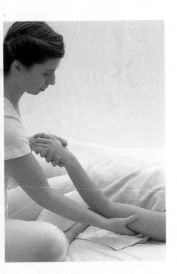

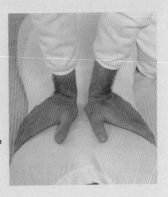

◁ The shiatsu practitioner works sensitively and intuitively, aiming to restore balance within the partner's body.

healing energy

The aim of shiatsu is to balance the body's "Chi" energy levels. The rocking, kneading and stretching techniques are most effective in unblocking the congested areas. If your partner has a low energy level, and is generally fatigued, then slow, deep, static and perpendicular pressure will be more effective in strengthening the energy flow. Holding certain points for one to ten seconds is a general guideline but use your intuition as to how long you hold.

practical points

A shiatsu session normally lasts up to an hour. It is advisable to wear loose clothing so that your movements aren't hampered. The receiver is also clothed, but should avoid wearing bulky or constricting clothes that would impede contact with the body. Generally, the therapist works on the whole of the body and having discovered your problems may suggest simple practical exercises for home use to help the process of recovery. The effects of shiatsu may be felt immediately or later on in the same day, but if painful reactions are later experienced then your practitioner should be contacted. There are no two people with similar mental and physical complaints and the number of sessions will depend upon the individual's needs.

Shiatsu helps to keep open the communication between body, mind, emotion and spirit.

the main techniques

palming

Palming is the simplest and most widely used technique in shiatsu. Palm pressure is gentle but firm, creating a supporting and soothing effect on any tense or vulnerable areas of the body.

Allow your hands to be relaxed so that your fingers can follow the contours of whatever part of the body you contact, then lean your body-weight through your palm, holding and waiting for the connection between your two palms. Lean back and without breaking contact, slide your hand along the body and lean forward again, creating stationary and perpendicular pressure.

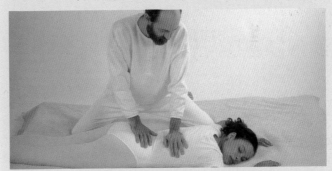

rocking

Use rocking on large areas to relieve tension. Placing your hands apart with palms down on your partner's body, rock slowly forward and back. The rocking should come from your own centre of balance, the *Hara*, which should control the movement.

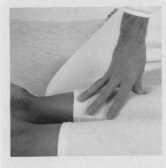

thumbing

Thumb pressure is far more precise and penetrating than palming, and is used for working the points along the meridians. Place your thumbpads on the points. Use your extended fingers for support, so that the thumb remains straight. Lean your body forward so that most of the pressure is transferred through the thumbs. Make sure your nails are quite short to practise this technique or you may hurt your partner.

Shiatsu Meridians

Shiatsu is a manipulative therapy which uses static pressure applied to specific points and lines all over the body. The lines are known as meridians. There meridian lines, which have been described as "channels of living magnetic energy", flow throughout the body and connect the main vital organs. It is this vital energy, known as "Chi", which keeps our bodies active, and the quality of our Chi depends upon our mental, emotional, physical and spiritual conditions. An imbalance in a person's vital energy levels may manifest itself as a back problem, headache, or in many other ways. By working along the meridians, the therapist summons energy to the place most vulnerable and disperses the trapped energy from the areas where it is congested, thus restoring balance to the whole body.

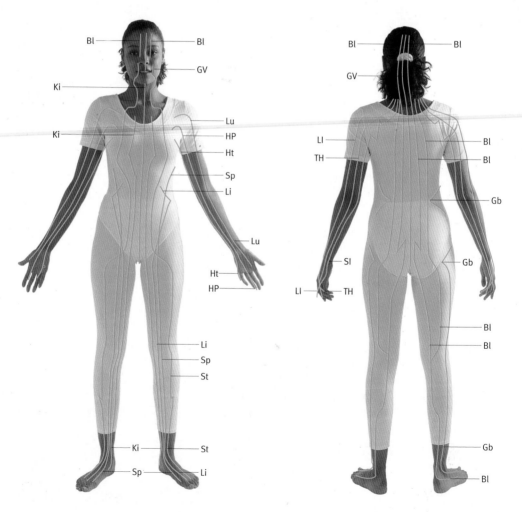

Simple shiatsu session

These sequences are arranged so that each technique can flow smoothly into the next. Ideally the whole treatment should be experienced as a complete uninterrupted unit, not as a collection of separate movements. To achieve this, always maintain contact with your partner and make the transition from one technique to the next with ease and fluency.

making contact with the yang

Position yourself at your partner's side. Take some time to centre yourself, clearing your mind so you can focus on your partner.

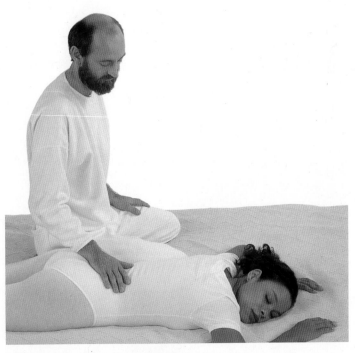

▷ **1** Gently and firmly lay your hand on the small of your partner's back. This contact is an important time for both receiver and giver to attune to each other's energy. Use this time to assess the needs of your partner; feel the quality of the energy, physically, emotionally and spiritually. This can focus your intention in all the techniques to follow.

working on the back

Once your partner is relaxed, you can begin the sequence with the back. This will encourage a sense of trust between you and your partner.

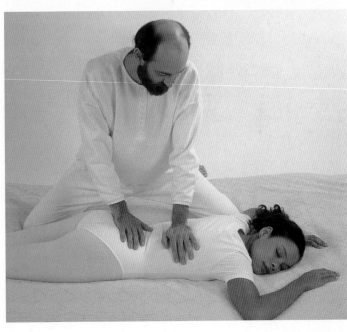

▷ **2** Turn to face your partner and place the heels of your hands in the space between the shoulder blade and spine. With your knees apart begin to rock back and forth from your *Hara* (centre of the lower abdomen) and let the movement transfer through your hands so your partner's entire body moves in a wave-like motion. Continue to perform the rocking technique, working all the way down to the sacrum (lower back), moving the hands down the back in sequence. Repeat two or three times and then repeat the same movements on the other side of the spine.

This rocking technique helps to disperse tension throughout the body, thus encouraging the energy to flow. It is useful to observe how your partner's body is moving. You will quickly be able to diagnose areas which may need more attention by simply observing which parts of the body are not moving as you rock.

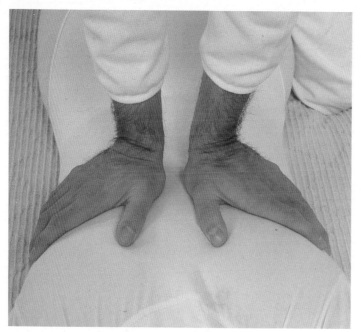

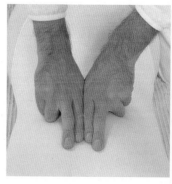

△ **5** Having relaxed the back you can now locate the bladder meridian, which has a structural and energetic relationship with the nervous system. Measure two fingers' width from the centre of the spine on each side and one hand's width down from the top of the shoulder.

△ **3** Come up on to one knee, keeping an open posture. Placing your palms no higher than shoulder-blade level, on your receiver's "out" breath, bring your body-weight forward applying perpendicular pressure to your partner's back.

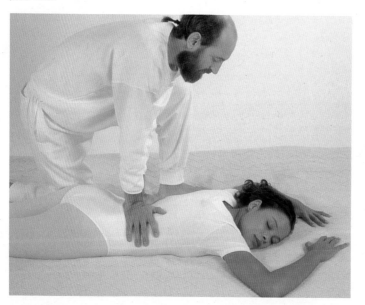

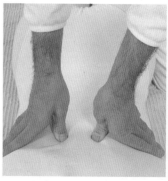

△ **6** Using the thumbs apply pressure at the points between the ribs. Thumb pressure is much more concentrated than palming. If you are unsure about how much pressure to use, simply ask your partner how it feels.

△ **4** Work down the back, moving a palm's width each time, and moving your body position to maintain perpendicular pressure. As you move below the ribs you may want to decrease the pressure slightly, as the internal organs are less protected here.

working on the legs

This sequence shows work on one leg only. When you have finished, move round and repeat on the other side.

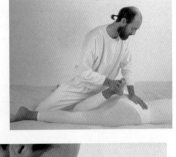

▷ **4** With one hand on the sacrum, use the other hand to bring the foot gently back toward the buttocks, taking into consideration the leg's stretching capacity. Hold for a few seconds and then release.

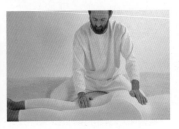

△ **1** Move your body down level to and facing your partner's legs. With your support hand on the lower back (sacrum), your messenger hand rocks and kneads simultaneously down the near-side thigh and calf several times.

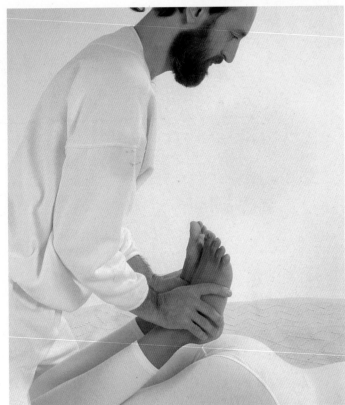

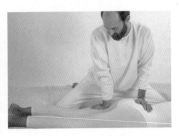

△ **2** Next palm down the leg, avoiding pressure on the backs of the knees.

△ **5** Clasp both feet together and bend the legs, bringing the feet toward the buttocks. Hold this position for a few seconds and notice which foot goes closest to the buttocks to assess pelvic balance.

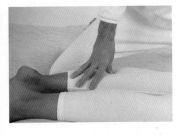

△ **3** Now thumb down the path of the bladder meridian. Depending on the length of the leg you may need to adjust your position. To avoid over-stretching, you can also move your support hand to just above the knee.

▷ **6** Cross this foot under the other foot and press them toward the buttocks on the "out" breath. Hold for several seconds then reverse the crossed legs and bend toward the buttocks once again. After these movements you will probably notice that the bending capacity of the legs has become more equal and the pelvis is more balanced.

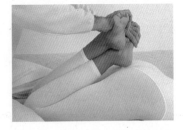

working on the feet

When "walking" on the feet make sure your position is well balanced as excess pressure or loss of balance may cause your partner pain.

Both the giving and receiving of pressure on the feet is very relaxing, and perfectly safe and easy to perform as long as you don't make any sudden or unexpected movements. Keep your body upright, centred and relaxed as if you were going for a walk.

If there is too much of a gap between your partner's ankle and the floor, or the feet don't turn inward symmetrically, you may have to leave this technique out.

As with all the techniques, remember to observe your partner's facial expressions and breathing. These are obvious indications of how the receiver is feeling. Don't forget at any time that it's a human being you are working with, not just a body.

General pressure to the soles of the feet helps to stimulate your partner's internal organs through the reflex areas and meridians. Walking on the feet is particularly good for grounding someone with too much mental activity.

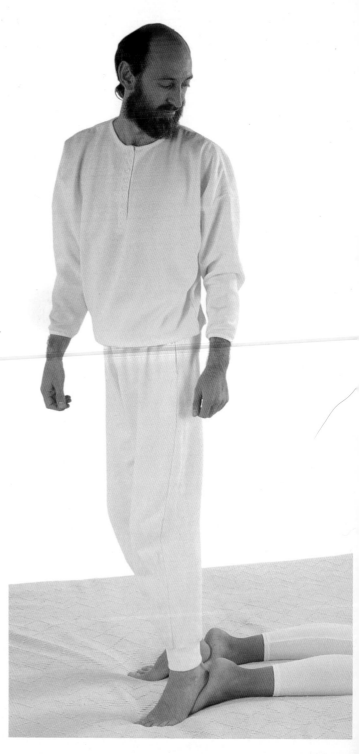

▷ **1** Turn around so that your back is facing your partner and stand on both their feet. Begin shifting your weight slowly from foot to foot, controlling the movement from your hips.

▽ **2** Keep in one position and shift your weight back and forth from left to right several times and repeat on various areas of the feet.

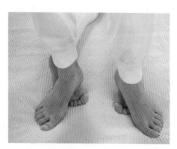

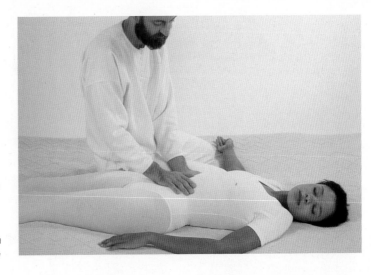

making contact with the yin

Gently assist your partner to turn over into the supine position (on their back). Lying in this position we can be psychologically, emotionally and physically open, but we can also feel quite vulnerable. It is important to bear this in mind as you work to establish reassurance and trust.

▷ **1** Position yourself at your partner's side. Place one hand on your partner's waist, and the other hand on the abdomen with the heel of the hand just below the navel, on your partner's *Hara*. Take a moment to listen with your hand to the rhythm of your partner's body. Feel the rise and fall of your partner's breath. Share the breath. This establishes a level of trust so that you will be sensitive to any vulnerabilities or pains that might become manifest. Gently palm around the abdomen in a clockwise direction. If you can coordinate your movements with your partner's "out" breath you should find that your partner gradually allows you to apply more pressure.

working on the legs

Use some basic shiatsu techniques to increase mobility and flexibility in the legs.

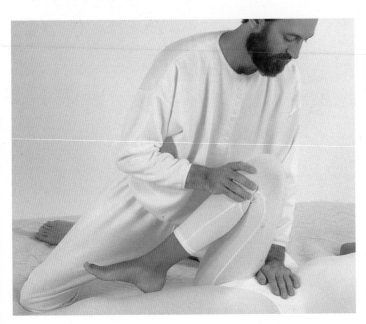

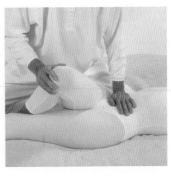

△ **2**,▽ **3** Rotate the leg out from the body, focusing on the hip joint. Start with small circular movements and, releasing the leg as much as possible, gradually increase the rotation to the fullest range.

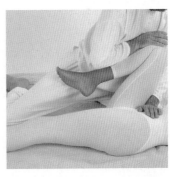

△ **1** Change your position to face across your partner, placing your uppermost hand on the *Hara* (lower abdomen). Place your other hand on the inside of the knee allowing your fingers to curl under the joint. Leaning back, simply allow your body weight to lift the leg. There should be very little effort involved in this. As the leg comes up, slide your hand from the inside of the knee to the upper shin.

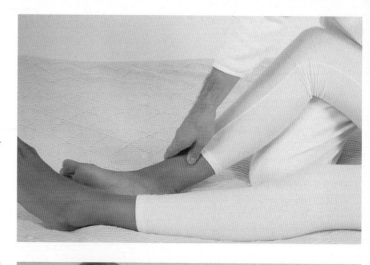

▷ **4** Place the leg so that it rests comfortably with the toes at the level of the opposite ankle, with the spleen meridian uppermost. You may prop it up either with your leg or a cushion underneath. Palm up the inside of the calf along the *Yin* meridians to the knee. Thumb up the calf from the ankle to the knee.

▽ **5** Use your forearm to continue the pressure up the thigh. Rotate the leg once again then move down to your partner's feet.

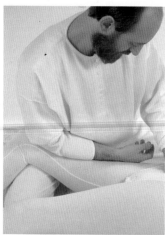

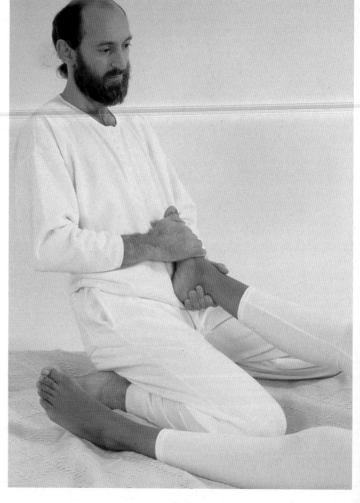

▷ **6** Cup underneath the ankle in one hand. Place the other hand on top of the ankle. Bring your *Hara* into contact with the sole of the foot. Grasp it firmly and rotate your body from the hips. As you move, your partner's body will move with yours.

Repeat all the techniques on the opposite leg and complete this section of the sequence with your hand back on your receiver's *Hara*.

caution
Do not give shiatsu on the spleen meridian during pregnancy if miscarriage is likely. Do not work below the knees in any pregnancy.

shoulders, arms and hands

Gently open out the shoulders and stretch the arms with these simple movements.

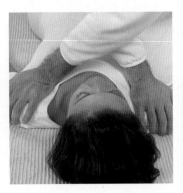

△ **1** Kneeling up, bring your free hand to your partner's furthest shoulder. Place your other hand on the near shoulder. Your arms should now be crossed. With your receiver's "out" breath, lean forward on your hands, opening up the shoulder and chest area.

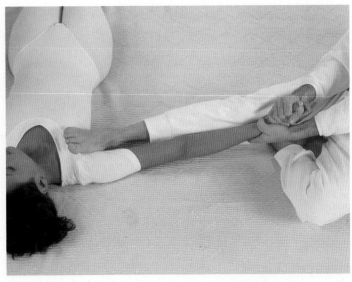

△ **3** Grasp the wrist and move your body so that your outstretched leg is parallel to the arm, your foot resting comfortably against the upper torso. Gently lean back, stretching the arm, giving counterpressure with your foot.

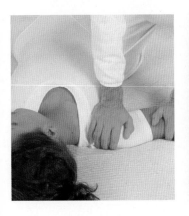

△ **2** Maintain the support of the shoulder nearest you. With the other hand, as in the treatment of the legs, begin by gently rocking and kneading the arms from the shoulder to the hand. Position the arm at right angles to the body with the palms facing up. Then palm down the arm, avoiding pressure on the elbow joint. Follow by thumbing down the middle of the arm to the palm along the heart protector meridian.

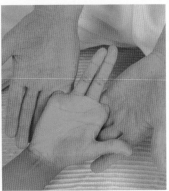

△ **4** Link your little fingers inside your partner's index and little finger to stretch open the palm.

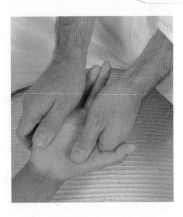

△ **5** Your thumbs are then naturally placed to work into the palm with circular movements.

One of the great benefits of shiatsu is that it encourages self-awareness. It is often in the still moments of a session, when we are just being with our partner, that both giver and receiver can have the most profound insights.

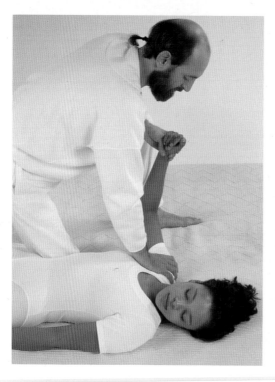

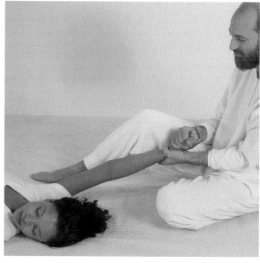

△ **6** Place the support hand on the shoulder, tucking your thumb into the armpit. Hold the wrist, lift and loosen the shoulder joint.

△ **8** Move your body so that by gently leaning back your partner's arm is stretched, using a two-handed grip to the wrist.

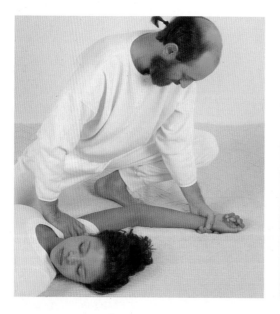

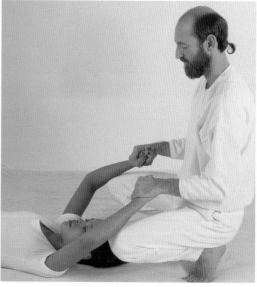

△ **7** Step forward with your outside leg, stretching your partner's arm to the floor above the head.

△ **9** Pick up your partner's other hand and rest the forearms on your knees.

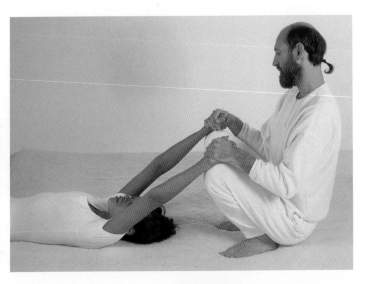

◁ **10** Lean back, allowing your knees to slide up the forearms to the wrists. On the "out" breath, this makes a powerful stretch for the shoulders and chest.

Repeat all the techniques on the opposite arm: stretching, rocking, kneading, palming, thumbing and massaging the hands.

▽ **11** To finish, return to the *Hara*. Simply holding for a minute or two gives your partner time to feel the changes that have occurred.

Break this final contact very slowly and if appropriate cover your partner with a blanket. Give your partner some time to experience how he or she feels.

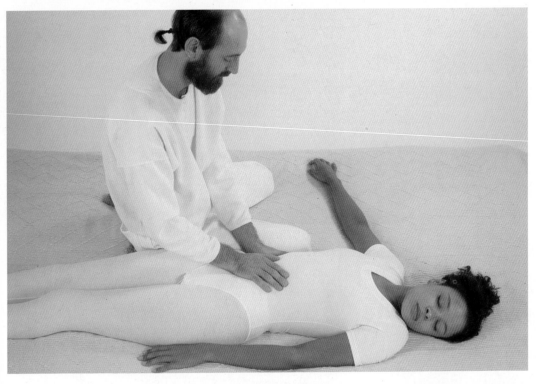

DoIn exercises

The term "DoIn" literally means self-massage, and involves a combination of different techniques to improve the circulation and flow of Chi throughout the whole body. The following exercises can be used not only to revitalize your tired muscles and low spirits, but also to relieve a stiff, tense body and a stressed mind. Starting your day with a DoIn session will quickly awaken your body and mind. You will soon notice the benefits.

the preparation

Prepare yourself by gently shaking your limbs and body. Shake your arms and hands to help release any tension in your upper body. Now gently shake your legs and feet as well. Place your feet shoulder-width apart and unlock your knees. Straighten your back to allow a better energy flow, relax your shoulders and then close your eyes. Take a minute to focus internally, and get in touch with how you and your body are feeling before starting the DoIn routine.

Note that when doing this exercise it is vitally important that you become aware of

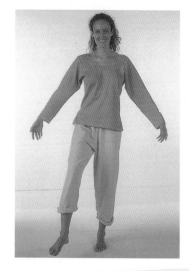

△ Prepare yourself for a DoIn sequence by shaking your limbs to get the energy flowing.

any areas that might be in any discomfort, and that you try to empty your mind completely of any disturbing or distracting thoughts. It takes time to learn how to do

the latter, and you will eventually succeed. What counts in the end is that you do not let tension ruin the effects of the DoIn.

the best way to complete

After having worked through your whole body as described in the following pages, stand up and gently shake out again. Now place your feet shoulder-width apart and bend your knees slightly. Imagine a string passing through your spine, from the tail bone to the top of your head. Stretch the string and feel your spine straighten up to allow better Chi flow. Close your eyes for a moment and see how you feel after your DoIn session. Try to remember how you felt at the beginning and compare that with the sensation you have now. Open your eyes again and to complete your session, practise breathing deeply.

You can do this DoIn exercise as often as time permits. Ideally it should become a part of your daily routine, being practised early in the morning and again perhaps later in the evening. You will quickly notice and appreciate the benefits.

neck

A stiff and aching neck is all too common a condition, particularly for people who work for long periods of time at a computer. It can be relieved quite quickly using some very simple DoIn techniques. Try to relax yourself physically before you begin. If you have long hair it is better to put your hair up so that you can easily reach your neck.

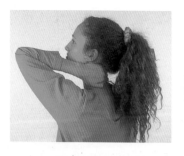

△ **1** Using one hand, place the palm across the back of your neck and firmly massage in a squeezing motion. This will increase the flow of blood and Chi to the area, release stagnation, and remove waste products such as lactic acid.

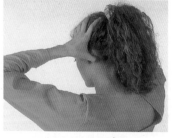

△ **2** With your thumbs, gently apply pressure to the point at the base of the skull, directing the pressure upwards against the skull.

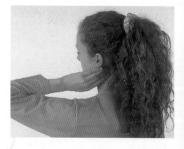

△ **3** Use your fingers and rub across the muscle fibres at the base of the skull. This technique will release the muscles and tendons in the area, and will also help to relieve headaches and any level of pain in the shoulder.

head and face

This routine is particularly good if you feel a cold coming on, or already have one. The movements are designed to ease discomfort and congestion and speed recovery. The tapping on your head part of the routine will also wake up your brain and stimulate blood circulation. Perform the actions slowly and with care.

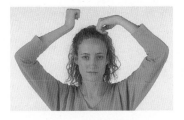

△ **1** Open your eyes and make a loose fist with both hands. Keep your wrists very relaxed and gently tap the top of your head.

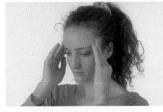

△ **5** Bring your fingers up to your temples. Drop your elbows and massage your temples, using slow circular movements.

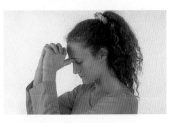

△ **9** Bring your thumbs to the inside of the eyebrows. Allow the weight of your head to rest on your thumbs.

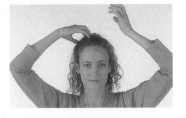

△ **2** Slowly work your way all around the head, covering the sides, front and back.

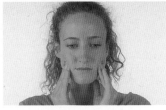

△ **6** Using the same motion, massage down the sides of your face until you reach your jaw.

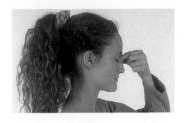

△ **10** With your index finger and thumb, pinch the bridge of your nose and the corners of your eyes.

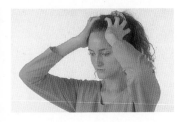

△ **3** Pull your fingers through your hair and over your scalp, stimulating the bladder and gall bladder meridians on the top and side.

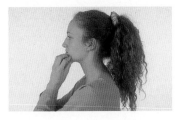

△ **7** Squeeze along the jawbone with the fingertips, working outwards from the centre. This is a very good technique for trying to relax.

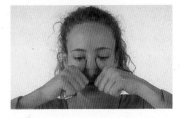

△ **11** Apply your thumbs to the sides of your nose. Breathe in as you stroke down the sides of your nose.

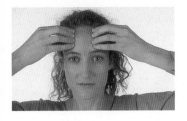

△ **4** Place the pads of your fingers on your forehead, and apply a little pressure and stroke out from the centre to the temples.

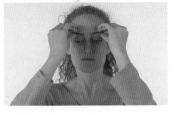

△ **8** Using your index finger and thumb, squeeze your eyebrows starting from the centre line and moving slowly and laterally.

key tips

Although Doln exercises are specifically designed for self-help, they can just as easily be carried out by another person, particularly if you are feeling too lethargic to do it yourself. If working on a partner, always communicate with them to make sure that you are applying the right amount of pressure.

shoulders, arms and hands

Meridians run down the arms and the hands, and various points can be stimulated in this area. Major pressure points are known by names, and these are included here. Please note that a number of these points are sometimes used in childbirth to speed up labour and therefore should not be used during pregnancy. See individual cautions about this.

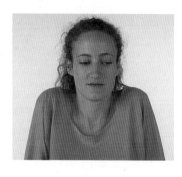

△ **1** Lift up your shoulders and breathe in. Breathe out, letting your shoulders drop and relax. Repeat.

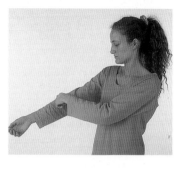

△ **4** Straighten your arm, open your palm and tap down the inside of your arm from the shoulder to the open hand. Good for the heart meridians.

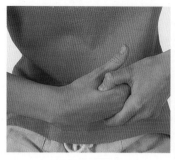

△ **7** Stimulate the "Great Eliminator" on the large intestine meridian, in the web between the index finger and the thumb. Press for a count of three. **Caution** Do not use during pregnancy.

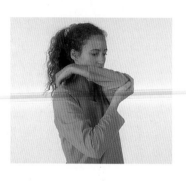

△ **2** Support your left elbow and with a loose fist begin tapping across your shoulder.

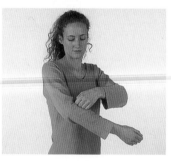

△ **5** Turn your arm over and tap up the back of your arm, from the hand to the shoulders. This technique stimulates the meridians for the intestines. Repeat three times.

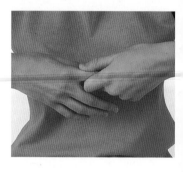

△ **8** Carefully squeeze and massage the joints of each finger using your index finger and thumb. Repeat as often as you find necessary.

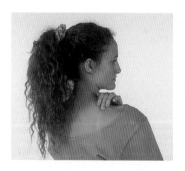

△ **3** Press your middle finger into the shoulder's highest point, which is known as the "Shoulder Well". **Caution** Do not use during pregnancy.

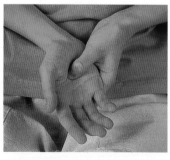

△ **6** Use your left thumb to work through your right hand, gently massaging the centre of your palm to relieve general tension and revitalize you spiritually.

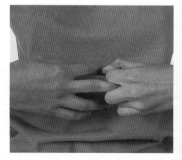

△ **9** Gently pulling out the fingers will stimulate the starting and end points of all the meridians. This is a great way to release any stress and tension in your hands.

chest, abdomen and lower back

Working on this area stimulates some important organs, including the lungs and the large intestine. Opening out your chest will increase the blood flow throughout the body and improve overall well-being. Remember to breathe deeply as you work to enhance the effects of the massage. Take care when massaging the abdomen.

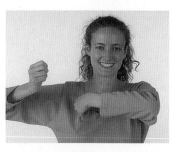

△ **1** Open up your chest, and using either a loose fist or flat hands for comfort, tap across your chest, above and around the breasts. This will stimulate your lungs and strengthen your respiratory system.

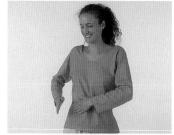

△ **3** Proceed down towards your abdomen, and with open hands tap round your abdomen, clockwise, for about a minute.

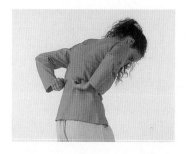

△ **5** Place your hands on your back, just below your ribcage. Start to rub the area until you feel some warmth. This will stimulate your kidney energy.

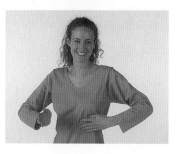

△ **2** Take a deep breath in as you open your chest again; then on the out breath tap your chest and make a deep resounding "Ahhh…" sound.

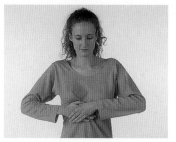

△ **4** Place one hand on top of the other, and then make exactly the same circular motion around your abdomen for about another minute.

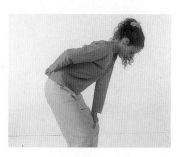

△ **6** Place one hand on your knee. Using the back of your other hand, tap across your sacrum bone at the base of the spine. It activates the nervous system.

legs and feet

Finish the DoIn sequence on the legs and feet, sitting to reach the lower legs and feet. Finding the pressure points will come more easily with practice. These exercises are excellent for revitalizing tired legs and can be done quickly at any time of day. Once you have completed your DoIn self massage, rest for a few moments, taking some deep breaths.

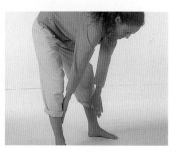

△ **1** Tap down the backs of your legs from your buttocks to your heels, following the flow of energy. Tap up the insides of your legs, stimulating your liver.

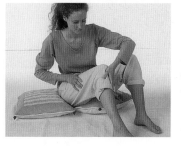

△ **2** Sit down on the floor, and measure four finger widths down from the knee-cap on the outside of your leg. Place your thumb on this point on the stomach meridian and press.

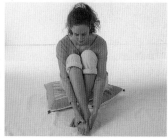

△ **3** On the dorsal part of your foot between the big toe and the second toe is LIV3, "Big Rush", which is good for alleviating cramp. **Caution** Do not use this particular point during pregnancy.

System calmers with a partner

If you notice that your partner looks listless, is feeling tired and stressed, is experiencing tension in the upper body, or suffers from shallow, rapid breathing, the following treatment will be very beneficial. It will aid relaxation and promote much deeper breathing, facilitating a more efficient energy distribution to all parts of the body. The treatment is quickly and easily given.

a calming back treatment

Timing your movements to your partner's breathing will increase the calming effects of this sequence, so spend a few moments tuning into their breathing pattern before you begin.

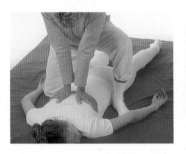

△ **1** To prepare for treatment, kneel by your partner's side and place your hand at the base of the spine. Concentrate on how your partner feels. Then place your palms on either side of your partner's spine. Crouch down if it feels easier.

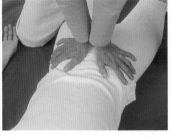

△ **3** Start at the top of the back between the shoulder blades. Work your way down towards the sacral area. Repeat this step three times. Always keep your elbows straight, and use your body weight as you work.

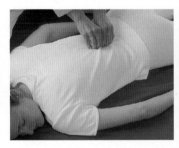

△ **5** This technique allows you to focus specifically upon the spinal column. You still need to rock; however, this time the spinous processes are gripped between the fingers and the thumbs. Applying a positive (firm) contact, gradually work the hands along the full length of the spine, moving it from side to side. This action is good for loosening the muscles and stimulating the nervous system.

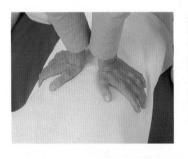

△ **2** Ask your partner to breathe in; on the out breath lean into your hands and apply pressure to your partner's back. Ease the pressure to allow your partner to breathe in again. Move your hands down and press on the next exhalation.

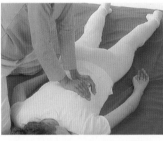

△ **4** Kneel at 90 degrees to your partner, place your palms in the valley (on the opposite side of the spine) formed by the spinous processes (spinal bumps) and the broad muscles running on either side of the spine. Rock the body with the heels of your hands. As you rock, you can move your hands down the back, one following the other. The rocking should be continuous and rhythmic. Repeat three times. Do both sides, working from the opposite side of the body.

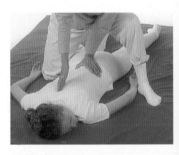

△ **6** Place your left hand on your partner's sacrum. Using the edge of your right hand like a knife, perform a sawing action down either side of the spine. Work both sides alternately, repeating the sequence three times.

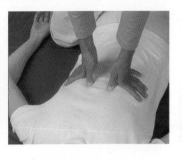

△ **7** Run your hands along the spine to feel the undulations of the spinous processes. Bring your thumbs sideways, two fingers' breadth from the dip between the two spinous processes. Apply perpendicular pressure.

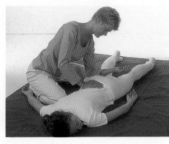

△ **10** Note the position of the support hand and keep the hands relaxed as you roll your forearm right across the surface of the buttocks.

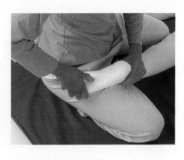

△ **13** Place your partner's foot in your lap and using your thumb apply pressure to the pressure point "Gushing Spring", which lies on the kidney meridian, one-third of the distance from the base of the second toe to the base of the heel.

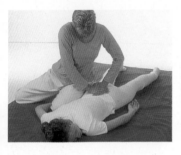

△ **8** Put one hand on top of the other and place your hands on your partner's sacrum. Lean forward to apply pressure to the sacrum, focusing all your energy into the base of the spine.

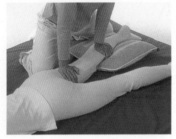

△ **11** Adjust your position so that you can move down the leg. Support your partner's lower leg with a cushion beneath the shin. One hand remains on the sacrum or is placed on the back of the thigh. Starting from the back of the thigh, gradually work down the leg, applying pressure with your thumb.

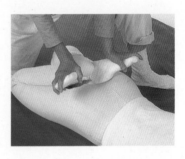

△ **14** Cross your partner's ankles and bring them slowly towards the buttocks. Do this stretch twice, the first time placing the more flexible leg in front (nearest to the buttocks), then reverse the position.

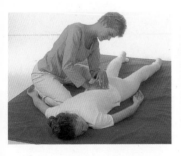

△ **9** Turn around to face your partner, spread your knees and, using the fleshy part of your forearm in a penetrating and rolling action, apply pressure across the buttocks. Stay on the same side to work both buttocks.

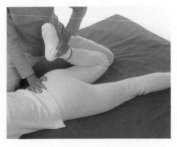

△ **12** Take hold of your partner's ankle and bend the leg towards the buttock. Adjust your position to allow you to use your body weight to achieve the stretch. Now move yourself all the way down to the feet. With both hands, take a firm hold of the ankle, lean back and stretch out the leg to its full length.

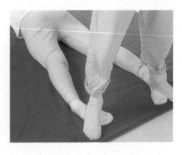

△ **15** Stand up and walk on the soles of your partner's feet using your heels. Have their feet turned inwards and apply pressure to the soles but place no weight at all on their toes.

Nervous system calmers: self-help

Stress can have quite a significant and dramatic effect on the nervous system, and badly affect a wide range of functions, including breathing. One excellent way to get you back on track is to balance the energy in the bladder channel through the following exercises and the shiatsu treatment of the back. Both techniques are designed to calm your nervous system.

the back and spine

By gently twisting, stretching and relaxing the spine you are encouraging the central nervous system, which runs the length of the spine, to relax the whole body.

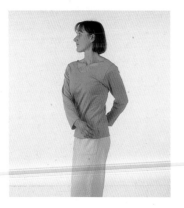

△ **1** Stand with your feet shoulder-width apart and knees bent. Keep your back straight. Let your arms hang loose at your sides. Swing them from side to side.

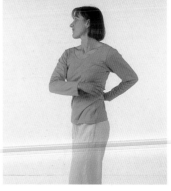

△ **3** Bring your arms a bit higher up so that you now feel the twist in the middle part of your back. This will loosen up the thoracic vertebrae and the diaphragm.

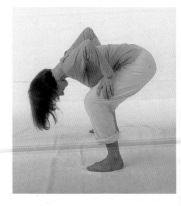

△ **5** Bend your arms and slowly bring your upper body down towards the floor. Keep looking at the ceiling until you no longer see it. Relax the head downwards.

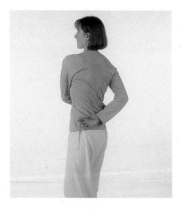

△ **2** Swinging your arms will create a twist in your spine, gradually loosening up the joints between the lumbar vertebrae and allowing for more relaxed and flexible movement.

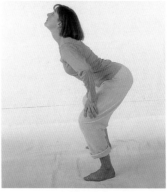

△ **4** With your feet wider than shoulder-width apart place your hands on your legs, above your knees, and straighten your back. Sway back and look up.

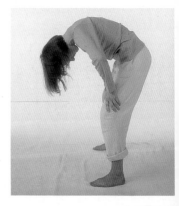

△ **6** Pull your abdominal muscles in and gradually roll up your spine, allowing the head to come up last. Lift your head and straighten your spine. Return to the sway back position and repeat the whole movement about ten times.

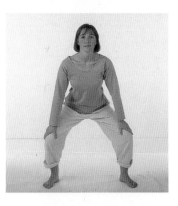

△ **7** Return to the sway back position shown in step 4, and hold for a short while.

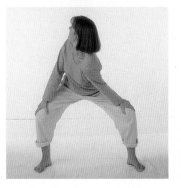

△ **8** Breathe in and, on the exhalation, drop the left shoulder down as shown. Keep your elbows gently locked and look up to the ceiling over your right shoulder. Feel the twist in your spine. Repeat on the other side.

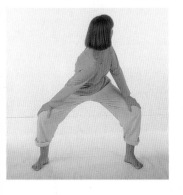

△ **9** Repeat three or four times on each side. Come back to the starting point. Relax your upper body and roll up your spine to a standing position.

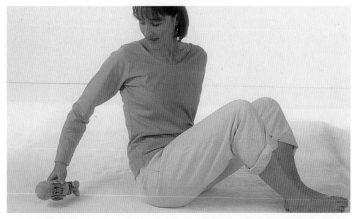

△ **10** To treat your back further in case of pain and tension, or whenever you feel in need of general relaxation, try using tennis balls as extra help. Put two tennis balls into a sock and knot the top. Lower yourself on to the tennis balls, which should be placed on either side of the spine. This is where your bladder meridian is located. Start from the area between your shoulders, or anywhere where you feel any pain and discomfort.

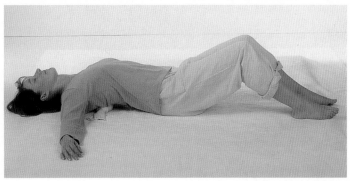

△ **11** Breathe deeply and allow your back to sink on to the balls. The balls will mould themselves to the contours of your back and stimulate your bladder energy. Keep the balls in one place until you feel the muscles relax and then slowly roll the balls to the next area "in need". Work this area in the same way, using your breath to enhance the relaxation. Give yourself 10–15 minutes, working down the whole spine. Afterwards your spine will feel open and relaxed against the floor. You will have a sensation of warmth down your back.

▷ **12** When you have finished these spinal exercises it is good to lie down on the floor and relax with your lower legs resting on a chair. This relaxes the lumbar area of your back and realigns the whole spine. Close your eyes, allow your breathing to slow down and feel the energy moving from the top of your spine down to the sacrum like a wave. Stay in this position for 10–15 minutes.

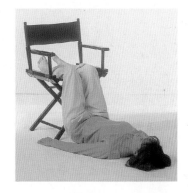

This relaxation exercise works directly on the nervous system, calming it down, and you can use the exercise at any time when you feel stressed.

Breathing enhancers with a partner

Correct breathing is the first, fundamental technique that keeps us going. Surprisingly, when things get stressful we do not always breathe as we should. Deep, relaxing inhaling is replaced by short, shallow gasps for air, and the whole body quickly suffers. The following techniques are aimed at the upper part of the body, helping you feel calm, relaxed and in control again.

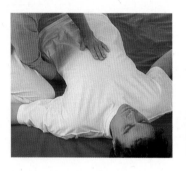

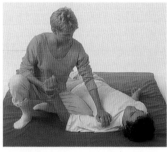

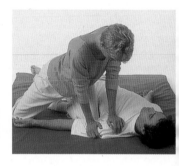

△ **1** Place one hand underneath your partner's back in the area opposite the solar plexus, and the other hand on top covering the area just below the sternum (breastbone). Focus into the area between your hands and encourage your partner to do the same. Feel the Chi from the breath of your partner reach this space, slowly allowing it to open and expand. You will gradually feel the tension go and the muscles relax to allow a deeper and more relaxed breathing.

△ **3** Keep your left hand on the shoulder and take a firm hold of your partner's hand with your right hand. Lift the arm from the floor, shake it out, and then finally allow it to relax again.

△ **5** Place your partner's arm at a 45-degree angle to the body. Use one of your hands to support the shoulder while the other hand palms along the arm. Stay on the thumb side of the arm to activate the energy in the lung meridian.

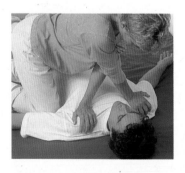

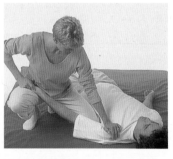

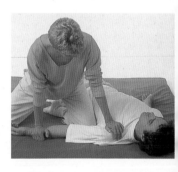

△ **2** Cross your arms over and place the palms of your hands on your partner's shoulders. Ask your partner to breathe in, and on the out breath bring your body weight over your hands, stimulating the first point of the lung meridian and gently opening the chest. Repeat this three times.

△ **4** Firmly hold on to the thumb and give the arm and the lung meridian a good revitalizing stretch. You can repeat this technique several times.

△ **6** Continue all the way down to the thumb (end point of the lung channel). Avoid applying any direct heavy pressure over the elbow joint.

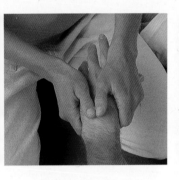

△ **7** Using your thumbs, massage the whole of the dorsal side of your partner's hand.

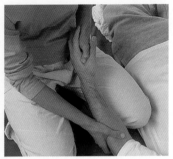

△ **10** Locate the "Great Eliminator" in the web between the index finger and thumb. Stimulating this point with gentle pressure from your thumb will relieve headaches and help clear any mucous congestion taking place in the lungs.

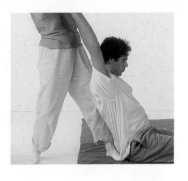

△ **13** Stand behind your partner. Take hold of the hands, gripping around the thumbs, and as you both exhale, lift up from your knees and lean backwards until your partner feels the stretch.

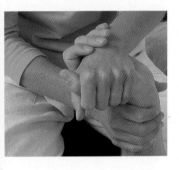

△ **8** Loosen up the wrist joint by slowly rotating the hand. Support your partner's wrist with one hand and grip their hand with your other hand as you do this.

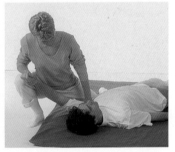

△ **11** Hold your partner's arm by the wrist and support the shoulder with your other hand. Step forward and rotate the arm into an overhead stretch. Before you step forward, you need to apply pressure to the supporting hand at the shoulder. Maintaining this pressure ensures a strong stretch. Step back, allowing the arm to return to the starting position.

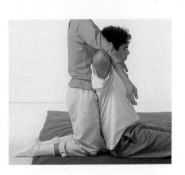

△ **14** Kneel down behind your partner and ask them to clasp their hands behind their neck. Bring your arms in front of your partner's arms, and on the out breath gently open up the elbows to the sides.

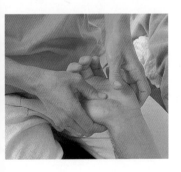

△ **9** Open up the palm of the hand and gently massage. Apply pressure to the point in the centre of the palm, "Palace of Anxiety", a very good point for calming and releasing tension.

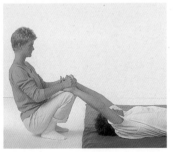

△ **12** Place both hands on top of your knees and stretch the arms by leaning backwards. Let go of the arm you have treated and move over to the other side. Repeat the whole sequence working on the other arm.

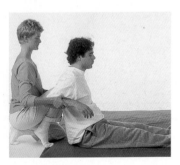

△ **15** Bring one knee up to support your partner's lower back. Take hold of the lower arms, and on the out breath bring the elbows towards each other behind your partner's back.

self-help breathing enhancers

The lung energy controls our intake of fresh air and Chi from the external environment. However, when your stress levels are high for a period the bronchial tubes expand to let in more air and the end result is that we tend to "over-breathe", or hyperventilate. By working on the lung meridian and practising these breathing exercises, you will facilitate deeper, more satisfying breathing.

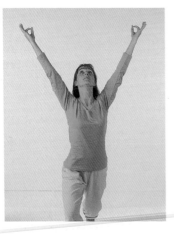

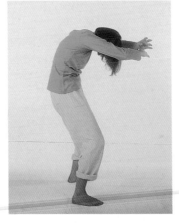

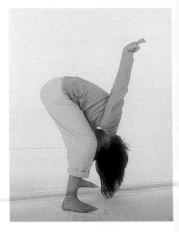

△ **1** Link your index finger and thumb on both hands. Step forward with your right foot and reach to the ceiling. Step back, relax the arms and repeat with your left foot. Repeat 3 or 4 times on each side.

△ **3** On the exhalation, cross your arms over in front of you and relax your head down. Keep your knees bent, press back the area in between your shoulder blades. Repeat four or five times.

△ **5** On the exhalation, bend forward and stretch your arms over your head. Breathe in and feel the stretch along the back of your legs, back and arms. Slowly exhale. Stay down and repeat twice more.

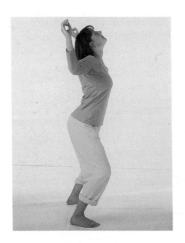

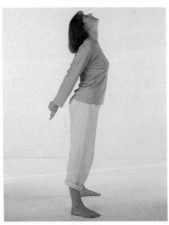

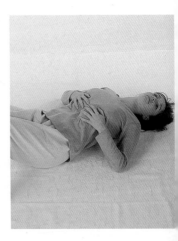

△ **2** Stand with your feet apart. Lift your arms to the sides with elbows bent, and make loose fists. Take a deep breath in, opening your chest by bringing your arms back as far as is possible.

△ **4** Stand with your feet shoulder-width apart and knees bent, and spread your feet slightly apart so that your toes point out. Hook your thumbs together behind your back, and inhale as you look up.

△ **6** Lie down with a rolled-up towel along your spine, allowing the head to drop back on to the floor or a pillow. Place your fingers along your ribs, gently pressing as you breathe out.

Immune system reivers

The immune system includes your spleen, thymus gland and lymph nodes. It is responsible for moving proteins and fats around the body and for filtering body fluids. The main function of the immune system is to protect the body from disease. White blood cells destroy foreign bodies such as bacteria and carry them away via the lymphatic and circulatory systems. Periods of stress weaken the immune system. These simple shiatsu techniques will help awaken and strengthen the immune and lymphatic systems.

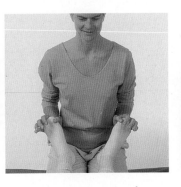

△ **1** Ask your partner to lie down on their back with straight legs. Place your palms over the soles of your partner's feet. Intermittently rock the feet towards the head in a rhythmic motion of about two movements per second for 3–4 minutes.

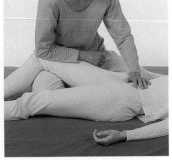

△ **3** Place your partner's foot against the opposite inside ankle so that the leg is bent, exposing the inside leg. Ask your partner to inhale and gently use your forearm to stretch open the spleen meridian on the out breath.

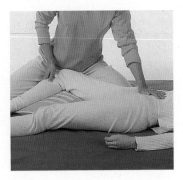

△ **5** At the top of the shin bone on the medial side of the leg is a powerful pressure point on the spleen meridian. Press this point to treat abdominal and menstrual pain, or local pain in the knee.

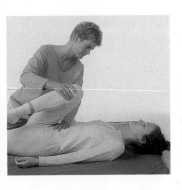

△ **2** Bend your partner's leg and move yourself up to the side. Hold the leg just below the knee. Slowly rotate the hip joint, moving from the centre of yourself. Keep a fixed distance between your chest and your partner's knee.

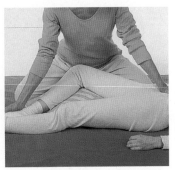

△ **4** Support the lower leg with a cushion and, starting from the inside of your partner's big toe, use your thumb to apply perpendicular pressure along the medial part of the foot.

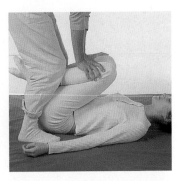

△ **6** Rotate the leg you have worked on and then bend the other leg as well. Come to a standing position, bring your feet close to your partner's hips for support and gently bring the knees to the chest. Ease up on the stretch and rotate both legs. Move over to the other side, stretch out the treated leg and repeat the sequence on the other leg.

Working on the digestive system

The stomach and spleen energy channels are associated with the highly important functions of ingestion and digestion of food. In traditional Chinese medicine, the stomach corresponds to the entire digestive tract, from the mouth to the small intestine, and it creates Chi energy. The following exercises are aimed at fine-tuning and improving the health of your digestive system.

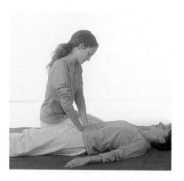

△ **1** Kneel at your partner's side and take a few moments of stillness to "tune in" and observe your partner. Be aware of any tension and note the breathing rate: fast and shallow indicates tension; slow and deep shows relaxation.

Trace the borderlines of your partner's *Hara* (vital body centre). Start at the ribcage just below the breastbone and move slowly out to the pelvis.

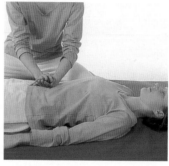

△ **3** With one hand on top of the other, make a rocking and pushing type motion like rolling dough, from one side to the other, and pull back using the heel of the hand. Repeat for relaxation.

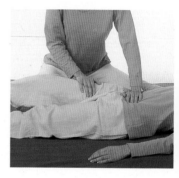

△ **5** Stretch your partner's leg out, and place your knee underneath your partner's knee for support, or use a pillow. Apply palm pressure along the outside frontal edge of the leg following the stomach meridian. Start from the top of the thigh and work to the foot. Repeat three or four times.

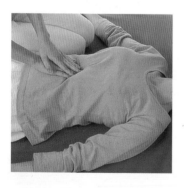

△ **2** Using two hands, one on top of the other, apply finger-pad pressure in a clockwise movement around the *Hara,* as shown. Where you find tension, apply gradually deeper pressure to dissolve it.

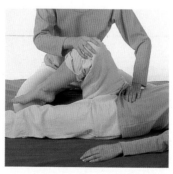

△ **4** One hand holds the right leg just below the knee. Move from your own centre, using your whole body, not just your arm muscles, to rotate your partner's leg. Keeping a fixed distance between your chest and your partner's knee will help to ensure a balanced rotation of the hip.

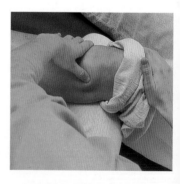

△ **6** Stimulate "Leg Three Miles" on the stomach meridian, using thumb pressure. The point is located four fingers' width below the knee-cap on the outside of the shin-bone. The name refers to this point's remarkable effect. It has been used since ancient times to build up endurance.

Circulatory system enhancers

The heart and heart protector channels are the central focuses for regulating circulation, according to traditional Chinese medicine. However, heart energy can be weakened in several circumstances. One excellent way of tackling the problem is by using wonderfully specialized shiatsu techniques which will help both calm the mind and ease such circulatory problems.

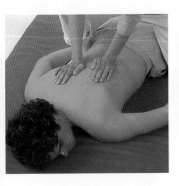

△ **1 To improve general circulation:** use both palms in a technique known as palm rubbing to apply pressure quite firmly and rub down either side of the spine.

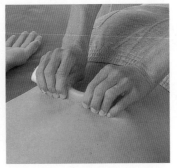

△ **3** Roll the skin by pinching and taking hold of the skin on the lower part of the spine (lumbar area). Lift the tissue and gradually "roll" it up the spine. Repeat three or four times. Then roll the skin from the spine, the centre line, out towards the sides of the back.

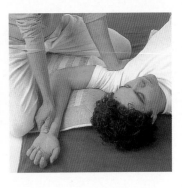

△ **1 To expose the energy channel:** place your partner's arm with the hand above the head, palm facing upwards. Support your partner's elbow with a cushion, and kneel beside your partner.

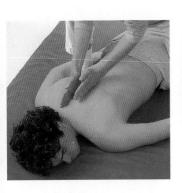

△ **2** Then, using the little finger side of your hands, vigorously rub down either side of the spine a few times until the area begins to redden.

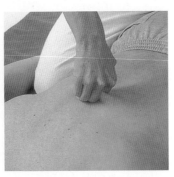

△ **4** Pinch the skin using your index and middle fingers to take hold of the tissue. Twist and lift the skin at the same time. Work within your partner's pain threshold. Cover the whole back using this technique. You will see the area redden as the circulation improves.

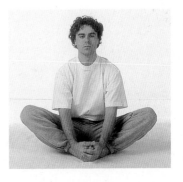

△ **1 To balance the energy in the heart meridian:** sit on the floor, bend your knees and bring the soles of your feet together in front of you. Hold on to your ankles and straighten your spine. Inhale and lean forwards, keeping your back as straight as possible. Breathe out as you bring your head towards your feet and your elbows in front of your legs. Open up the axilla (armpit) and relax.

Tension relievers

Surprising though it may sound, when you are under stress your centre of gravity tends to lurch and shift from the abdominal area up to the chest, causing tension levels to increase in the neck, shoulders and face. It often also results in a feeling of great heaviness across your shoulders. Imagine how wonderful it is to lie down, close your eyes and allow someone to touch and manipulate these tender areas sympathetically, in exactly the way you need to provide instant, soothing and long-lasting relief.

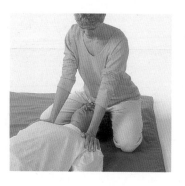

△ **1** Kneel at your partner's head, place your hands on the shoulders and tune in. Be aware of their breathing and state of relaxation before you start. Ask your partner to breathe in, and on the exhalation apply a bit of pressure to the shoulders by leaning into your arms. Repeat a few times. This encourages deep relaxation.

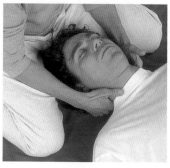

△ **3** Move your hands to the neck. With your thumbs on the side and fingers underneath, stretch out the neck by gently pulling away. Repeat a few times until you feel the neck muscles relax.

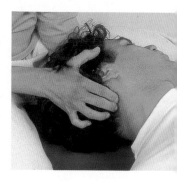

△ **5** Turn the head to one side and support it with one hand. Use the finger pads of your other hand to "rub" across the muscle fibres. Treat the other side of the head in the same way.

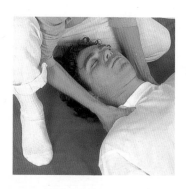

△ **2** With your fingers underneath and thumbs on top, gently and firmly massage the shoulders using a kneading action. Feel the tension in the muscles relaxing and the tissue gradually softening.

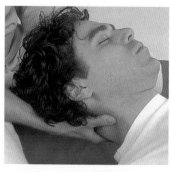

△ **4** Now, gently lift your partner's head off the floor and, supporting the head on your forearms, firmly squeeze the muscles of the neck. Be careful not to squeeze too hard.

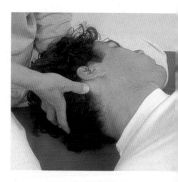

△ **6** With your partner's head turned to the side, press the points along the base of the skull. Start at the ear and work towards the spine. Turn the head and treat the other side in the same way.

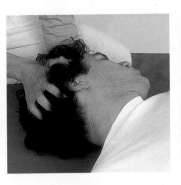

△ **7** Rub all over the scalp using your fingertips, and then run your fingers firmly through the hair. Repeat several times.

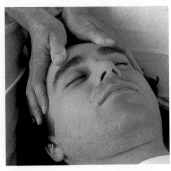

△ **10** Apply a bit of pressure and stroke your thumbs out towards the temples. Repeat three or four times. This will ease tension in the head.

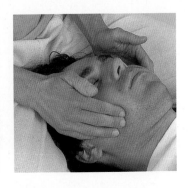

△ **13** Massage the side of your partner's face, moving down to the jaw. This treatment will relax the whole body as well as the face.

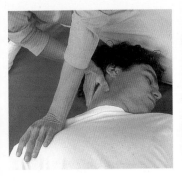

△ **8** Turn your partner's head to one side and support it by placing one hand under the skull. Stretch the neck out by gently pushing the shoulder away.

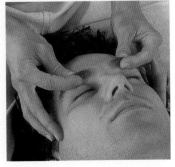

△ **11** Use your index finger and thumb to squeeze your partner's eyebrows. Work from the centre out to the sides. Repeat a few times to clear sinus problems.

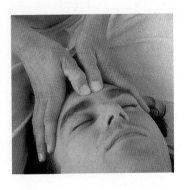

△ **14** Come back to the starting point at your partner's forehead. Apply some pressure and stroke out to the sides.

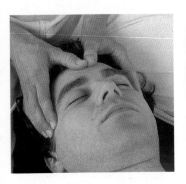

△ **9** Start treating the face by placing your thumbs gently on the midline of your partner's forehead, with your fingertips to the side.

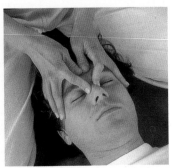

△ **12** Using your index fingers, stroke along the side of the nose to help clear nasal congestion. Come all the way up to the bridge of the nose.

key tips

When giving tension relievers, try to take a little time to relax yourself fully. Commence the techniques from a position of well-being and strength. Listen to some calming music, make sure that the room is warm and dry, and when you are feeling entirely comfortable, begin. Since this is an intimate kind of massage, it is also important that the subject feels completely at ease with you. A little deep breathing before the first exercise will help induce a marvellous, soothing feeling of harmony. It will certainly make all the difference. Once you feel ready, you may begin.

Foot Massage
Principles

Anyone can learn to give pleasurable foot treatments
to themselves and others. This chapter covers the basic
techniques of massage, aromatherapy and reflexology,
and offers some classic types of routine. There is
also advice on how to prepare for a treatment
– from warming up the hands to creating
a healing atmosphere at home.

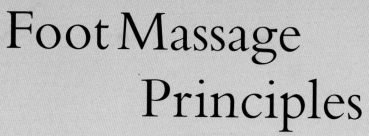

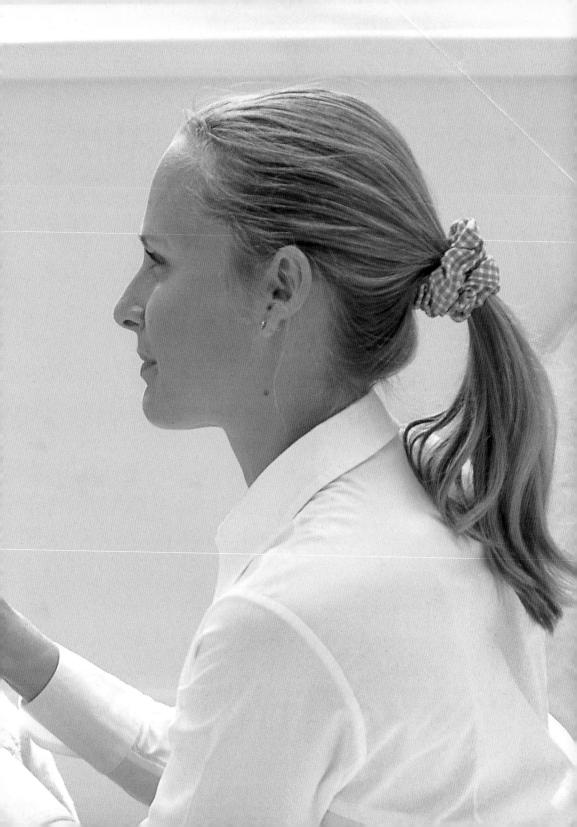

Foot massage principles

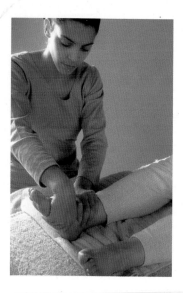

◁ Foot massage techniques are broadly similar to those used on other areas of the body, with some minor adaptations.

Most massage practised in the West is Swedish massage. This was developed in the late 18th century by the Swedish gymnast, Per Henrik Ling. The therapy aims to bring about therapeutic results by manipulating the body's soft tissues: the muscles, skin, tendons and ligaments. A Swedish massage therapist will usually treat the whole body, but a treatment focusing on the feet and legs is also highly effective.

A variety of techniques are used, including stroking, kneading and fast rhythmic movements. These are delivered in a continuous flowing sequence. Oil is usually smoothed into the skin before and during the massage, to prevent pulling.

aromatherapy massage

In aromatherapy massage, oils extracted from plants are diluted in a carrier oil or cream, and then worked into the skin using Swedish massage techniques. The oils have delightful fragrances, which heighten the pleasure of the massage. They also have healing properties. Different oils can be used

There are many different ways of working on the feet. It is worth spending the time to learn and assimilate fully the basic techniques of one method before going on to the next. That way, you will become adept at giving treatments.

therapeutic massage

Massage developed from our natural instinct to use touch to relieve pain: for example, we automatically rub an aching area, stroke a painful limb or hold an injured hand. Massage is highly relaxing to receive, making it an effective antidote to stress-related problems. For this reason, it has become very popular in recent years.

There are more than three thousand massage movements in common use, but you do not need to know more than three or four of them in order to give an effective foot treatment. The basic techniques are very easy to learn, and can be used at home to promote general well-being.

▷ Essential oils can be added to foot creams for a healing and nourishing treat. Rose cream, for example, makes a superb moisturizer.

the birth of aromatherapy

Essential oils were originally used in cosmetics. In the early 20th century, a French chemist called René-Maurice Gattefossé discovered by accident that the oils also had healing properties. While working in his laboratory he burned his hand. To ease the pain he plunged his hand into a bowl of cool lavender oil. He was impressed by the effect that it had in relieving pain, reducing redness and speeding up the skin's healing process. He went on to investigate the therapeutic properties of the oils, coining the term "aromatherapy" in 1928.

The use of essential oils combined with massage was developed by Marguerite Maury, who worked with Gattefossé. She brought the idea of the everyday use of essential oils, to enhance health and well-being, to the wider world.

▽ All kinds of plants yield essential oils with a wide range of healing properties. Roses are good for skin complaints.

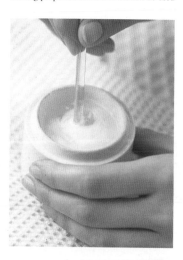

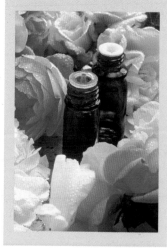

to induce feelings of calm, to boost energy or to treat minor ailments and relieve pain.

Aromatherapy foot massage is a highly enjoyable and easy way of using the therapy for self-help. You can also add the oils to baths and foot baths, incorporate them into nourishing creams for the feet and legs, or add them to compresses to help soothe away troublesome aches and pains. This book includes many suggestions for using essential oils, as well as recipes for luxurious or therapeutic aromatherapy home treatments.

reflexology

The therapy known as reflexology is a form of natural healing that focuses on the feet. It is based on the belief that there are specific reflex points on the feet which correspond to all the organs, systems and structures of the body. In reflexology, the points are stimulated by means of gentle finger-pressure. This helps to promote self-healing and good health in all kinds of ways.

Reflexology is a holistic therapy: it works on the whole person – the mind, body and

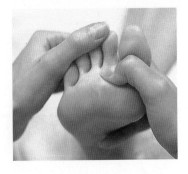

spirit – rather than focusing on a specific condition or on a set of symptoms. Although reflexologists can detect specific problems, their main aim is to bring the whole body back to a natural state of balance and well-being. Over time, this can help to eliminate problems caused by specific disease.

acupressure

Like reflexology, acupressure is used to stimulate the body's own natural self-curative powers. Acupressure is similar to

◁ In both reflexology and acupressure, specific points on the foot are said to correspond to other parts of the body. Pressing these points stimulates healing, and can be used to treat anything from a sore throat to digestive problems and backache.

acupuncture in that they both use key energy points on the body – including many on the feet and legs – in order to bring about healing. However, while acupuncturists use special needles to stimulate the energy points, acupressure involves the use of finger or thumb pressure to work the points. Sometimes, the heels of the feet can be used for stimulation instead, or as well as, the fingers.

Acupressure can help to reduce tension, increase the circulation, and encourage the body and mind to relax. It helps to strengthen our resistance to disease, by relieving built-up stress and tension. One great advantage of the therapy is that it can be used as a quick fix, which can be done anywhere and at any time.

lymphatic drainage

One of gentlest forms of massage, lymphatic drainage massage works on the lymph system. Since lymph vessels are close to the surface, there is no need for heavy pressure. The body's lymphatic system is a secondary circulation system that supports the work of the blood circulation. The lymphatic system has no heart to help pump the fluid around the vessels, and therefore it must rely on the activity of the muscles to aid movement.

Lymphatic massage involves using sweeping, squeezing movements along the skin. The action is always directed towards the nearest lymph node: the main nodes used when treating the foot are located in the hollow behind the knee. Lymphatic drainage massage is hugely beneficial in helping to eliminate waste and strengthen the body's immune system.

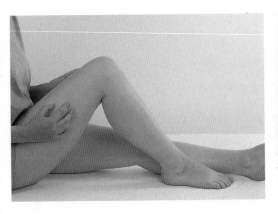

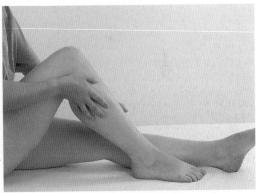

△ **1** To improve lymphatic drainage to the feet and legs, try a daily skin "brush", using your fingertips. Begin by working on the thigh. This clears the lymphatic channels ready to receive the lymph flood from the lower legs. Briskly brush all over the thigh from knee to top, three or four times.

△ **2** Work on the lower leg in a similar way. Brush either side of the leg from ankle to knee, then treat the back of the leg. Follow this by brushing along the top of the foot, continuing up the front of the leg to the knee. Brush over each area twice more, making three times in total. Repeat on the other leg.

Caring for our feet

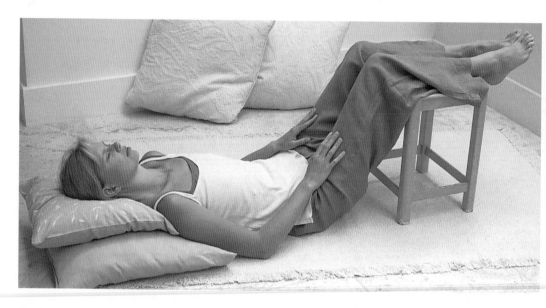

Our feet are an amazing construction. Twenty-six ingeniously shaped bones are bound together with bands of ligaments to form the basic structure of each foot. This structure is very strong – strong enough to bear the weight of our entire body – yet it is also remarkably supple. The foot is capable of making many intricate movements. Its dexterity is made possible through the actions of numerous small joints, as well as the 30 tiny muscles in the foot and by the leg muscles.

There are about 7,200 nerve endings in each foot, making it highly sensitive to touch. The nerve supply comes from the sciatic nerve passing from the spinal nerve through the buttock and branching down the back and side of each leg to the foot.

helping the circulation

The foot is richly supplied with blood vessels. However, since it is at the end of the body and does not have its own pump, it depends on muscular activity of the foot and leg to keep a good return flow of blood to the heart. You can help the circulation in

your feet by taking regular exercise – such as a daily walk – and by keeping your feet and toes moving whenever you are sitting down or standing up for long periods.

It is also beneficial to put your feet higher than your heart as often as possible – at least once a day. This will encourage any pooled blood to drain back down the legs. Regular massage will also keep the circulation of blood and lymph functioning well. This helps to remove any toxins from the feet, and also brings nutrients to them.

It is particularly important to put your feet up when you are pregnant, since you are particularly susceptible to varicose veins at this time.

pamper and protect

Our feet take a lot of punishment, and most of us take them for granted. Having a regular foot-care session can help to keep your feet healthy and prevent any problems

△ Take time every so often to rest your feet above heart level. This helps to relax the muscles here and can be very soothing. It also lets blood drain away, which can help to prevent varicose veins and swollen ankles. Keeping fresh blood circulating will also help to nourish the skin.

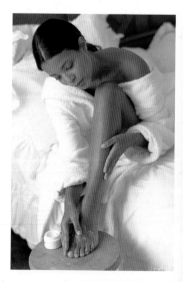

▷ Pamper your feet on a regular basis; they take a great deal of punishment and richly deserve as much time and attention as you can manage.

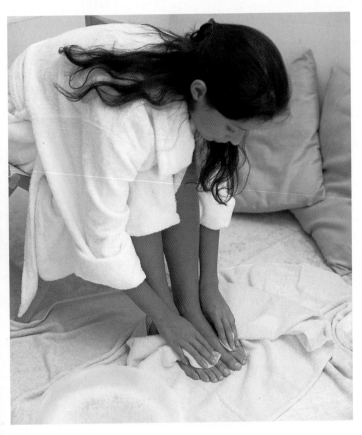

▽ The healthy foot is one that displays no signs of infection, skin breaks or ingrowing toe nails. Ideally the inner arch will be raised slightly off the ground as this is used as a shock absorber while walking and running.

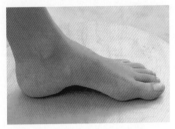

△ Drying your feet thoroughly is an important part of good foot care and foot health. Special attention should be paid to drying the areas between the toes – allowing moisture to build up here can lead to problems such as athlete's foot.

from arising. For a simple pamper, try soaking the feet for ten or fifteen minutes in warm water. Remove any hard skin with a pumice stone, then cut your toe nails. Always cut straight across rather than trying to shape the nail. This will help to prevent ingrowing toenails, which can be very painful. Moisturizing your feet daily will help to keep the skin soft and supple.

It is a good idea to visit a chiropodist for a professional pedicure at least twice a year. You should also act quickly if you notice flaking skin between the toes (athlete's foot), or a dark mark on the sole (a verucca) to prevent these problems from spreading. Seek medical advice if you develop any unusual symptoms on the feet.

the right shoe

You should avoid wearing high-heeled shoes since these distort the natural shape of the feet. The ideal shoe is not flat, but has a low heel.

Wearing badly fitting shoes puts unnecessary pressure on the feet, and it may lead to aching, blisters or bunions which are unsightly and can be painful. The idea that new shoes should hurt is a myth. Correctly fitting shoes should be comfortable from the first time of wear; they should not need to be "worn in".

Always try to buy new shoes in the afternoon. Our feet tend to swell slightly as the day progresses, and whenever they become hot. Shoes that you buy in the morning may feel tighter later in the day, and may restrict the blood and lymph flow to our feet and legs.

It is quite common for one foot to be slightly larger than the other. It is therefore important to try both shoes of the pair before making a purchase. Always buy the size that fits your larger foot, and buy foot pads or insoles, if necessary, to create a more comfortable fit for the smaller foot.

shoe-related allergies

Many chemicals are used in the adhesive, dye, rubber, tannins or metal commonly found in footwear. A small number of people suffer from allergic reactions to their shoes. It would be almost impossible to produce a shoe that is allergen-free because different people are allergic to different substances.

If you experience redness, itching or soreness in the feet, consult a doctor. He or she will be able to refer you to a dermatologist (skin specialist) if an allergy is suspected.

The dermatologist will usually perform a skin test to identify the substance or substances causing the allergy. You can then seek out footwear that is free of this particular chemical. If staff at the store cannot help, it is usually possible to check this information with the manufacturer.

Setting the scene

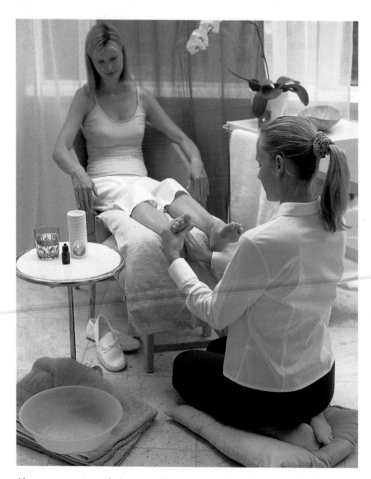

◁ Keep your massage space clean and attractive. Using matching towels will help to create a luxurious and professional atmosphere. Be sure to get everything ready before you start massaging, so that you do not have to stop halfway through the treatment.

Always try to create a relaxing atmosphere in the room where you are treating, whether it is yours or someone else's. Ideally, the area should be warm, inviting and quiet. A few simple preparations will help to give any room a suitably supportive atmosphere for relaxing massage or reflexology work.

First of all, make sure that you are somewhere private, and that you won't be disturbed during the treatment or immediately afterwards. Turn off any phones, including mobiles, close the door and shut the windows if there is noise outside. Ignore the doorbell if it rings while you are treating, or make a previous arrangement with another family member to deal with any callers. Make sure that nobody else will come into the room while you are treating; interruptions will break your concentration as well as the relaxing flow of the massage.

clear away clutter

Tidy and clean the room, and clear away any clutter. You want as few distractions as possible when you are massaging.

Decide where you are going to massage. The floor is a good option because there is usually plenty of room to move about. It can be hard on your knees, so make sure that you have a few floor cushions to hand. The person you are massaging should sit in a comfortable arm chair with their legs supported on a small table or stool. You want to be able to reach their feet without bending or twisting in any way.

Have any massage oils and equipment that you will be using to hand. You'll want two or more towels; at least one to place under the foot being worked and another to keep the resting foot warm.

Sitting or lying down for any length of time can cause some loss of body heat, so make sure the room is warm. On cool days and evenings, you may like to offer the person a light blanket to keep him or her feeling warm and secure.

creating atmosphere

Where possible, have soft lighting. Turn off bright lights that are positioned directly overhead or in direct line with eye contact – either yours or the person you are treating. A couple of lamps will usually give

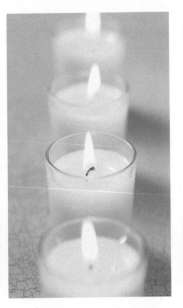

△ A few candles will help to create soft relaxing lighting in the room. Scented candles will often help to lift the mood, too.

enough light, and you may also like to light a few candles in the room. A flickering candle helps to create an atmosphere that is calm and cosy.

Flowers always look attractive. If you have dried or fake flowers, try adding a drop of essential oil to three or four cotton buds and place them in the arrangement. Rose, jasmine, neroli, violet and ylang-ylang are good oils to try: they give appealing, slightly heady, floral aromas.

Other ways to introduce pleasant smells into the area are by using scented candles or by burning an essential oil in a vaporizer. You could also use an essential oil room spray half an hour before treatment. However, don't use a strong scent, since some people may find it off-putting.

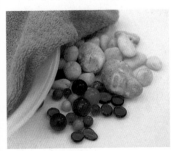

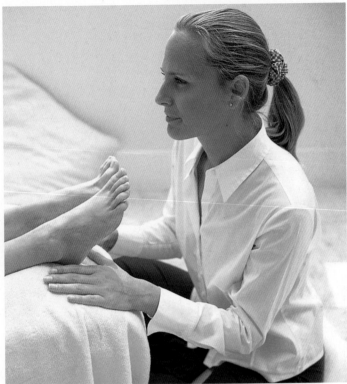

Most people like music, but tastes vary, so choose soft instrumental music that is relaxing to mind and body, and keep the volume low so that it is not intrusive. Always ask if silence is preferred.

preparing yourself

Once the room is ready, prepare yourself. Wash your hands and check your nails are well trimmed. There should be no danger of them catching the recipient's skin.

Spend a few moments centring yourself before you start the massage. Sit comfortably with both feet flat on the floor. Relax your shoulders and face, then breathe slowly and deeply for a few moments. Posture and breathing are vital for an effective massage treatment. To warm up your body carry out some stretching sequences combined with

◁ Suggest that the receiver has a footbath before you treat them, particularly if he or she has come at the end of the day. Place a layer of marbles or pebbles in the footbowl. The receiver can roll their feet backwards and forwards over them for a relaxing mini-massage.

△ Always make sure that you can reach the person's feet easily. You should be able to keep your back straight as you work.

deep breathing exercises. Relax and warm your hands with a quick self-massage to ensure they are supple and soft.

When all is ready and you are about to start, see if you can feel the healing energy of your hands. Bring the hands together in a prayer-like position, but pull them apart just before they touch. Do this two or three times before you start. You may feel a slightly pulling or tingling sensation as you do so – this is the energy of your hands.

post-massage

After the massage or treatment, let the person relax for a few minutes. You may decide to leave the room for this, or simply to sit quietly beside him or her.

Drink a glass of water, and offer one to the receiver as well. Suggest that he or she spends the next hour or two quietly, in order to appreciate fully the relaxing effects of the foot treatment.

Foot massage strokes

You can give an excellent massage using just a few simple actions. Each movement can be performed twice or more, and your favourite few movements could be done three, even four times.

When you are learning new massage techniques, it is a good idea to try them out on yourself first. Practise until you become familiar with the different actions involved, and see how the movement feels when you vary the pressure. Always pay full attention to what you are doing. You will find that, if your attention wanders, your touch is unlikely to feel good. Feel your way into your hands and focus on the sensations here.

It is often helpful to massage without talking, except for when you are asking for or giving feedback. It is also much easier to concentrate on exactly what you are doing if you are quiet, and this will also help both you and the recipient to relax.

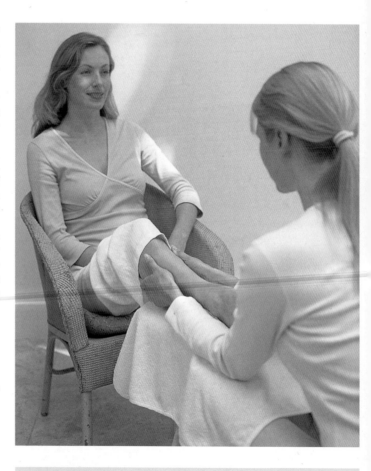

▷ If you are massaging someone else, make sure that he or she is comfortable, and that you are too. You will find it easier to concentrate if you maintain a good posture. Keep your back straight and your head balanced throughout the massage; imagine your head is connected to the ceiling and being pulled upwards. This posture will help you to use your body weight, giving depth to your movements.

getting feedback

People like different pressure. When you work on yourself, you get instant feedback about whether you are working at the correct level of firmness. When you work on other people, you have to monitor their reactions. Ask for feedback, but don't assume that you are getting it right just because the person doesn't tell you otherwise. Be aware of the person's general posture – if he or she is tense, you may be pressing too hard.

Always keep the pressure lighter on the top of the foot. The bones are closer to the surface than those on the sole, so it is easier to cause bruising and pain in this area.

massage aids

There are many aids now available for massage in general, and some can be suitable for use on the feet. Most masseurs say that it is better to use your hands if you are treating another person. However, some gadgets may help with self-treatment.

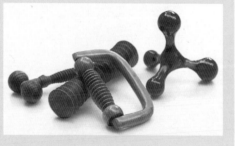

△ You may need to experiment with a few different massage aids to see what suits you best.

basic strokes

Always pay equal attention to both feet when you are massaging. You should start on the right foot, then move on to the left. The right side of the body is said to relate to your physical self; treating this one first will begin to relax muscle tension throughout the body, and will also boost the circulation and elimination processes. Treating the left foot will work on a physical level, too, but it will also help to release built-up tension in the sensitive emotional inner being.

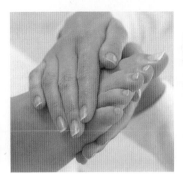

△ **Effleurage (stroking)**
Place your hands across the foot at the base of the toes. One hand should be on top and one below so the foot is sandwiched in-between them (sandwich hold). Slide your hands down the foot from the toes to the heel, then up from the heel to the toes. Repeat this movement twice more, or until the person feels relaxed. Use light pressure to start with, increasing it as you go. You usually start and finish a routine with effleurage, and it is also a good linking technique.

▷ **Knuckling (kneading)**
Make your hand into a fist. Press into the sole of the foot, using the flat part of the fingers from the knuckle to middle joint. Turn the fist as you press, so that you make a slight rotational movement. Cover the whole area from heel to toe. This movement is good for warming up the muscles, opening up the foot and releasing tension.

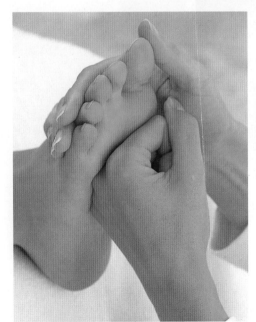

▽ **Thumb circling**
Place the thumbs on the foot, one slightly higher than the other. Then, use the pad of alternate thumbs to massage the area all over, making small rotational movements. This movement is used for fleshy areas. It is good for the circulation and for warming the muscles of smaller areas.

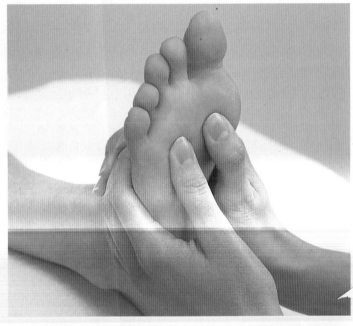

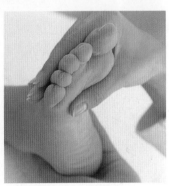

△ **Foot rotation**
Wrap your fingers around the top of the foot near the toes, and use your other hand to cup the heel. Slowly rotate the foot clockwise, then anticlockwise. Repeat, so you have rotated the foot in each direction twice. This movement loosens the ankle joint. It is important that you do not push the ankle further than its limits. Take particular care if treating someone with arthritis, diabetes or a foot disorder.

Spreading

▽ **1** To spread the top of the foot: place the thumbs and the heels of your hands on top of the foot, letting your fingers curl round to hold the sole. Pull the thumbs across the top of the foot towards the edges, keeping your fingers in position. Then return your thumbs to the starting position.

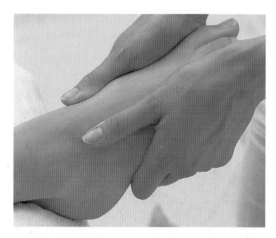

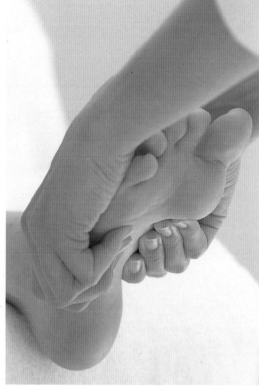

▷ **2** To spread the sole of the foot: keep your hands in the same position as before but reverse the action, so that you pull your fingers to the edges of the sole, leaving the thumbs in position. Start near the toes and work down the foot to the heel. This action works in a similar way to knuckling. It stretches the muscles and brings oxygen and nutrients to the area by improving blood flow.

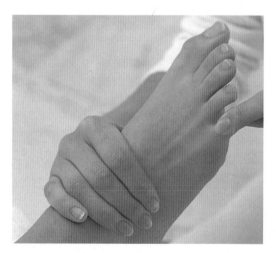

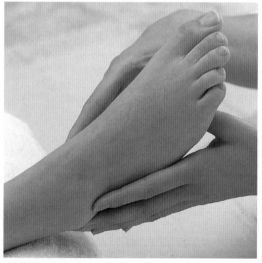

△ **Toe rotation**

Support the foot by placing your fingers across the top of it and curling your thumb underneath. Use your thumb and forefinger to grasp the base of the big toe. Gently rotate the toe in a clockwise direction, then anticlockwise. Work each toe in turn, ending with the little toe. This action helps to mobilize the joints and also improves the supply of nutrients and oxygen to the toes. Work gently, and take extra care if treating someone with arthritis.

△ **Circling the ankle**

Circle around the inside and outside of the ankle bone at the same time, using the pads of your fingers. You can work quite strongly, provided that the person has no problems in this area. Work in a clockwise direction, then in an anticlockwise one. This movement helps to relax the ankles and improve mobility.

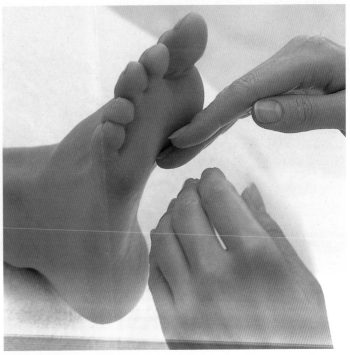

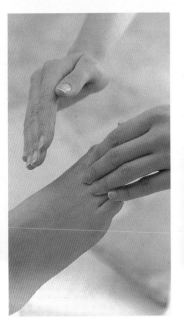

△ **Percussion (tapping)**

1 Use the tips of your fingers to tap all over the top of the foot. Work using alternate fingers. Do not tap too hard: the action should be pleasurable, and not a shock to the system. You can also use this movement on the sole of the foot.

△ **2** To perform percussion on the sole: use the back of the hands to strike the sole lightly all over. This action is stimulating; it helps wake up the foot and increases the circulation. It is a good movement to do if the foot is cold. Be gentle if the person has arthritis, diabetes or a foot disorder.

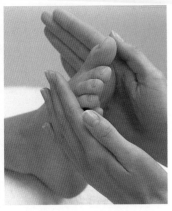

△ **Push-pull**

Place one hand on the outside of the foot and the other on the inside, so that the foot is gently wedged in-between them. Using the heel of the hands, pull one side towards you and push the other side away. Repeat, but this time reverse the action. Do this push-pull action twice more. This is a general movement which helps to open and relax the foot.

baby massage

Foot massage is a wonderful way to soothe and give pleasure to your baby. Always work very gently, massaging one foot at a time. As with adults, do the right foot first, then go on to the left. Try the following routine, or make up your own variation.

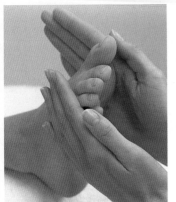

△ **Babies love to be touched – in fact, they cannot thrive without it.**

- Cup your left hand around the baby's right ankle, holding the foot in a confident way. Use the tips of your fingers to stroke the sole from heel to toe. Then stroke the top of the foot from toes to ankle. Do as many strokes as are needed to cover the area.
- Use two fingers to stroke the inner side of the foot, working from the big toe to the heel.
- Use two fingers to stroke down the outside edge of the foot in the same way.
- Use your right thumb to stroke across the sole, just below the ball. Start from the big toe side and stroke to the outer edge. Do this three times.
- To finish, gently hold the base of the big toe between your thumb and first finger. Gently stroke down to the tip of the toe. Repeat on the rest of the toes, ending with the little one. Then do the whole routine on the left foot.

Using oils in reflexology

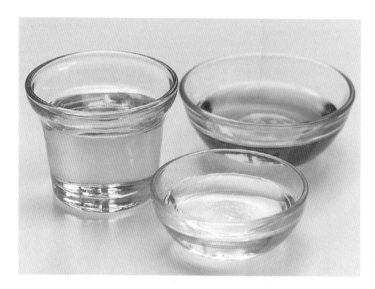

△ Many oils can be used as carriers, as long as they give good slip. Almond oil (front) is gentle and is suitable for most skin types, including very dry or dehydrated skin. Grapeseed (left) has almost no smell, so it is ideal for blending with essential oils. Olive oil (back right) is easy to get hold of, but it does have a strong smell that is difficult to disguise.

Using oils and creams to massage helps to keep skin soft, supple and moisturized, and prevents the build-up of hard skin. On a practical level, oil or cream helps to give "slip" so that your hands glide over the feet rather than dragging and stretching the skin. Oils and creams also give you the chance to incorporate essential oils, with their varied healing qualities, into the treatment – simply by adding some drops of essential oil to the cream or to an oil such as almond, grapeseed or olive. These three oils are popular choices for using on their own; they are known as "carrier" oils if drops of essential plant extract is added to them.

If your skin is dry, dehydrated or mature, it is best to use a massage cream instead of a carrier oil. The creams are heavier, take longer to be absorbed and leave a protective film on the skin, which helps to trap moisture, preventing further dehydration. It is rather like covering food with cling film in order to prevent it from drying out. Massage base creams are available from most drugstores and natural health stores, or you can make your own using one of the recipes in this book.

getting ready

Begin by pouring a little oil, just a drop or two, into the palm of one hand. If using cream, just one or two small blobs are sufficient. Rub your palms together, then move your hands, one over the other, in a hand-washing motion. This distributes the oil all over the back of your hands, your fingers and cuticles, which has the extra benefit of making them soft and supple. Add a little more massage medium into one palm, then gently bring your palms together, so you evenly cover both hands. The medium should not run all over the area but be just enough to give slip and shine. You are now ready to massage.

While working, observe the skin for changes in texture (from slippery to dry) and a gradual reduction in shine. At this point, add more massage oil or cream in the same way as described above.

If you are using a blend of different oils, it is worth making up enough to last for a few treatments and storing it in a clean, screwtop container. For an average-sized person, you will use about 10 ml (2 tsp) of oil or cream for each massage involving the feet, and a little more when you are also massaging the lower legs.

using essential oils

Essential oils are made from natural plant ingredients and are a gentle and effective way to boost general health and treat minor ailments at home. However, it is very important to treat these oils with respect, as you would with any chemical or drug.

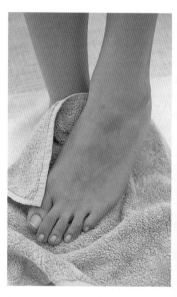

△ Massage oil into the skin until it is well absorbed. Give the feet a quick wipe at the end of an oil-based treatment to ensure that there is no slippery residue left. You can use the sole of one foot to rub the towel over the top of the other, so that you do not have to bend down.

The benefits of reflexology

Reflexology works quite simply, and in a highly effective, efficient way. It manages to relax and overcome any build-up of excess tension in the muscles. Consequently, during a treatment, all parts of the feet will be stimulated and the significant dual effect is to relax your muscles and also to increase the efficiency of the circulation to all parts of the body. You will quickly notice the positive effects of reflexology.

reflexology and you

Working along holistic principles, reflexology takes into account body, mind and spirit as they are all interrelated. Whatever happens to you will affect all levels of your being, whether you notice or not. If you feel under pressure or are stressed, the effect on your body will be detrimental, as your muscles remain tense and taut, constricting the circulation and nerves, and compromising their functioning. Similarly, if you have a physical accident or mishap, your feelings will be affected by the degree of pain you experience, the way in which the accident happens, and the effect it has on you afterwards.

Although you are working mostly on the feet in reflexology, you are affecting the whole of the body, both inside and out, through the treatment. This is achieved by working the reflexes to the internal organs and glands as well as to the surface of the body. It appears that you can have a more far-reaching effect by working the reflexes than by working directly on the corresponding body part. Such referral treatment, as it is sometimes called, is a highly effective way of stimulating the body's own healing powers into action.

Pain in the back, for instance, may be due to the onset of structural problems in which the bones are actually out of place and misaligned, and should be checked by an osteopath, cranial osteopath or chiropractor. If the pain results from muscular problems, or if manipulation has already been done

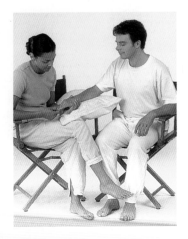

△ **Through working the hands (or feet) you are working the whole body.**

but muscular strain remains, the next step is to identify the muscles involved and then begin work to relieve the situation with massage and reflexology. As a follow-up treatment it is highly effective.

Massage has an immediate and profoundly relieving effect, but the pain and discomfort are likely to recur when the effects of the massage have worn off. Benefits resulting from working the reflexes to the relevant area of the back will last longer than those produced by working directly on the muscles themselves. This is because through the reflexes you are stimulating the body from within, rather than exercising and soothing the muscles from without. Stimulating the reflex to a troubled area will promote healing. Reflexology uses both massage and specific stimulation of the reflexes to achieve more long-lasting results than massage alone.

what treatments involve

Reflexology is not just a foot massage, but this technique is certainly incorporated. Sweeping whole hand movements on the whole foot will relax the entire person and

prepare the feet for reflex work. During the working of the reflexes, massage soothes and relaxes the area where congestion or discomfort is to be found. It actively links the treatment together into a continuous, flowing whole, and manages to relax and stimulate the whole of the body while various individual parts are being treated specifically. Equally beneficial are the whole hand massage movements which are used to complete a reflexology treatment, engendering a feeling of well-being in the entire person before the session ends.

A reflexology session can be both relaxing and stimulating for the patient. As muscle tensions are relaxed, and the nerve supply freed from constriction, the body slips into a deep state of relaxation. At the same time, the circulation is being stimulated to bring nutrients to all parts of the body, and to remove waste products that interfere with the healthy functioning of the parts and the whole. Energy is able to flow more freely around the body, and feelings of total well-being result.

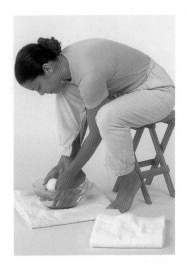

△ **Always wash your feet before any treatment to refresh the skin.**

Reflexology techniques

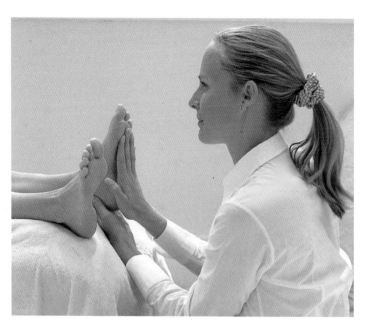

◁ Establish a connection with the person you are treating before starting a reflexology treatment, and always ask the recipient how he or she is feeling. Placing your hands on the soles of the feet before you begin is a reassuring and centring experience for both giver and receiver.

Reflexology is a method of self-healing that can easily be done at home. The basic movements are simple to learn. Once you have become familiar with them, you can use reflexology to treat minor ailments as well as to boost the general well-being of yourself and your family and friends.

When doing reflexology, wear comfortable clothing that does not restrict your movements: in particular, do not wear a tight top. Maintain good posture throughout; try to keep your back straight and your shoulders relaxed. Remember to breathe naturally and deeply – many people tend to hold their breath when they are concentrating.

What every reflexologist needs is a good touch. To a certain extent, this comes with practice. However, it is always very important to check the responses of the recipient, and to ask him or her for feedback. Practise the hand exercises given in this book regularly: this will help you to develop suppleness in your wrist and fingers.

Have a glass of water after giving a treatment. If you are treating another person, offer him or her a drink as well.

giving a treatment

Always start a reflexology treatment by giving the feet a gentle massage. This helps you to connect with the person you are treating, and it will help you to connect with your own body when self-treating. Massaging also gets the fingers mobile, and it encourages both you and the recipient to relax. The simple self-massage and relaxing massage treatments on the previous pages are good routines to do at this point. A short massage should also be given after the reflexology treatment.

You can either give the full reflexology routine – described on the following pages – or you can focus on a particular area of the body, or on a symptom. If doing a full treatment, remember to work gently, and do not repeat the routine more than once a week. If you are working on specific points rather than doing the full routine, then two or three treatments a week should be sufficient. Do not treat anyone with a major illness or severe problem, or a woman in the first three months of pregnancy.

getting the pressure right

Reflexology should neither hurt nor tickle – aim for firm, pleasurable pressure. The pressure will need to be varied depending on the size of the person's foot, his or her general health and individual tolerance level. In general, the pressure applied to bony areas such as the top of the foot should always be lighter than that applied to fleshy areas, such as the heel or ball. The pressure used when treating a child or an elderly person should always be significantly lighter.

Start off using a light pressure, then gradually increase to tolerance level. Do not overtreat particular points – keep to the number of times suggested.

hand preserver
This great lotion can be used every day to keep your hands soft.

ingredients
- 15ml/1 tbsp avocado oil
- 15ml/1 tbsp almond oil
- 15ml/1 tbsp petroleum jelly or glycerine
- 1ml/⅛ tsp vitamin E oil
- 10 drops essential oil. Use any one or a combination of these: rose, sandalwood, geranium, lavender, neroli.

Combine the ingredients in a small bowl. Transfer to a 50ml (2fl oz) screwtop jar.

basic techniques

Anyone giving a reflexology treatment needs soft skin, so moisturize daily. Always check that your nails are clean and short before treating. This is even more important for reflexology than for massage since you press into the skin.

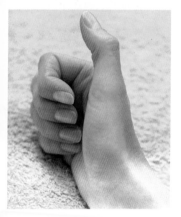

△ **Thumb walking or crawling**

Hold your thumb straight up in front of you, then bend it from the first joint and straighten it again – this is the basic technique used in thumb walking. Place the thumb on the skin, and use alternate bending and straightening movements to "walk" across the area. This has been likened to the crawling movement of a caterpillar.

▷ **Rotation on a point**

This movement is used for sensitive reflexes. Place the pad of your thumb on to the reflex point, then use your other hand to bring the foot slowly into the thumb. Rotate the foot in a circular movement around the thumb.

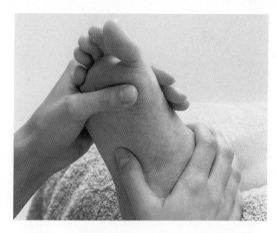

▷ **Pinpoint, or hooking**

This is used for small reflexes or those that are difficult to locate. Place your thumb on the point, and apply pressure. Now, keeping the pressure steady, move the thumb on to the uppermost tip in a "hooking" action. Move the thumb back to the original position.

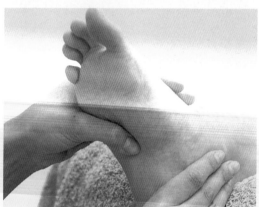

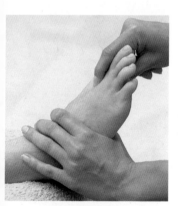

△ **Finger walking or crawling**

This technique is the same as the thumb-walking technique described above, but you use the index (first) finger instead. The action is used on the top of the foot and other areas where the flesh is thinner and less pressure is required. You can use another finger if you find that easier.

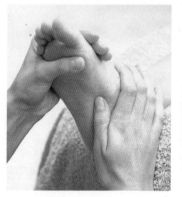

△ **Holding and supporting**

One hand is used to support while the other works the reflex. Always support the foot while you are working. Position your working hand close to the holding hand: this allows you to support and control the movement of the foot. It also gives the recipient a feeling of security.

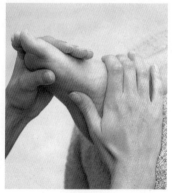

△ **Pressure circles on a point**

Hold the foot comfortably with one hand and place the flat pad of the working thumb on the reflex. Press into the area and then slowly circle your thumb gently on the point. This movement is usually used for very sensitive areas.

Warm-up foot massage

It is always of great benefit to the patient if their feet are massaged right at the beginning of a reflexology treatment. This gives them time to get used to your touch, and to leave behind the cares of the day. Their overall mood is extremely important, and you should do your best to make sure that they are feeling relaxed. Give another massage at the end of the reflex work.

the first steps

Massage prepares the feet for reflex work: it warms and relaxes the tissues, accustoms the receiver to your touch and soothes and relaxes the whole body. Massage will also loosen tensions in the muscles and stimulate the blood supply to and around the feet. Consequently, when the reflex points are worked the tissues will not be strained, and they will respond fully. Do not miss out this stage, as it is extremely important.

During treatment use plenty of massage to link the movement from one reflex area to the next, to soothe and relax the foot in between working the points, which may produce sensations of tenderness.

oil and massage treatments

When you have covered all the reflex points, end with a massage on both feet to instil a sense of deep relaxation. Use 2–3 drops of essential oils mixed in with some almond oil. Do not use the oil beforehand because once on your hands it will counter any accurate hand reflexology movements.

When it comes to massage movements, note that there is no one set sequence. The prime object is to fit movements together in a way that is customized to your individual needs. They should feel good to you and to the person you are working on. The first few movements are good as an introduction, and you should always rotate the ankles as this frees up the blood and nerve supply through the ankle to the foot.

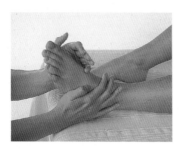

△ **1** Stroking movements, or effleurage, are just as they sound, sweeping and soothing, and are good all over the foot. Use them wherever appropriate.

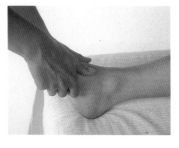

△ **3** Repeat the second movement, gradually working your way from the top of the foot down towards the ankle with each subsequent repetition.

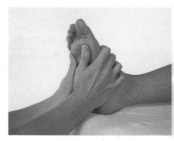

△ **5** Finally, massage into the ball of the foot with both of your thumbs.

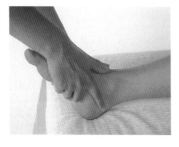

△ **2** To make spreading movements on the top of the foot, draw your thumbs off sideways, keeping your fingers still.

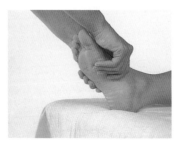

△ **4** To cover the sole of the foot, start in the same position as before, but this time draw your fingers off sideways, keeping your thumbs still.

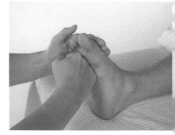

△ **6** To knead, use a movement like kneading dough and work into the sole of the foot using the lower section of your fingers.

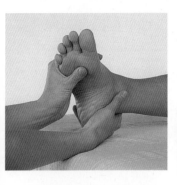

△ **7** To rotate the ankle, rotate the foot clockwise several times, feeling gently as you proceed so that you do not force stiff ankles, but you do manage to exercise the joint.

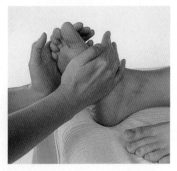

△ **10** With your hands in the same starting position, this time move them alternately up and down from the top to the sole of the foot so that the foot tips from side to side. Do be very careful not to twist the ankle.

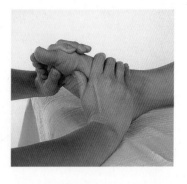

△ **13** To relax the diaphragm, hold the foot and bring it down on to the thumb of your other hand, and lift it off again. Next, move your thumb one step to the side and repeat the movement.

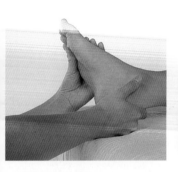

△ **8** Repeat the ankle rotation, but this time in an anti-clockwise direction.

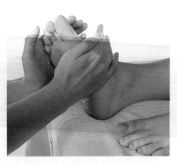

△ **11** With your hands palms up on either side of the foot, move them quickly to and fro, to exercise and loosen the ankle. When this movement is done correctly, the foot will waggle around.

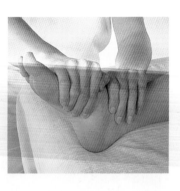

△ **14** To make a spinal twist, the hand on the ankle remains still while the other, lower hand moves to and fro across the top of the foot, round the instep and finally back again. Repeat several times.

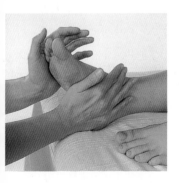

△ **9** To make vigorous, fast movements, massage both sides of the foot, running your hands freely up and down the whole length of the foot. Repeat this technique several times.

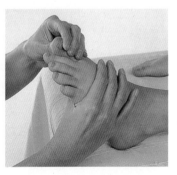

△ **12** To rotate the toes, begin with the big toe, holding it securely but not too tightly and gently rotate. Repeat this movement carefully with each toe. Support the foot with your other hand.

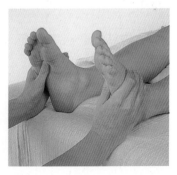

△ **15** For good breathing and to relax the solar plexus reflex, place your thumbs in the natural dent. As your partner breathes in, press in with your thumbs and as they breathe out, release them.

A complete reflexology treatment

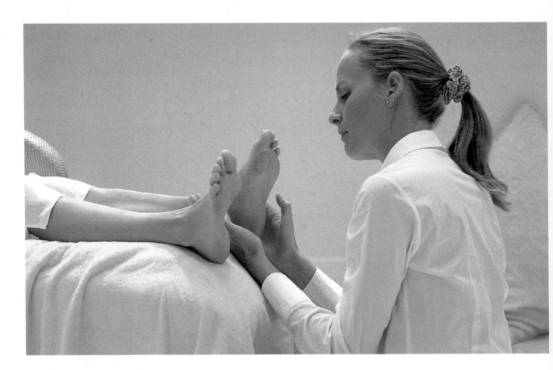

A full reflexology routine treats the whole body, and can be a great way to enhance general well-being, and boost energy. Reflexology treatments work best if the recipient is mentally and physically relaxed, and if he or she is breathing well. For this reason, the first movements in the routine work on the diaphragm and solar plexus reflexes. These points are powerful relaxants which encourage natural, deep breathing. The third movement in the routine treats the head and brain. Stimulating this reflex helps to clear the mind, and also prepares the brain to receive and send messages to and from the rest of the body.

Although each reflex point relates to a specific organ or part of the body, it will also have an effect on other areas. For this reason, it is important that you work round the foot in the exact order given. Be sure to treat all the reflex points on both feet. Ideally, you should perform reflexology on the right

foot first (unlike massage, where it is not so important which foot is attended to first).

Reflexology can be very powerful, so it is important that you do not repeat a movement more than the amount of times specified here. You should also not give more than one treatment to the same person – or to yourself – in a week.

△ This is a long routine so make sure that both you and the person you are treating are comfortable. In particular, it is important that the feet are at the right height so that you do not have to bend to reach them. The recipient can lie on a couch, or sit in a chair with the feet propped up on a footstool, with you sitting or kneeling directly in front.

in the hands
The hands, as well as the feet, contain a stylized "map" of the body. Reflexologists tend to treat the feet because they are more sensitive, but the hands can be easier to use for self-treatment. A person's hands may also be used for treatment if they are very frail or have a foot problem.

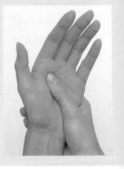

▷ The point being pressed here is connected to the solar plexus. It is an excellent reflex to stimulate if you are feeling anxious or stressed. Breathe deeply as you work it.

holistic reflexology routine

Before starting the treatment, give the person a short foot massage. This helps to release tension in the foot, and allows the person to get used to your touch. You may use a massage oil or cream, but you should blot this off with a towel to prevent your hands from slipping when you are working on the reflexes. At the end of the treatment, massage the feet again. This time, you can leave the oil or cream to sink in. Here the right foot is treated first, then the left.

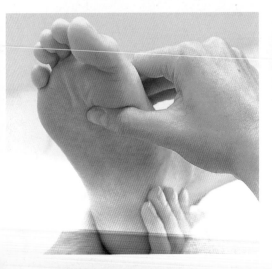

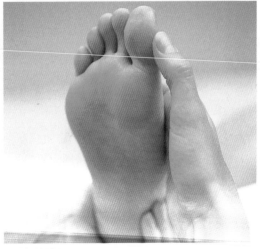

△ 1 Diaphragm (sole)

Cup the right heel in your left hand. Place your right thumb on the edge of the foot, so that it is on the big toe side just below the ball. It should be pointing across the foot, towards the inside edge. Now walk the thumb across the sole in a crawling motion, remaining just below the ball. Repeat the movement once more.

△ 3 Head and brain (big toe)

Continue cupping the heel. Use the right thumb to crawl up the outside of the big toe, going over the top and down the inner edge, in a large horseshoe shape. Then crawl up the back of the big toe from the base to the top. Do as many crawls as necessary to cover the entire surface area.

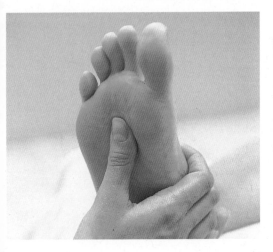

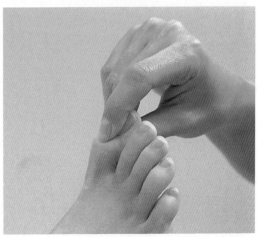

△ 2 Solar plexus (sole)

Repeat the action described in step 1, but this time stop when you reach the point directly below toes two and three. Turn the tip of your thumb so that it points towards the toes and press three times on the solar plexus reflex. Then continue the crawl to the outer edge of the foot. Do this movement twice.

△ 4 Face (front of big toe)

Continuing to cup the heel, use the right index finger to crawl down the front of the big toe (finger walking). Use your thumb to keep the toe steady as you do this. Crawl from the top of the toe to the base, and do as many crawls as necessary to cover the entire surface area.

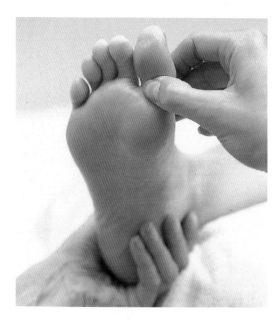

△ **5 Front and back of neck (base of big toe)**
Place your index finger on the base of the big toe, at the edge of the foot. Finger-walk around the front of the big toe, until you reach the join between the big and second toes. Now use your thumb to crawl around the back of the toe, again starting from the edge of the foot and stopping at the join between the toes.

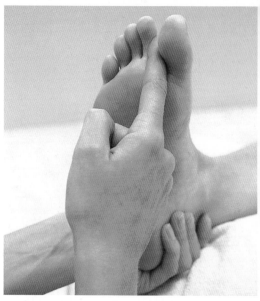

△ **7 Cranial nerves (four small toes)**
Place your right index finger in-between the big and second toes, angling it towards the second toe. Finger-walk up the second toe and down the other side, making a horseshoe shape. Finger-walk over the next three toes in the same way. Now repeat the whole movement.

treating between meals

You should not give reflexology to someone who has eaten a heavy meal within the last two or three hours. On the other hand, a person should not have reflexology treatment on an empty stomach, as their energy levels will be depleted and they will not respond to the treatment as well as they should. If the person that you are treating has not eaten for several hours, or if he or she is hungry, offer a small snack such as juice and biscuits before starting the routine.

▽ **A glass of orange juice and a couple of biscuits will help to boost the person's energy before a reflexology treatment.**

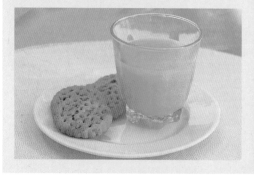

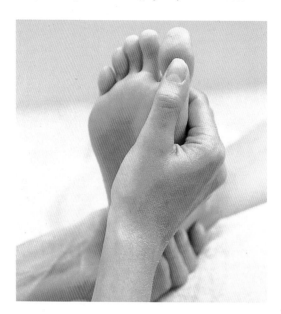

△ **6 Pituitary (back of big toe)**
Continue cupping the heel. Place your right thumb in the centre of the widest point on the big toe and press deeply on the reflex here three times. **Do not work this point on a woman who is pregnant.**

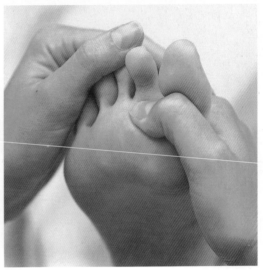

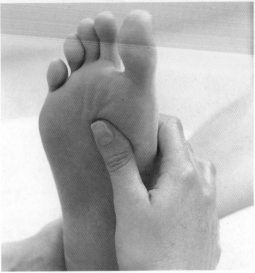

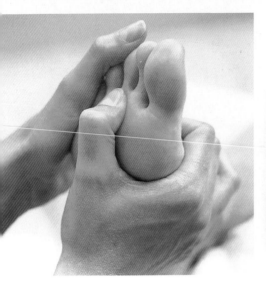

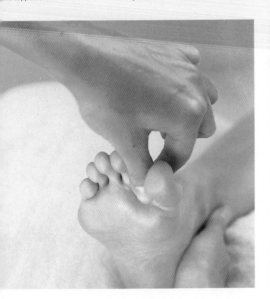

△ 8 Sinuses, teeth and gums (back and front of four small toes)

Support the toes with your left hand. Thumb-walk up the back of each toe: start at the base and crawl up the centre-line to the top. Repeat the movement, but pause when you reach the fleshy bulb of each toe, press in and slide the thumb up to the top. Now, use your index finger to walk down the front of each toe – start at the top and support the base of the toe. Do as many crawls as needed to cover the area.

△ 10 Eyes and ears (under the toes on the sole)

Use your left hand to hold the tops of the toes and bend them back slightly; this exposes the ridge on the sole underneath the toes. Starting on the inner edge of the foot, use the right thumb to crawl along the ridge to the outer edge. Exert a good downward pressure as you thumb-walk. The eye reflex is located under toes two and three, while the ear reflex is under toes four and five.

△ 9 Lymphatic glands (webbing between toes)

Support the foot by cupping the heel. Use your index finger and thumb to pinch and release the webbing between the big and second toes. Repeat on the webbing of the other toes in turn, working gently. Now place your index finger between the big toe and second toe. Slide the finger down the groove on the top of the foot, by a distance of about half its length. Draw back along the same groove.

△ 11 Thyroid, parathyroid, thymus (sole)

Cup the heel in your left hand again. Use the thumb of the right hand to crawl along the diaphragm line, which runs across the foot at the base of the ball: start at the inner edge of the foot and thumb-walk until you are directly in line with the point between the big and second toe. Turn the thumb to point upwards, and thumb-walk up until you reach the base of the toes.

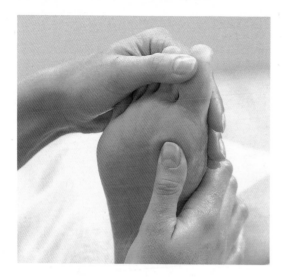

△ **12 Oesophagus, chest, lungs, heart, shoulder (sole)**

Now gently grasp the top of the toes. Place your right thumb on the diaphragm line at the edge of the foot; this thumb should be pointing up, towards the big toe. Using your thumb, make crawling movements up the ball of the foot to the base of the big toe. Do as many crawls as necessary to cover the area. Now, work in the same way to cover the area of the ball of the foot from toe two to toe four. Finally, cover the area under the little toe.

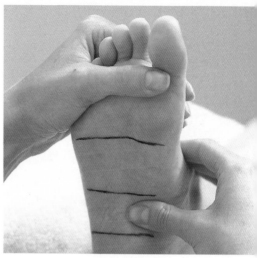

△ **14 Lower abdominal area (sole)**

Here you work in the same way as for Step 13, but you cover the area between the arch (waist line) and the edge of the heel pad (the pelvic floor line.) Again, crawl with the right thumb across the foot as many times as necessary to treat the area. Do the movement twice. The reflex for the small intestine is in this area.

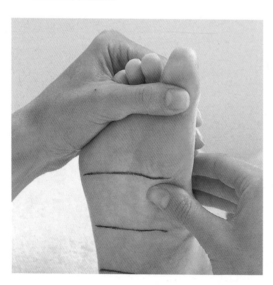

△ **13 Upper abdominal area (sole)**

The upper abdomen reflex is located between the diaphragm line and the waist line, which is in the arch of the foot (marked above). Use the right thumb to crawl across the foot from the inner edge to the outer edge. Repeat the movement as many times as you need to in order to cover the entire area twice. The reflexes for the liver, gall bladder and duodenum reflex are in this area on the right foot; the stomach, pancreas and spleen reflexes are on the left foot.

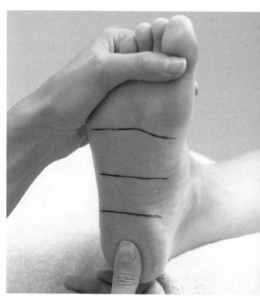

△ **15 Lower back pelvic and sciatic (sole)**

Continue to support the foot at the toes. Start at the back of the foot, and use the right thumb to crawl up through the heel pad, stopping when you reach the soft flesh. Use as many crawls as needed to cover the entire pad, always working in the same direction. Now, place the thumb on the inner edge of the heel, so that it points across to the outer edge. Crawl across the heel as many times as necessary to cover the entire area.

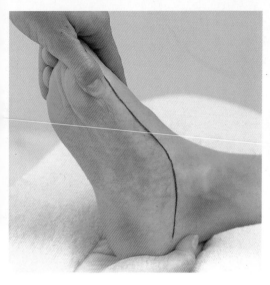

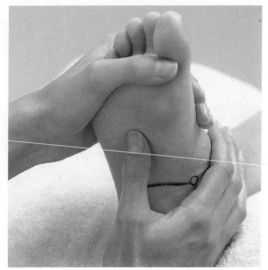

△ 16 Spine (inner edge of the foot)

Cup the heel with your right hand. Crawl the left thumb down the inner edge of the foot. Start from the first joint of the big toe and work to the heel, following the bone (as marked above). Change hands and crawl back upwards, this time pressing upwards into the bone as you crawl. Do the movement twice in both directions. Most conditions benefit from work to the spine, because nerves run from here to all areas of the body.

△ 18 Kidney (sole)

Support the foot by gently holding the base of the toes. Put your right thumb on the waist area, which crosses the centre of the arch; the tip should be pointing towards the join between toes two and three. Make one tiny crawl up the foot; this is the kidney reflex. Press twice, rotating the thumb as you do so (pressure circling). Release the pressure for a second, then make two further pressure circles on the same point.

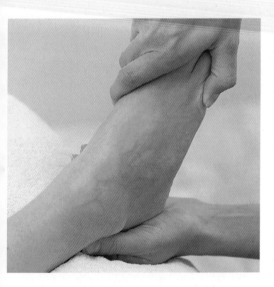

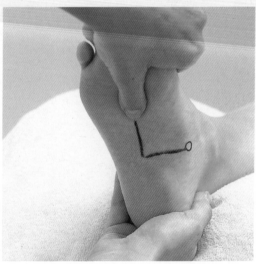

△ 17 Shoulder, hip and knee (outside edge of the foot)

Now cup the heel firmly but gently in your left hand. Thumb-walk right down the length of the outside edge of the foot, from the base of the little toe to the heel. Then work back up to the toe along the same line. Do this movement twice in both directions. It is important to work this area of the foot thoroughly as you are treating three very different parts of the body.

△ 19 Ureter and bladder (sole)

Now use the right hand to cup the heel. Turn the left thumb to point towards the heel and crawl down the ureter reflex to the line where the heel pad and the soft flesh of the foot meet (as marked). Now, turn the thumb again and crawl up on to the inner side of the foot. You will reach a soft, fleshy mound, which is the bladder reflex (circled). Press on this point three times.

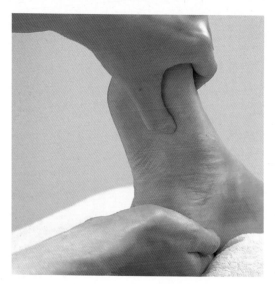

△ **20 Adrenal gland (sole)**

Continuing to cup the heel with the right hand, place your left thumb on the kidney reflex again. Move the thumb across the foot so that it is directly below the second toe. Turn the thumb around so that it is pointing towards the heel, then hook into the flesh and pull back towards the toes. Do three distinct hook-in and back movements on this point.

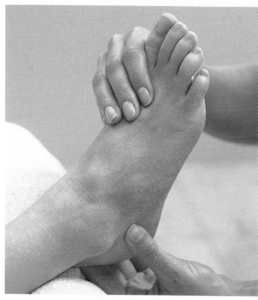

△ **22 Ovaries (female) or testes (male) (outer edge of foot)**

Find the same midpoint on the outer side of the foot. Press in the same way. (You may find it easier to swap your hands over.) **Stroke rather than press this area if you are treating a woman who is pregnant.**

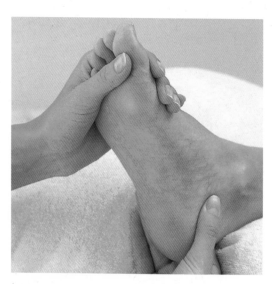

△ **21 Uterus (female) or prostate (male) (inner side)**

Hold the toes with your one hand (whichever feels easiest to you). With the other hand, place the thumb midway along an imaginary line running between the ankle bone on the inside of the foot and the back corner of the heel. Press this point three times. As you press, rotate the thumb slightly (pressure circling) so that you are covering an area the size of a large coin. **Gently stroke rather than press the area if you are treating a woman who is pregnant or has an IUD fitted.**

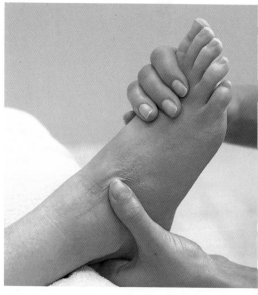

△ **23 Fallopian tube (female), vas deferens (male) (top of foot)**

Continuing to hold the toes with one hand, use the thumb of the other hand to crawl across the top of the foot on the crease line between the leg and foot. Work from the outside ankle area to the inner ankle area. Repeat.

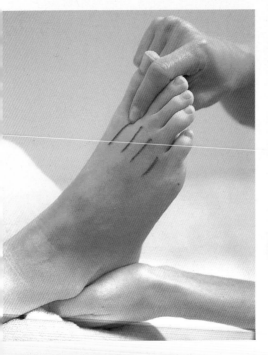

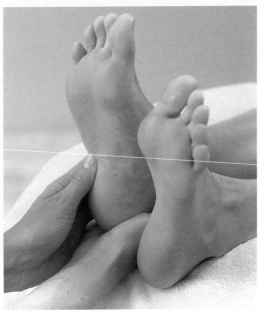

△ 25 **Colon/large intestine** (soles of both feet)
Start at the edge of the right heel, in line with the join between toes four and five.
Thumb walk up the right sole to the middle of the foot. Now thumb-walk across
both feet until you are in line with toes four and five on the left foot. Crawl down to
the left heel pad, then a little way across the foot until the thumb is in line with
toes three and four. Turn the thumb to point towards the heel and make three deep
pressure circles here. Crawl to the inside of the left foot, make two pressure
circles, then crawl down about two-thirds of the heel – to the anus reflex. Make
three deep pressure circles. Repeat the movement three times.

△ 24 **Breast area** (top of foot, at base of toes)
Cupping the heel in your left hand, use the index finger of the right hand to crawl
down the top of the foot from the base of the toes to a point corresponding with
the diaphragm line (the base of the ball). Now, crawl backwards over the same
area. Do as many crawls as needed to cover the breast reflex, which starts
between the big and second toes and ends between the fourth and little toes.
Repeat steps 1–24 on the left foot, then bring both feet together to finish.

treating with care

Being able to offer friends and family a reflexology treatment
is very satisfying. However, it is important to be sure that
you are treating people safely and responsibly. Always ask if
someone has any major illnesses. If so, it is probably wisest
to offer a gentle massage rather than reflexology. Similarly, if
the person is experiencing any severe or unusual symptoms,
advise him or her to get a diagnosis and treatment from a
doctor before giving reflexology. People with conditions such
as arthritis can benefit from reflexology, but they should
ideally check with their doctor before receiving treatment,
and you should always work very gently.

If treating a woman, check whether there is any chance
that she is pregnant. Do not treat a pregnant woman in the
first three months, or if she has experienced any problems.
Some points must not be pressed at all during pregnancy.

▷ **Reflexology can help to alleviate some of the common symptoms of
pregnancy. However, you should not treat if the pregnancy is unstable.**

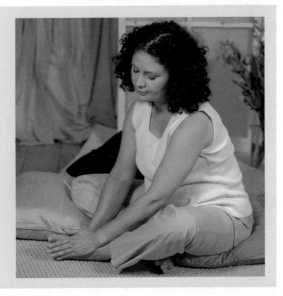

Foot Massage Routines

Your feet can transport you into realms of pleasure. They are one of the most sensual and sensitive parts of your body, and a loving touch applied here can be wonderfully relaxing, energizing or stimulating. Here are some fabulous foot treatments that will soothe your spirits, and restore your soul.

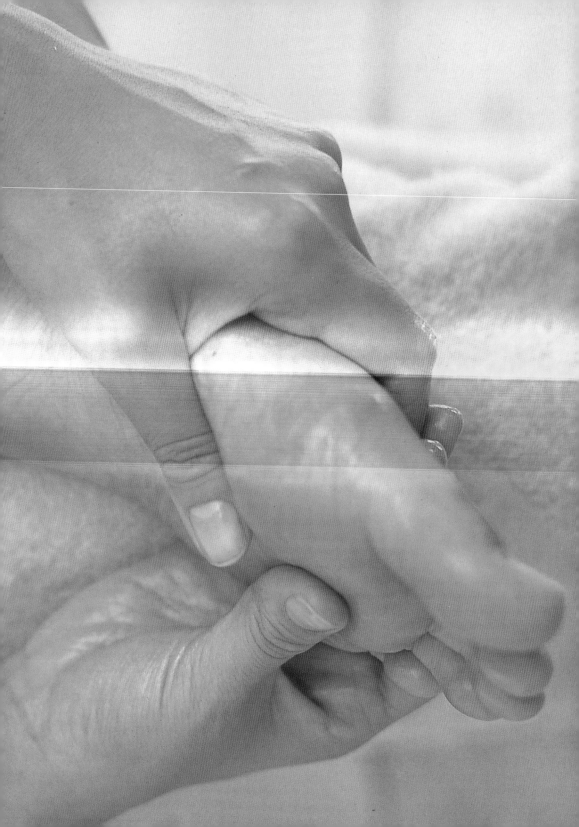

Simple self-massage

All that is needed for a simple self-massage treatment is an understanding of a few basic strokes. After that, it is a matter of practice so that you become comfortable with the different techniques involved.

Self-treatment is a great way of learning massage, because you have your own physical responses to guide you. It is important to get yourself into a relaxed position: you should not need to twist your back or the knee in order to reach the foot. If you are comfortable, you will find it much easier to detect the subtle differences between different strokes and types of pressure, and your reactions to them. You will instantly know when you have got the technique right, and when your touch is sufficiently sensitive and pleasing.

Once you have mastered the basic routine described here, you will be able to adapt the techniques to suit your particular needs and your different moods. You'll also find it much easier to learn the other treatments in this book.

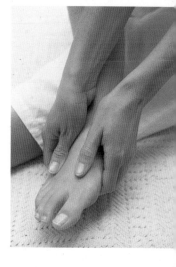

easy self-treatment

This is a quick, simple and effective massage that helps to soothe tired muscles. It can be used at any time as a treatment to relax and refresh the feet, as a quick pick-me-up or as a way to boost your vitality and energy. You can use a cream or massage oil if you like. This basic massage is best done while sitting on the floor, with the resting leg stretched out in front of you.

△ 3 Place your foot on the floor, beside the knee. Hold the foot so that your fingers curl round the sole and your thumbs and heels are on top. Spread the top of the foot by sliding the thumbs apart, applying firm pressure and keeping your fingers in place.

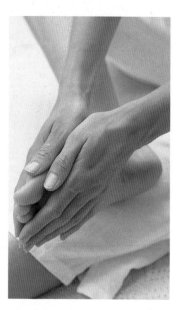

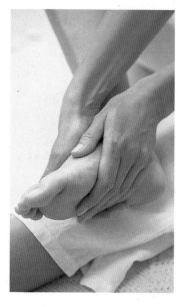

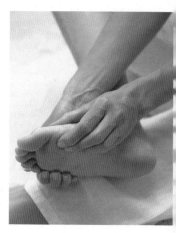

△ 1 Bring your right foot to rest on your left knee; make sure that you are sitting in a comfortable position. Start with gentle stroking. Grasp the foot between your hands, in a sandwich hold, then slide them up the foot, from your heel to the toes.

△ 2 Keeping the foot in the same position as before, slide your hands in the opposite direction – down the foot from the toes to your heel. Keep the pressure steady and firm. Now repeat these up-and-down sliding movements two more times.

△ 4 Now lift up your foot and place it on your knee again. Place your hands in the same position as in step 3. Now, pull the fingers slowly outwards so that you stretch and spread the sole of the foot. Apply firm pressure as you do so.

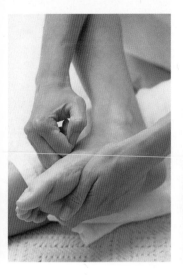

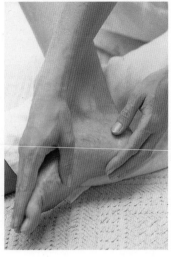

different strokes

When giving yourself a foot massage, take the opportunity to experiment. Try out different strokes, levels of pressure and combinations of the two. People vary considerably in what strokes they like best, and in particular how much pressure they enjoy. What you like can also change depending on your mood and the part of the foot being worked. As a general rule:

Fast strokes are stimulating and energizing.

Slow rhythmic strokes have a hypnotic, relaxing effect.

Deep pressure can be used to release muscular tension, relieve stress or to enhance vitality.

Gentle pressure is soothing and has a calming effect on both the mind and the body.

△ **5** Support the sole of the foot with your left hand. Make a fist with your right hand. Use your knuckles to apply light pressure to the top of the foot, making circular movements. Now support the top of the foot with your right hand. Use the knuckles of the left hand to work the sole, applying deeper pressure.

△ **7** Continue to support the heel of your foot with your left hand. Place the right hand over the top of the foot, placing your thumb on the sole. Now, gently stretch and push the foot downwards. Again, stretch only as far as feels comfortable. Do steps 6 and 7 once more.

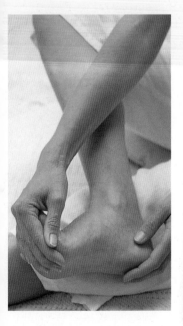

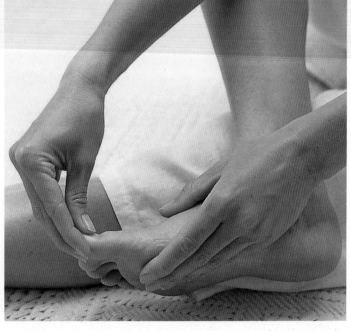

△ **6** Hold the heel of your foot with your left hand, then grasp the ball with your right. Pull the ball of your foot gently upwards so that you stretch the sole. Make sure that you stretch the foot only as far as feels comfortable.

△ **8** Support the foot near the arch with your left hand. With your right hand, hold the big toe near the main joint. Gently rotate the toe first in a clockwise direction, then in an anticlockwise direction. Repeat the action on each toe, finishing on the little one. Now, repeat steps 1 to 8 on your left foot.

Soothing relaxer

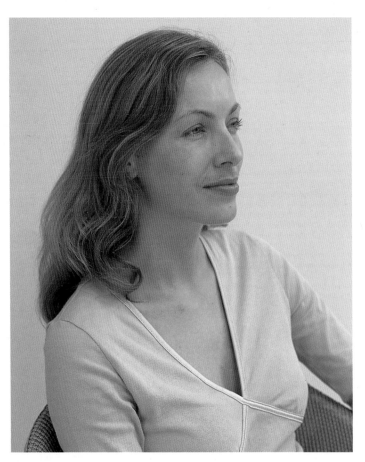

calming massage routine

If you like, you can incorporate this massage into a longer pamper treatment for the feet. You may also like to use some favourite aromatherapy oils to heighten the effects. Neroli and sandalwood or rose and bergamot would be excellent soothing blends to use. Take some time to relax afterwards, too – perhaps with a cup of herbal tea.

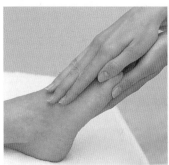

△ **1** Start with the right foot. Hold the foot between your hands – place one hand lengthways over the top of the foot, with the other underneath it. Slide the hands up the foot to the toes, then back down again. Repeat the action at least three times, increasing the pressure as you go.

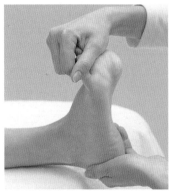

Self-treatment is wonderfully soothing. However, nothing you do to yourself can quite match the sensation of leaning back and letting someone else do the work, as in this routine. There is something utterly relaxing about having your feet massaged; tension seems to drain out of the whole body almost as though a tap had been opened. Perhaps because the feet are so far away from your head, it feels easy to let your mind release worries and anxieties, too.

teach a friend

A relaxing foot massage is a wonderful gift to be able to offer others. It's also worth persuading a friend to learn this short routine, so that you can benefit from it.

△ **This treatment should leave you thoroughly relaxed. Take some time to sit quietly after the routine. If you are giving it to someone else, leave them alone for five or ten minutes so that they appreciate the full effects.**

Anyone can do it even if they have never learned massage techniques before.

There is no need to make any special arrangements in order to do this massage. It can be done anywhere, and works well if the person is sitting on the sofa watching TV or if you are in the garden on a warm, sunny afternoon. You can use it to give a friend a pick-me-up after a late night, and it can also be done in the morning to set someone up for a long, stressful day.

△ **2** Support the heel of the foot in your left hand. Gently grasp the toes with the other hand and then slowly push the top of the foot towards the leg. This gives the sole a good stretch, which helps to release tension. Do not push further than feels comfortable.

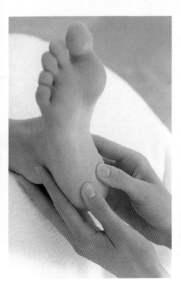

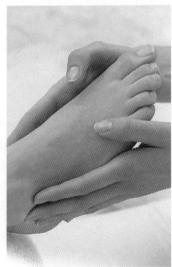

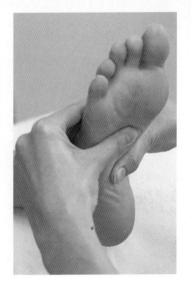

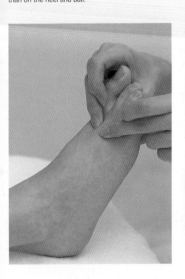

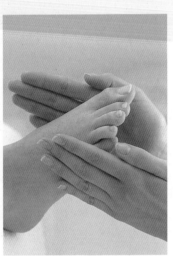

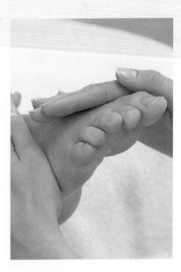

△ 3 Place both of your thumbs on the heel of the foot, with one thumb positioned slightly higher than the other. Now start to massage, by making tiny circles with the thumb, using alternate thumbs. Work your way right up the foot, to the top of the sole, and remember to use much lighter pressure on the arch than on the heel and ball.

△ 5 Place both of your hands on either side of the foot, in such a way that your fingertips are positioned next to the ankle bones. Now, using firm (but pleasurable) pressure, massage in a clockwise direction around both ankle bones at the same time. Repeat the movement, but this time working in an anticlockwise direction.

△ 7 Now place your thumbs on the sole so that they point in opposite directions. Wrap your fingers around the top of the foot to keep it steady. Slide the thumbs up the sole, making a criss-cross movement – so that first the left thumb slides above the right, then the right one slides above the left. Start at the toes and work down the foot; then work back up to the toes.

△ 4 Massage the top of the foot, using your two middle fingers to make tiny circular movements. Start in the groove between the big and second toe, and work down the entire foot to the ankle. Repeat the movement, this time starting in the groove between the second and third toes. Work across the foot in this way until you reach the little toe.

△ 6 Place your hands either side of the foot, so that it is wedged in-between them in a sandwich hold. Using a gentle push-pull action, pull one side of the foot towards you and push the other side away at the same time. Repeat, but this time reverse the action so that you push the first side away, and pull the other towards you. Do the movements twice more.

△ 8 Finish the massage by making feather-light strokes on the top and sole of the foot, using alternate hands. Cover the whole area two or three times, or longer if you feel that the person is really benefiting from this relaxing action. Now repeat the whole sequence on the left foot.

Start the day massage

The ancient Greeks believed that a daily massage was one of the best ways of keeping the body healthy. Few of us have time for a full treatment, but a quick self-massage for the feet is a great way to start the day. This routine is designed to be relaxing yet invigorating – a real wake-up call.

▽ It's worth getting up 15 minutes early so that you can enjoy a relaxing start to the day. A foot massage doesn't take long, but it can make all the difference to the way you feel.

wake-up routine

Ideally you will be relaxed before starting this sequence. However, don't worry if you wake up feeling anxious; you will find it almost impossible to remain so once the massage is underway. Start with the right foot, then repeat on the left.

▷ **1** To start, get into a comfortable position in a peaceful spot. Have a glass of juice and some fruit on hand to enjoy after the massage. Choose a favourite cream or essential oil blend to apply to the feet – they should have reasonable slip but should not be dripping.

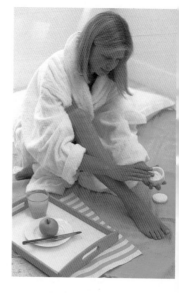

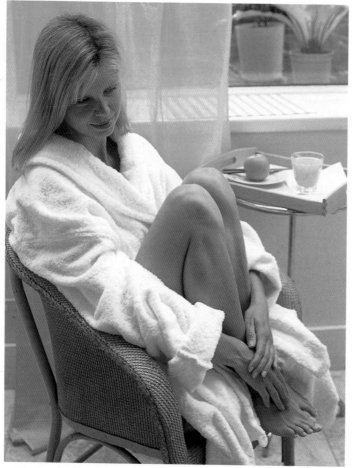

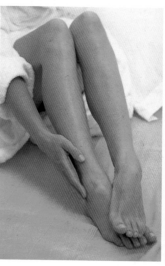

△ **2** Use your fingers to rub the cream or oil liberally over the top of the right foot. Then place your left foot on top, and use the sole to massage from the toes to ankle. Apply heavier pressure on the toes than to the top of the foot, which is more delicate. Take particular care around the ankle area.

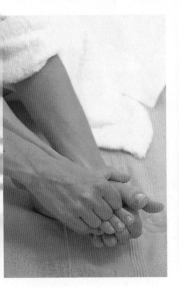

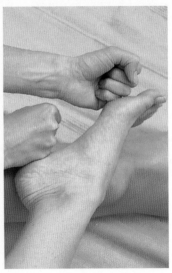

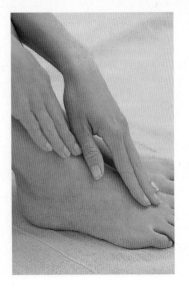

△ **3** Now smooth the cream or massage oil all over your toes. Make loose fists with both of your hands, and place the left one underneath your toes, with the right one on top. Slowly but decisively slide your knuckles across each toe in turn – from the big toe to the little one. You should keep the pressure firm, but it should not be painful.

△ **5** Rest the heel of the right foot on your left knee and apply the cream or oil to the sole. Make fists of both hands. Use the outside edge of alternate fists to strike the sole of the foot, starting at the toes and working towards the heel area. Hit the foot harder on the ball and heel than the arch, which should be struck only lightly,

△ **6** Add more oil or cream to your hands, then rub the palms together to spread it evenly. Use alternate hands to stroke the top of the foot, starting from the toes and working down to the ankle. Begin with a feather-light touch to encourage relaxation, and then increase the pressure to a strong energizing level. Keep it pleasurable at all times.

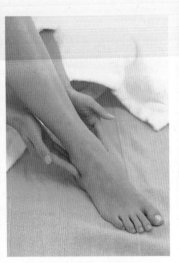

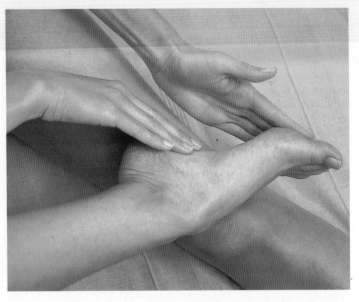

△ **4** With plenty of cream or oil on your hands, massage around both sides of the ankle at the same time. Work in a clockwise direction, making three distinct rotations. Repeat, this time working in an anticlockwise direction. If you are still feeling sleepy or if your ankles feel tight or tense, repeat the movement in both directions.

△ **7** Now rest the heel on your left knee, exposing the sole. Add a little more oil or cream to your hands and rub the palms together to spread it evenly through them. Use alternate hands to make long sweeping strokes down your foot from the toes to the heel. Again, start with light touch to aid relaxation, then gradually increase the pressure. Now repeat the sequence on the left foot.

Recharge your batteries

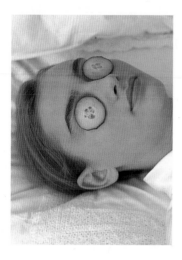

Most of us don't have enough time in our lives to relax and recharge. Ideally, we should stop and rest whenever we feel tired or low in energy, but we often need to keep going because of work, home or social commitments.

This treatment is designed to soothe and revitalize at the same time, so it should leave the recipient feeling refreshed and energized. It is an excellent treatment to do if someone is going out in the evening after

◁ Slices of cucumber or potato placed over the eyes while your feet are being massaged will enhance the general revitalizing effect.

a hard day at work, or in the middle of a busy or stressful week.

The routine can easily be adapted for self-treatment – and used as an instant pick-me-up wherever you happen to be. It is great for days when you can't stop – but feel you can't go on.

the power of silence

Try to work in silence except when you need to ask for and receive feedback – a few minutes of calm can help to increase the restorative effect of this massage. The person you are treating may like to cover his or her eyes with slices of cucumber or raw potato; these will have a restorative effect, and closing the eyes will also reduce any temptation to chat.

Give the recipient a glass of water to sip before and after the massage – dehydration can increase feelings of fatigue. It is also good to eat a small snack – a piece of fresh fruit would be ideal – to boost energy levels. If possible, he or she should take a short walk in the fresh air after doing the routine.

revitalizing routine

Make sure the recipient is sitting comfortably. Suggest that he or she takes a few moments to relax the shoulders and face muscles, and to take a few deep breaths before you start.

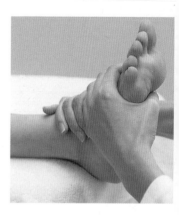

△ **1** Stroke the sole and top of the right foot, using alternate hands. Cover the foot three times or more. Now place your thumbs on the sole and the fingers on the top, one hand slightly above the other. Move the hands in opposite directions, in a gentle twisting action – as if wringing out a wet cloth. Start near the ankle and work up to the toes, then work back down the foot. Repeat the action once more.

tonic massage cream

This thick cream works well with the revitalizing routine, and it is suitable for any skin type. Made in the following quantity, it will last for about 12 treatments. You can substitute other essential oils for the peppermint and petitgrain if you like. Try cypress and lemon to aid detoxing, rose and mandarin for total indulgence, or rosemary and geranium for an uplifting effect.

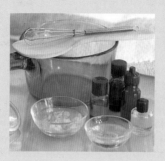

△ **You can make a superb massage cream using just a few natural ingredients.**

ingredients
- 20ml (4 tsp) almond oil
- 40ml (8 tsp) avocado oil
- 20ml (4 tsp) rosewater
- 5ml (1 tsp) lecithin granules
- 10g (¼fl oz) beeswax
- 8 drops each petitgrain and peppermint essential oils

Put the almond oil, avocado oil and beeswax into a ceramic or stainless steel jug. Stand in a saucepan that is half-filled with water. Heat on a low temperature, stirring occasionally until the wax melts. Remove the jug from the water. Add the lecithin and beat the mixture vigorously, then stir in the rosewater. Allow the mixture to cool (but not to become completely cold). Now mix in the essential oils. Scrape the cream into a clean, screwtop jar.

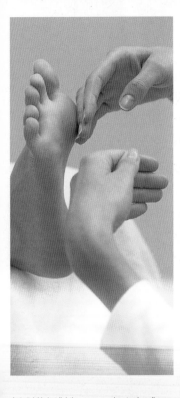

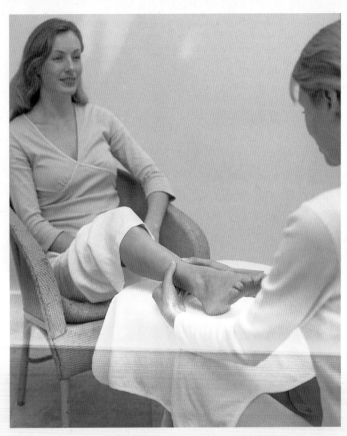

△ **2** Briskly but lightly, use your palms to slap all over the top of the foot, working from the ankle to the toes. Then use the back of your hands to slap all over the sole – the pressure can be heavier here. Do this a few times. It helps to increase the circulation, removing toxins and bringing nutrients and oxygen to the area.

△ **4** Place your thumbs either side of the shinbone. Use the tips to massage, making little circles. Work up the leg from the ankle to the knee. Slide the hands back down to the ankle, without applying any pressure. Repeat.

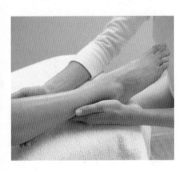

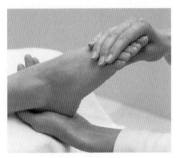

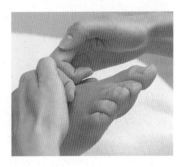

△ **3** Hold the foot behind the ankle to keep it steady. Cup the other hand around the calf muscle, then squeeze and release. Start from just above the ankle and work up the leg to just below the knee, squeezing every part of the muscle. Now slide your hand back to the ankle and work up the leg in the same way twice more. Tension often collects in the calves, and this is a good way to release it.

△ **5** Cup a hand around the heel to support the foot, while resting your other hand against the base of the toes. Gently push the foot away from you three times – remember that you should never push it further than it will go naturally. Now do a forward stretch (shown): place the hand on top of the foot near the toes and pull them gently towards you. Do this pulling movement three times.

△ **6** Curl your fingers to make very loose fists with your hands. Rest the flat area between the top two joints of each fist on top of the foot, and use to massage, making small circular movements. Start near the toes and work down the foot to the ankle, then work back up again. Repeat. End the routine by stroking the sole and top of the foot, as in Step 1. Repeat the whole sequence on the left foot.

And so to sleep

When you sleep well, you wake up feeling refreshed and ready for the activities of the day. Sleep is also essential for good health: while we rest, the cells in our body repair and regenerate, our detoxifying organs do their work unimpeded, and our blood pressure drops. All this helps to combat stress and improves our ability to fight off illness.

Regular sleep is a key element of a healthy lifestyle, along with exercise, a good diet, and drinking plenty of water. Exercising helps tire you out, so it can aid sleep, as can certain foods such as starchy carbohydrates.

getting into a routine

Your sleep is likely to be better if you have a regular routine before bedtime. Having a warm bath and a warm, milky drink each night will help you to relax. If you do these things each evening, you will start to associate them with bedtime, and this will get you in the right frame of mind for sleep.

A foot massage is another great way of relaxing. It is particularly good if your mind is buzzing with thought, because it redirects your attention from the head to the feet – the grounded part of your body.

sleep enhancer

This is a very simple self-treatment routine that you can do before bedtime. You use the feet to massage each other, so that there is no need for you to bend down. An oil-based spray is used, so that you can massage without pulling the skin. You can do the routine sitting on your bed, but put a towel down to protect the cover.

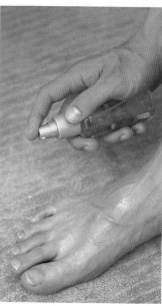

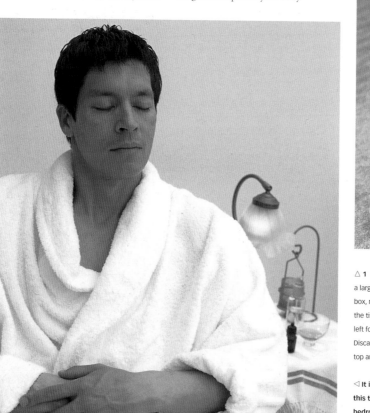

△ **1** Place a large towel underneath your feet. Spray a large, clean tissue with the sleep-time oil spray (see box, right), then spray the top of your right foot. Drop the tissue on top of the foot, and use the sole of the left foot to wipe it all over the top of the right one. Discard the tissue. Repeat on the left foot, so that the top and sole of both feet are lightly perfumed.

◁ It is good to get ready for bed before doing this treatment. Ideally you should do it in the bedroom, either sitting in a comfortable chair or lying down in bed, in which case you can go straight to sleep afterwards. If you find yourself getting sleepy, do not feel you have to finish the routine but simply let yourself drift off.

sleep-time oil spray

This oil spray uses chamomile and lavender oils, which are prized for their relaxing and sedative properties. Neroli and marjoram can also be used, if you prefer their aromas. You can adapt the spray for other occasions by changing the oils: a combination of bergamot, clary sage, geranium and lemon, for example, will make a cleansing spray that is great after a workout and shower.

ingredients

- 25ml (5 tsp) grapeseed oil
- 25ml (5 tsp) almond oil
- 20ml (4 tsp) jojoba oil
- 10ml (2 tsp) rosewater
- 10ml (2 tsp) glycerine
- 20 drops each lavender and chamomile essential oils.

Mix the first five ingredients together, then stir in the essential oils, mixing well. Transfer to a clean 100 ml (3 ½ fl oz) spray bottle. Shake before use.

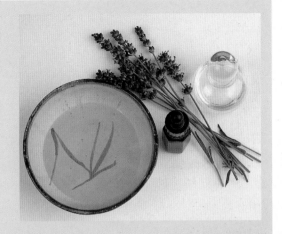

△ Essential oil distilled from lavender is well known for having a calming effect and for promoting deep, peaceful sleep

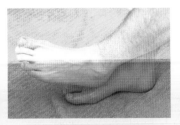

△ **2** Bend your right knee so that the right foot lies flat on the floor or bed. Use the heel pad of the left foot to massage the right toes. Work up and down each toe in turn.

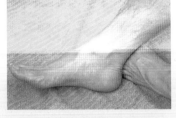

△ **4** Push the left foot around to the back of the right heel, as shown. Now use the toes and the top of the left foot to massage all round the right outer ankle – a quick and easy self-massage technique.

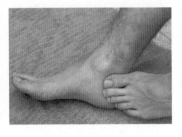

△ **3** Slide the left heel up to the right inner ankle. Use the left heel to massage all around and on top of the ankle bone. Then massage all over the same area with the toes of the left foot. Try to establish a soothing rhythm to the movements. The beauty of these kinds of self-massage techniques is that they can be done anywhere and at any time. So, you can easily try this kind of movement as you sit and watch television or sit on an aeroplane, for example.

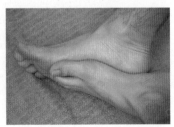

△ **5** Turn the right foot so that it is resting on its outer edge. Use the sole of the left foot to massage up and down the sole of the right. Now repeat steps 2–5 on the left foot. To end, rub the soles of the feet on a towel to ensure they are free from any residue of oil. If you are sitting up, close your eyes, lean back into the chair and relax for ten minutes. If you are in bed, then simply switch off the light and get into your normal sleeping position.

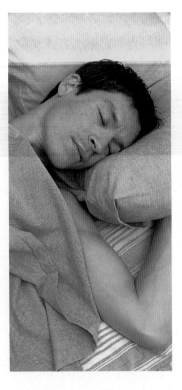

△ **How much sleep you need depends on how old you are and also on your individual constitution. Babies sleep up to 16 hours a day, while older people may need only six hours a night. Most adults need between seven and ten hours a night.**

Foot pamper session

Most of us neglect our feet – particularly in the winter months when they are not on show. Setting aside time for a regular treatment will help you to care for your feet and keep them healthy all year round.

This is a great routine to do at the weekend, or whenever you have some time to yourself. You'll need at least an hour to do it properly – or you can really indulge yourself and take two hours over it.

Think of a pamper session as a time to relax; working on the feet is a great way of taking your mind off day-to-day worries and allowing yourself to focus on feeling good. It is also great to share a pamper session with a friend – set aside an afternoon so that you can really indulge yourselves. You may like to give each other a foot massage at the same time, using one of the relaxing treatments in this book.

Doing a full pamper session once a month will greatly improve your feet's appearance, and will also soften the skin and help the circulation. It is also an excellent way of pepping up your feet at the start of the summer or before going on holiday. You can also shorten the routine and use it as a basis for a mini-pamper session. You may like to do this each week, to keep your feet looking and feeling good in-between full pamper sessions.

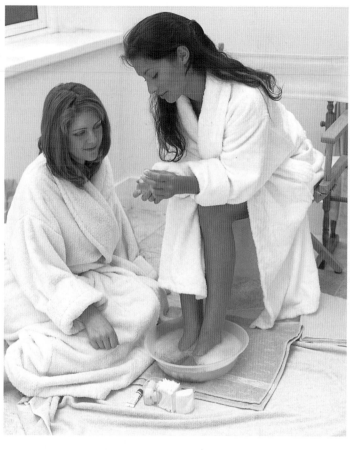

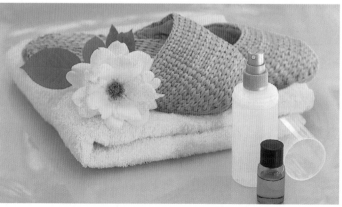

△ Instead of meeting a friend in a bar or restaurant, suggest that you spend an afternoon or evening enjoying a pamper session. It is a good way of spending some relaxed time together, and you could give each other a foot massage at the same time.

◁ Once you start the foot treatment, you won't want to stop, so get everything ready beforehand: lotions, oils, sprays and thick, fluffy towels. Make sure you have a pair of comfortable slippers to slip your feet into after the treatment.

foot care routine

This routine uses the luxury foot scrub described overleaf. If you don't have time to make it, buy one that includes essential oils so that you can benefit from their soothing properties. You'll also need foaming bath or foot gel, a large foot bowl, one large towel and two smaller ones, two plastic bags to slip your feet into, a pumice stone and other items for the pedicure.

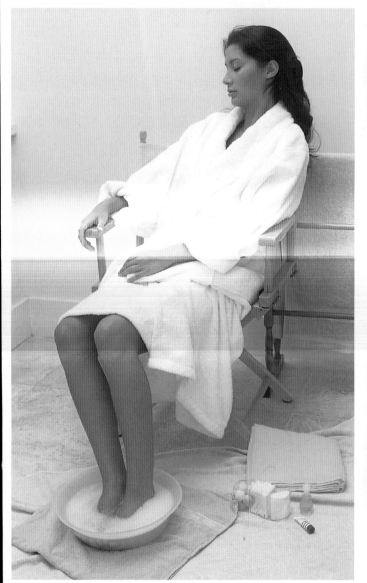

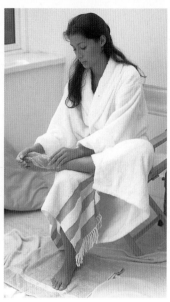

△ **2** Put a towel on one knee and rest the foot of your other leg on top. Massage the foot scrub all over the sole and toes: pay extra attention to any rough skin. Place the foot in a plastic bag and secure.

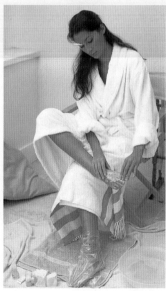

△ **1** Half fill a large bowl with warm water. Place the bowl on a large towel on the floor. Add a little foaming gel, and perhaps a couple of drops of essential oil which have been diluted in a carrier oil or in full-fat milk. Swish the water around with your hand to create plenty of bubbles and to release the aroma of the essential oil. Put both feet into the water, then sit back and relax as you soak them for a good five minutes. Remove your feet from the bowl and rub on the floor towel to remove most of the water.

△ **3** Repeat on the other foot. Relax for ten minutes, then remove the bags from your feet, sliding the bags down so that they remove most of the scrub. Dip your feet back into the water. This will now be cool, and will stimulate the circulation.

a
wn
ow
tion
the
area,

of the
nsive
only

grooming the feet

A pedicure will keep your feet looking great, and will also help to keep them healthy. You need a few special items in order to give yourself a pedicure. Once bought, they will last for ages, so it is worth the investment. Leave out the polish if you prefer to keep your nails natural.

what you need

• Nail polish remover – choose one with a conditioner.
• Cotton wool – to separate the toes while applying polish.
• Nail brush or orange stick (with the tip covered with cotton wool) – for cleaning under the nail.
• Hoof stick or cotton wool buds – to push back cuticles.
• Toe nail clippers – these are easier to use than scissors.
• Emery board – toe nails are harder than finger nails, so you'll need a strong one.
• Cuticle remover – to soften and loosen the cuticle.
• A base coat – to create an even surface.
• Polish colour of your choice.
• Clear top coat – to help seal the polish and prevent chipping.

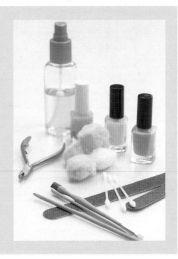

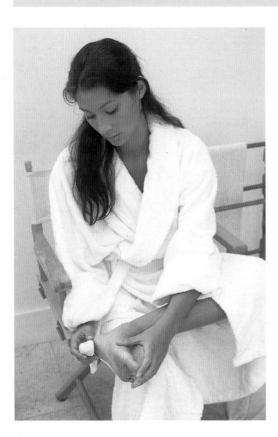

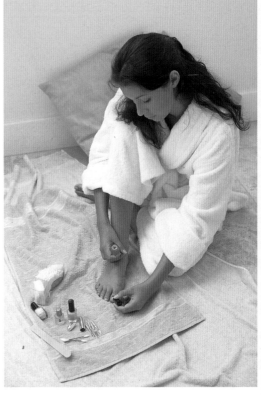

△ **4** Remove your feet from the bowl. Now deal with one foot at a time, placing the foot on your opposite knee. Take the pumice stone and rub over the sole. Use firm pressure on the heel and ball, and very light pressure on the arch. Now, very gently, rub the pumice all over the top of the foot. This improves skin texture and brings nutrient-rich blood to the surface, which will help improve the appearance.

△ **5** Trim the nails straight across, then smooth the edges with an emery board. Use a cotton-wool bud to apply cuticle remover, wait a few minutes, then gently push the cuticle back with a hoof stick. Soak the feet again, then carefully clean under the nail. Dry the feet, then apply base coat, polish and top coat; use cotton wool to separate the toes and allow each layer to dry before applying the next.

luxury foot scrub

This grainy scrub is an excellent cleanser and exfoliator for the feet. The oils and glycerine have a nourishing, moisturizing effect, while the Fullers earth and salt help to soften and deep-cleanse. The essential oils are added for an aromatic, feel-good factor. Choose whichever oils you like best, or use the blends suggested.

This scrub can be used whenever you feel that your feet need a bit of a boost. It should be applied after a warm bath or shower when the feet are damp but not sopping wet. For the best results, though, use it as part of the full pamper session, as described on these pages.

ingredients

- 5ml/1 tsp almond oil
- 5ml/1 tsp jojoba oil
- 5ml/1 tsp glycerine
- 5g/1 tsp each Fullers earth and rock salt
- 10ml/2 tsp foaming foot or bath wash
- 2 drops mandarin and 1 drop geranium essential oils – you could also use lavender and lemon here.

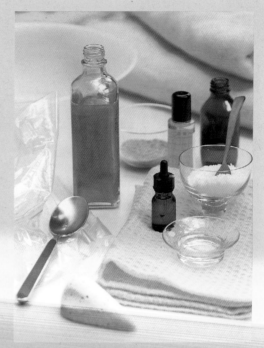

In a small, clean bottle, mix together the foaming wash, essential oil and glycerine. Shake and set aside while you prepare the other ingredients. Put the Fullers earth and rock salt into a medium-sized dish and mix together well. Add the almond and jojoba oils, and mix well. Add the glycerine mixture to the bowl, and mix all the ingredients together with a metal spoon. You should now have a paste with a runny consistency, which can easily be applied to the feet.

▽ Always soak your feet before applying the foot scrub. You can use a foot spa if you have one. This will give a strong massage at the same time as you soak. However, be aware that foot spas are not advised if you have high blood pressure.

△ To make the luxury foot scrub, you'll need a mixing bowl that is large enough to hold all the ingredients, a metal spoon and a small clean bottle. Other equipment used in the pamper routine includes a pumice stone, a couple of freezer-type bags to put on your feet and three towels, one large one to protect the floor and two smaller ones for resting and rubbing the feet.

▽ A mini pamper session can be achieved by soaking the feet in warm suds for ten minutes. Use a loofah or nail brush to scrub and deep cleanse, then pumice all over the soles of the feet. Pat them dry, then give a quick massage using a blend of neroli and lemon essential oils well diluted in almond oil.

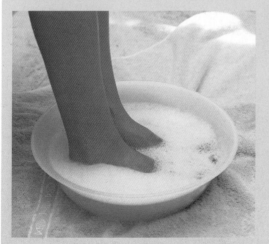

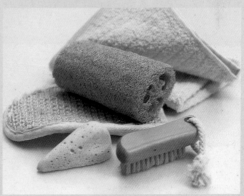

Detox treatment

Fast foods, sugary or salty snacks, alcohol, coffee and tea all contain toxins, which can build up in the body and cause us to feel lethargic and unhealthy. Even if you have a healthy lifestyle, you are still exposed to poisonous substances in the atmosphere. The air that we breathe contains chemicals, gases and dust particles, and it can pollute our land, water and food.

The body is a highly efficient machine, and it is constantly working to remove toxins from the circulation. However, an unhealthy diet, stress or late nights all put the body under pressure, and can affect how well its elimination systems work. Regular exercise supported by a healthy diet and a weekly detox massage regime will help improve your circulation, eliminate waste from the muscles and keep the detoxifying organs in good working order.

It is also important that you drink plenty of water. We lose fluid daily through the natural elimination processes of urination, defecation and sweat. This fluid needs to be replaced. To maintain good health and an efficient detox system we should drink at least three large glasses of water each day.

the role of the feet

The feet are the most distant part of the body – that is, they are furthest away from the heart, the main circulation organ. Toxins and wastes therefore tend to collect in the feet, particularly around the joints. Regular foot massage helps to break down and eliminate these toxins, and also to mobilize the joints. At the same time, it improves the circulation. This has a knock-on effect throughout the body, aiding the natural purification processes.

cleansing routine

It takes only a few minutes to do this simple routine, but it can have a highly beneficial effect on your general well-being. Use gentle strokes at first, to help relax the foot, then increase the pressure as you go on. If you like, use a massage cream or an oil of your choice.

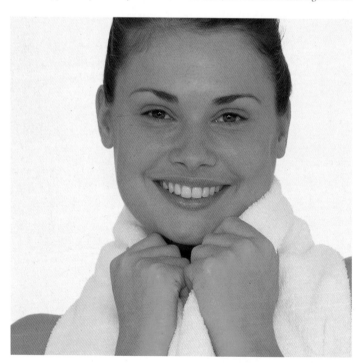

△ You can include the foot detox routine in a fuller programme of cleansing and relaxing. Dedicate some time – perhaps a full day – to enhancing your well-being. Enjoy some brisk exercise, such as running or fast walking, as well as some gentle stretches. Drink plenty of water and eat small, healthy meals consisting of whole grains, fresh vegetables and fruit.

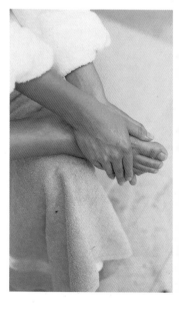

△ 1 Bring your right foot to rest on your left knee. Place your right hand across the top of the toes and your left hand underneath them, with the fingers of both hands pointing towards the outside edge. Gripping the foot between the hands, in a sandwich-like hold, slide both hands down to the heel then back to the toes. Do the movement three times in each direction. Repeat on the left foot.

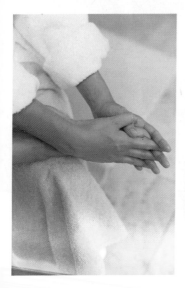

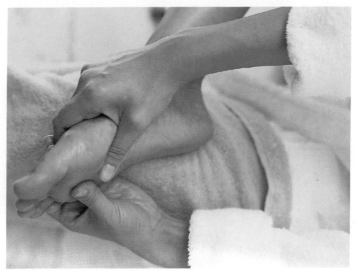

△ **2** Put your left hand on the right sole, fingers towards the toes. Place your right hand on the top of the foot in a similar position. Link the fingers of both hands across the tops of the toes. Now gently pull the hands apart, sliding one down the sole and the other down the top. Do this three times. Then, repeat the movements on the left foot.

△ **4** Place the thumbs of each hand across the sole of the right foot, so that they point towards opposite sides of the foot. Start off as close to the toes as you can. Using a strong pressure, slide your thumbs backwards and forwards across the sole, pulling out to the edge of the foot each time. In this way, work down the foot to the heel, then back up to the toes. Do this three times; this movement helps to improve circulation and eliminate waste. Repeat the whole movement on your left foot.

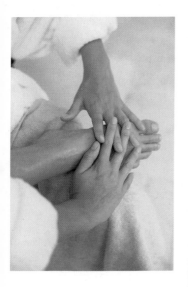

what is detoxing?

Toxins can build up in the body, causing us to feel tired and drained. Detoxing is a way of cleansing the body of these impurities by helping the body's natural elimination processes. Most people benefit from the occasional detox – having a healthy day once a month can be a great way to keep energy levels up. It will also benefit your skin, hair, nails and general well-being.

how to detox

There are different approaches to detoxing. The most extreme one is fasting – abstaining from all foods and drinking only water, herbal tea and juices over a short period.

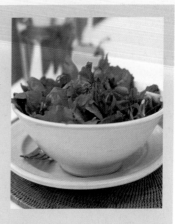

△ **Raw, fresh foods play a vital role in any body-cleansing programme.**

Fasting tends to slow the digestive system, so it can be counter-productive and is not recommended for most people. Your body is more likely to benefit from a gentle programme that does not place it under pressure. A detox is best done over a day or two. During this time eat little and often, having only fibre-rich, healthy foods such as raw or lightly cooked fruits, vegetables and grains. Do several sessions of gentle exercise and get lots of rest. Drink plenty of water to help flush toxins away. You can also drink fresh juices, and herbal teas. Massage speeds the detox process, and brings a pleasurable, relaxing element to the day.

△ **3** Link your fingers together over the top of the right foot. Keep pressing down into the foot at the same time as you pull your fingers apart and draw them towards the edges of the foot. Work in this way from toes to ankle, then work back to the toes; this helps to eliminate waste. Repeat on the left foot.

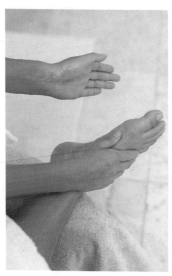

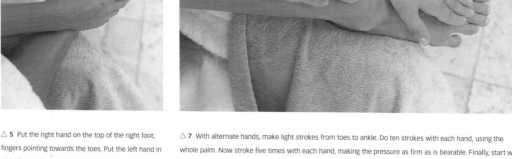

△ **5** Put the right hand on the top of the right foot, fingers pointing towards the toes. Put the left hand in a similar position on the sole. Using alternate hands slap the foot all over, moving up and down between the heel and toe to boost the circulation. Pressure should be harder on areas where the skin is thick. Slap all over four times, then repeat on the left foot.

△ **7** With alternate hands, make light strokes from toes to ankle. Do ten strokes with each hand, using the whole palm. Now stroke five times with each hand, making the pressure as firm as is bearable. Finally, start with the fingers interlaced between the toes. Do five medium-pressure strokes with each hand. Repeat on the left.

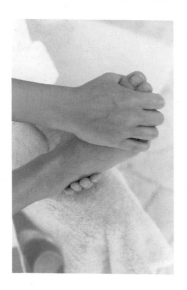

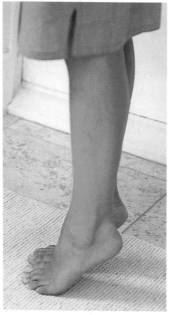

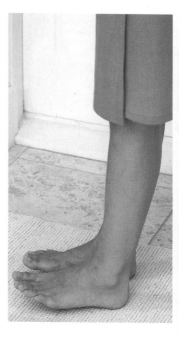

△ **6** Hold the toes of the right foot in your right hand and cup the heel in your left hand. Circle the foot, rotating it from the ankle three times clockwise, then three times anticlockwise. This action helps to mobilize the joints. Rest then repeat. Do not force the ankle beyond its limits. Repeat on the left.

△ **8** Stand up straight. Keep breathing as you lift both heels off the ground and hold them there for a slow count of ten. Return the heels to the floor and count to five. Do this muscle stretch three or four times, depending on your fitness level. You can rest your hands on a chair back if you feel unsteady.

△ **9** This movement stretches the tendons as well as the muscles. Standing upright, firmly press your heels into the floor as you lift the forefoot and toes off the ground. Hold to a count of five, return feet to start point. Rest to a count of five. Do the movement three times. Again, use a chair if you find this difficult.

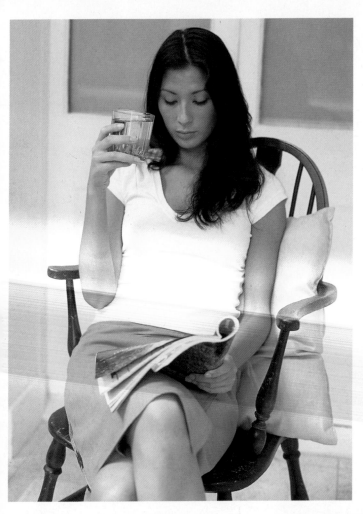

◁ **10** When the massage is over, sit down quietly. Enjoy some peaceful time on your own or read a magazine or book. Spend at least 20 minutes relaxing. During this time, drink a large glass of water or fruit juice. This will help the elimination processes started by the massage routine.

after the routine

If possible, you should try not to do too much after doing the detox routine. If you have time, it is a good idea to combine this treatment with other health-enhancing activities. For example, you may like to do some gentle exercise – such as swimming, walking, yoga or Pilates. You could also go for a sauna; impurities are passed out of the body in sweat.

Make sure that you drink plenty of water. If you like, add a slice of lemon to zing up the taste; lemon has cleansing properties so this will aid the detoxifying process. Try not to eat any sugary, salty or processed foods, at least for the rest of the day. The best foods to help the body get rid of wastes are those that contain plenty of fibre. Eat fresh fruit and vegetables, in the form of juices, soups and salads, together with whole grains such as wholemeal bread, wholewheat pasta or wholegrain rice.

For the best results, you should do this detox routine every week or so. Combined with regular exercise, a healthy diet and drinking plenty of water, it will help to keep your system working well, and prevent the build-up of toxins in the body.

vitamin-packed juicing

Drinking freshly made juices is an easy way to up your nutrient intake and boost your energy levels without placing the digestion under any strain. Here are some good juices to try when you are detoxing, or at any time.

• Apple, orange and carrot: packed with vitamin C and energizing fruit sugars to give you a lift.
• Papaya, melon and grapes: papaya is soothing on the stomach, and this juice can also help the liver and kidneys.
• Carrot, beetroot and celery: a good juice to kickstart the system in the morning. Try using 100g (3¹/₂ oz) beetroot to three carrots and two celery sticks.
• Cabbage, fennel and apple: a cleansing juice with antibacterial properties. Use ¹/₂ a small red cabbage, ¹/₂ a fennel bulb, 2 apples and a spoonful of lime juice.

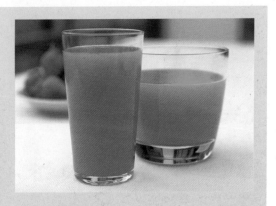

△ **Fruits and vegetables are packed with vitamins and nutrients. Use the freshest produce, and buy organic whenever you can.**

De-stress and unwind

The modern world presents us with more opportunities and choices than we have ever had before. With these new opportunities come new challenges, responsibilities and the need to make an ever-increasing number of decisions. Our everyday life now involves a multiplicity of claims on our time, involvement, commitment and energy.

It is not surprising, then, that we all feel overwhelmed occasionally. Stress has become one of the biggest health problems in the western world, and most of us are affected by it at some point in our lives. Sometimes, a little stress can be helpful; it may galvanize us into action, for example, or motivate us to finish a necessary task. All too often, though, it is counterproductive, and leaves us feeling exhausted, anxious and less effective than we might otherwise be.

the need for rest

The best antidote to stress is rest. However, when you are feeling tense, it can be hard to relax. The solution is to slow yourself down so that your mind becomes quieter and the tension drains out of your body.

There are many ways to do this, but giving yourself a foot massage is probably the quickest. Not only does it require you to focus on what you are doing, which always helps to clear the mind, but you are working on one of the body's most sensitive areas. It is almost impossible not to relax when your feet are being stroked and pummelled.

Do this routine in a quiet place where you won't be disturbed; close the door and switch off the phone. After the treatment, give yourself a few minutes simply to sit and listen to the sound of your breathing.

releasing tension routine

This de-stressing routine has been designed to help you to let go of strain and tension. Try to relax your whole body as you do it; this will enhance the effects. The routine could be practised each day – perhaps after work – but a one-off at any time will bring rewards.

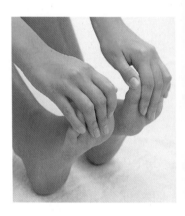

△ **1** Stretch both feet out in front of you, toes pointing upwards. Bend forwards and bring your fingers to rest on the ball of the foot, then pull your feet gently back towards you.

essential oils for de-stressing

Using an essential oil that has soothing and uplifting properties will heighten the relaxing effects of this routine. Add a few drops of your chosen oil to a carrier and massage into the feet at the start of the routine, or heat in a burner. Good stress-relieving oils include geranium, lavender, bergamot, jasmine, chamomile, neroli and rose. Choose one with an aroma that really appeals to you.

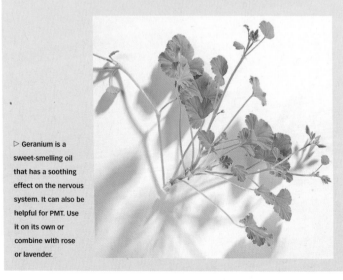

▷ **Geranium is a sweet-smelling oil that has a soothing effect on the nervous system. It can also be helpful for PMT. Use it on its own or combine with rose or lavender.**

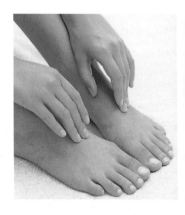

△ **2** Massage the grooves that start between the toes and run up the foot: use the two middle fingers of each hand to make small circles. Start between the two biggest toes, then do the others in turn.

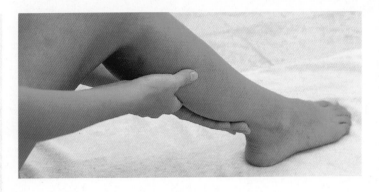

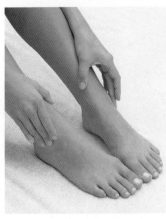

△ **3** Massage around both outer ankle bones at the same time, using the two middle fingers of each hand. Massage first in a clockwise direction, then in an anticlockwise direction. If an area feels tender or tight, repeat the movement in both directions. Do the same on the inner ankles.

△ **5** The next step is to massage the Achilles tendon and muscles of the lower leg. This helps to relieve tension in the feet and legs; it works best if you oil your hands first. Begin the massage on the right leg. Use alternate palms to work up from the back of the heel to behind the knee. Massage the area twice. Repeat on the left leg.

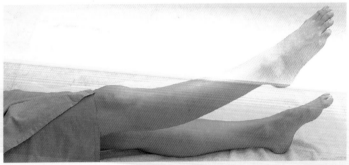

△ **6** Lie on the floor or sit on a chair. Stretch both feet out in front of you. Make scissor movements by crossing the right foot over the left, then the left over the right. Keep your feet and toes pointing straight up towards the ceiling. Work each leg ten times. Rest for a few moments, then repeat the exercise.

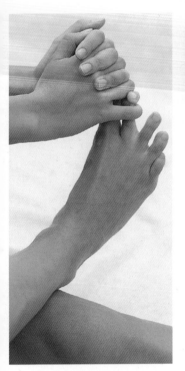

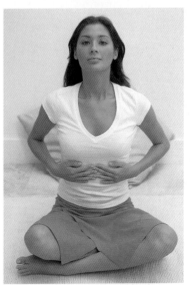

◁ **7** Sit in a comfortable position, eyes closed, fingers resting on your solar plexus. Allow your breathing to follow its own rhythm. Quietly repeat to yourself a meaningful two-syllable word, such as re-lax or hea-vy. This helps to soothe your mind while simultaneously encouraging your body to unwind and de-stress. Don't worry if you feel a little awkward or find this difficult at first. With practice, your voice will become calm and low, and your breathing deep and slow.

△ **4** Place one hand on the sole and the other on the top of the right foot. Cup your hands together, interlocking your fingers. Slide the hands over the tips of your toes, pulling and separating each one as you go. Repeat on the left foot.

Sports routine

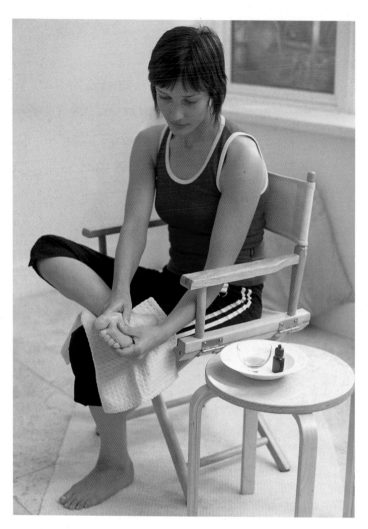

◁ If you wish to use oil for this routine, add a few drops to your palm. Rub the hands together to distribute the oil, then briskly rub all over the right foot and lower leg – you should add enough oil to create a light sheen but not so much that the skin becomes greasy. Oil the left side when you are ready to massage it. Afterwards, wipe off any excess with a towel before putting your shoes back on.

soothing foot powder

This is a great powder to use before or after doing sports. It will help to keep the feet dry and fresh. Tea tree is a vital component because of its antiseptic qualities, but you could use rosemary or sandalwood instead of the lemon – choose whichever has the most appealing aroma.

ingredients

- 150g (5oz) rice flour
- 150g (5oz) orris root powder
- 150g (5oz) bicarbonate of soda
- 5ml (1 tsp) boric acid powder
- 6 drops each lemon and tea tree

Mix together the rice flour, orris root powder and bicarbonate of soda. Add the boric acid powder and mix well. Drop in the essential oils, and stir well until they are thoroughly absorbed. Now transfer your powder to a clean, plastic shaker.

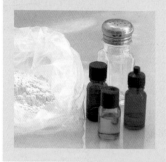

It is essential to warm up properly before doing any type of sport. Warming up helps to prevent cramp and reduces the possibility of aches and pains – you are much more likely to get injured if your muscles are cold.

Cool-down exercises after a work-out are also important. They give the body a chance to come back to a balanced state after its exertions. Warm-ups and cool-downs also help you to manage the transition between normal life and exercise and back again.

Massage is a valuable addition to your usual warm-up and cool-down routines. It is a good way of connecting with your body, and becoming aware of any held tension or awkwardness that you may be experiencing. It is also good to pay some attention to the feet, which bear the brunt of much of the exercise that we do.

before a work-out

This short routine is easy to do in the gym or at home. Start on the right foot, and then do the left. For the first two moves, sit down and bring the foot you are working on to rest on your knee.

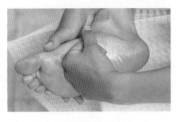 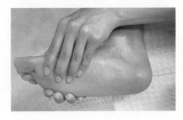 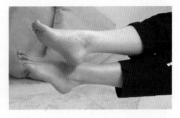

△ **1** Hold the top of your foot in your right hand and make the left hand into a loose fist. Use the flat area between the knuckle and first joint to knead the sole. Work all over the foot, starting at the heel. Use firmer pressure for the heel and ball, and light pressure on the arch. Massage the sole area three times.

△ **2** Place the thumbs on top of your foot, near the toes, and let the fingers of both your hands curl round the foot to meet in the middle of the sole. Keep your thumbs in position and press the fingers in deeply, then pull them out to the edges to spread the sole. Slide the fingers back to the middle and work in this manner down the foot towards the heel. Repeat.

△ **3** Sit down on the floor or on a very stable chair with your legs stretched out in front of you. If on the floor, raise your feet up. Now cross them alternately and rapidly, one over the other in a scissor-like action. Keep the feet straight and the toes pointing upwards. Do the movement at least ten times with each leg.

after a work-out

After exercise or a sporting activity, have a warm shower to help relax your muscles. If you are at home, it is a nice idea to soak your feet in a large foot bowl half-filled with warm water. Add 10ml/2 tsp of almond oil blended with two drops each of rosemary and tea tree. Dry your feet thoroughly before the massage.

▷ **1** Start with the right foot. Use the thumb and index finger of your left hand to pull your big toe straight. Hold to the count of five. Gently rotate it in clockwise direction, then anticlockwise. Do the same to all the toes in turn, ending on the little one.

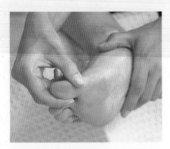

▷ **2** Using the back of the fingers, slap all over the foot. Start on the sole, then do the top of the foot. Repeat so that you cover the entire area twice. Make the slaps as heavy as is tolerable; they should be lighter on the top of the foot than on the sole. This is an excellent action for breaking down toxins.

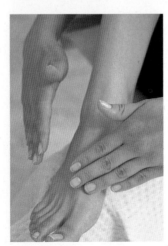

▷ **3** This movement is good for eliminating cramp in the calf. Put the first two fingers of the left hand on the Achilles tendon, then slide upwards to the base of the calf muscle. Press in and make deep circular movements on the spot. Continue to work in this way as you move up the leg, so that the entire muscle is treated. Slide your fingers back down to the Achilles tendon. Do the movement five times in total.

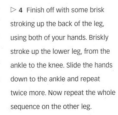 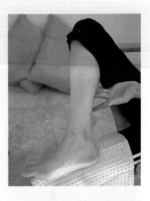

▷ **4** Finish off with some brisk stroking up the back of the leg, using both of your hands. Briskly stroke up the lower leg, from the ankle to the knee. Slide the hands down to the ankle and repeat twice more. Now repeat the whole sequence on the other leg.

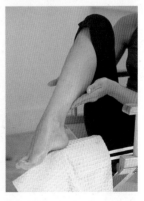

Take a break

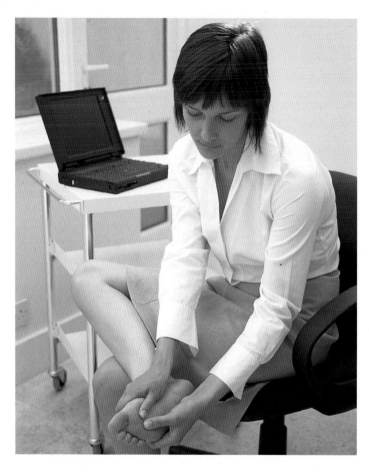

We often have to work or fulfil other obligations when we are feeling under par, because it just isn't possible to take a day out every time we feel a little unwell. Even on a good day, your energy will inevitably flag at various points.

Taking regular breaks from work is always beneficial – and, in the long run, will help you to work more efficiently. If possible, get some fresh air every day, perhaps taking a short walk during your lunch hour. Many office workers eat lunch at their desk, but it is important to get away and have a proper break. Make sure you have healthy food, such as fruit, to snack on at other times of day, too. This will stop you from relying on quick sugar fixes, such as chocolate and biscuits, to keep your energy up. You should also drink plenty of water – have a litre bottle to hand, and top up regularly.

Giving yourself a quick treatment can be a great way to revitalize body and mind. The treatments given here are easy to do in the office, or in a quiet area of any workplace.

◁ If you work in one place all day, such as an office, you may find that you feel low at certain times. If you also work on a computer, you are likely to develop tension in the shoulders and neck. Giving yourself a quick self-treatment will make you feel cared for, and will help to release tightness in the back of the body.

quick cure-all

The reflexology points that treat the spine also have an effect on the whole nervous system. Working these points may help to shift a headache, backache or shoulder tension, and it is a great way to give yourself a general boost.

Remove your shoe and bring one foot to rest on your left knee. Turn the foot to expose the inner edge. Starting at the base of the big toe, walk your thumb along the bone and down to the heel, using a caterpillar-like crawling motion. Now thumb-walk back towards the toes, but this time press up into the bone as you go. Repeat the movements on the other foot.

▷ The spine reflexes run along the inner edge of each foot. As you work the points, try to be aware of any areas of tenderness, and give them a gentle massage.

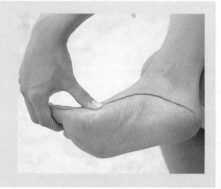

general pep-up

This easy revitalizing routine uses a combination of massage and reflexology. It's easy to do at your desk or in any quiet corner. Start with the right foot, then repeat on the left.

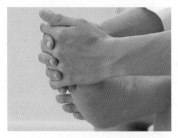

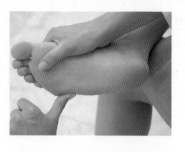

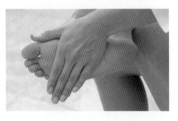

△ **1** Place your right hand over the top of the foot and your left hand on the base, in a sandwich hold. Gently slide your hands up from toe to heel and back again. Press the lower hand in so that the pressure is firmer on the sole. Do this three times, or more.

△ **3** Clasp your hands over the toes, so that they join directly over the little toe. Slowly pull along the top of the toes, allowing each one to open out as you go. This releases tension in the head area.

△ **5** Support the inner edge with your right hand, and use your left thumb to crawl down the outside edge. This works on the shoulder, hip and knee, relaxing the muscles in these areas.

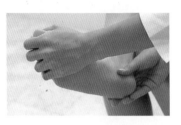

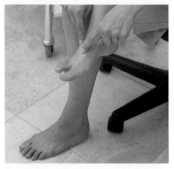

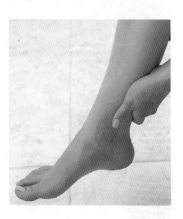

△ **2** Cup your heel in your right hand for support. Hold the top of your toes with your left hand and rotate the ankle gently. Do this first in a clockwise direction, then circle it anticlockwise. Repeat until you have done three circles in each direction.

△ **4** Move your foot so that you can reach the top easily; you may like to rest it on a stool. Use both index fingers to make tiny circles all over the top of the foot. Work from the base of the toes up to the ankles. Vary the pressure depending on how you are feeling; light pressure is very relaxing, heavier pressure will have an energizing effect.

△ **6** Massage the back of the leg, using alternate palms to stroke briskly from the top of the ankle to just behind the knee. This is a good energizing movement to end the routine. Now repeat the whole sequence on the left foot and leg.

relieving headaches, sore throats and neck tension

Here is a excellent treatment for headaches or sore throats that are related to tiredness, stress and tension. This will also help if you have tension in the neck. Do it on both feet.

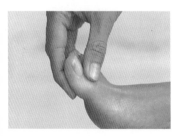

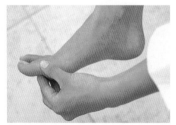

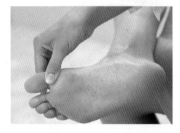

△ **1** Take off your shoes and raise up your right foot. Using your thumb and index finger, pinch your big toe all over. Do the sides, back and top. This action is good for the head and neck.

△ **2** Use your thumb to walk around the top of the big toe from the outside to the inside. This is a reflexology technique used to relax the throat area.

△ **3** Use your thumb to walk from the outside to the inside of the big toe, along the base. This helps relax the muscles at the back of the neck and base of the skull, which may be implicated in a tension headache.

Tonic for tired legs

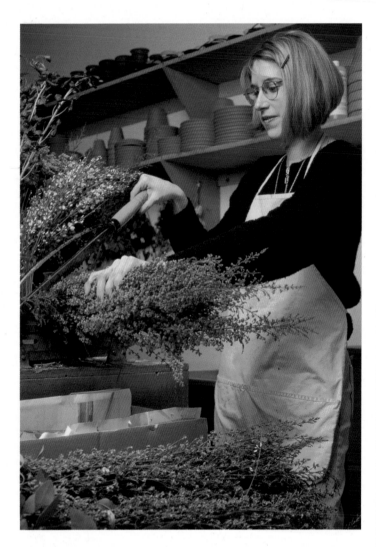

quick rejuvenating routine

These simple foot-and-leg exercises will help to keep your circulation moving and should be done at regular intervals. They are particularly effective at the end of the day.

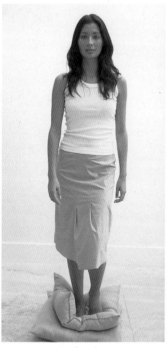

Standing on your feet all day long is not good for your circulation. The force of gravity means that fluid tends to pool in the ankle and feet area.

Muscles do not get a good supply of oxygen and nutrients unless they are moving. If you stand still for a long time, there will also be build-up of waste, which can make the muscle feel tired and achy. A sluggish circulation is the main cause of varicose veins. It also tends to make your skin very dry.

If you need to be standing for long periods, take regular breaks so that you can sit down. You should also keep your feet moving from time to time – walk on the spot, or go up on to the balls of your feet for a few seconds, then release.

△ **1** Stand on a beanbag, or a couple of cushions if nothing else is available (the many tiny beans used in a bean bag have a pleasurable massaging effect). Try to balance for a few moments. Move your feet one at a time, in a walking motion. This gets all the leg muscles working, and kick-starts the circulation. Have a chair or wall nearby in case you feel unsteady.

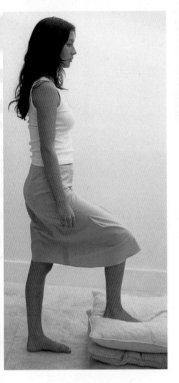

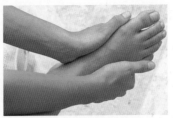

△ **3** Sit down, and rest the right foot on your knee. Place the thumbs on top of the foot, pointing towards the toes, and wrap the fingers round the sole. Draw the thumbs out to the edges of the foot. Return to the start position, and draw the fingers to the edges of the sole. Do this alternate spreading movement all along the foot, starting at the toes and ending at the ankle.

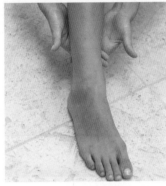

△ **2** You need a step for this exercise. The easiest place to do it is at the bottom of the stairs, or you could improvise with a stack of folded towels or cushions. Use alternate feet to step up. Do up to ten steps with each foot, depending on your fitness level. This also works the muscles, and helps to raise oxygen levels in the leg.

△ **4** Place your hands on the calf above the ankle area. Cross the back of one hand over the palm of the other, as shown, ready for the following step.

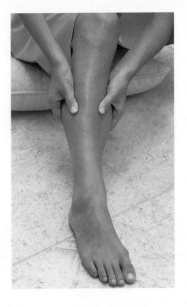

△ **5** Now grasp the sides of the calf muscle with your thumbs. Pull back the thumbs to squeeze the muscle between thumbs and fingers. Work up your entire calf muscle to just below the knee. Repeat.

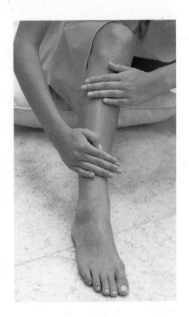

at the end of the day...

It is an excellent idea to rest with your feet above hip level for at least 15 minutes at the end of the day. A good way of doing this is to use the following modified yoga pose. Find a place next to a wall and put a folded blanket, rug or mat on the floor. Sit on the mat with the side of one buttock against the wall. Lie down and at the same time bring your legs up against the wall, then move onto your back. The backs of your legs should be flat against the wall, your buttocks should touch the base of the wall, and your body should be straight. Stay like this for 15 minutes.

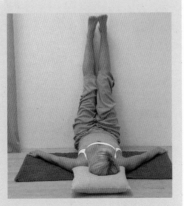

△ **As you rest in this circulation-restoring position, relax your arms and close your eyes.**

△ **6** Stroke up the front of the leg from ankle to knee, using alternate palms. Use soft pressure. If you wish, stroke a diluted essential oil into the leg in step 6 of the routine, shown here. Good oils to help the circulation and aid relaxation include a blend of geranium and rosemary. Repeat on the other leg.

Travel tips

Travelling is hard on the body. Whether in a car, train or aeroplane, we tend to sit in cramped conditions and often need to maintain the same posture for many hours.

A few simple techniques can make travelling more pleasurable, and reduce any negative effects on the body. First of all, make sure that your clothes are comfortable and do not restrict your movements.

If you are travelling by car, stop the vehicle and get out at regular intervals. Walk around for a few minutes; stretch your arms above your head and out to the sides and drop your neck towards each shoulder in turn. Raise and drop the shoulders a few times to relieve tension here.

On a plane or train, get up and walk down the aisle from time to time. Every half

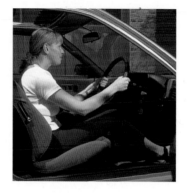

◁ Travelling often involves sitting in fixed positions in a cramped space for long periods of time. This is bad for all of the body, and it takes a heavy toll on the legs and feet. Make sure that you don't slump forwards, like this woman, but sit up straight. It may help to place a wedge-shaped cushion under the buttocks.

an hour or so, do some foot and leg exercises to keep the circulation moving.

On aeroplanes, the air is dry and your feet and ankles can swell. If you are flying,

it is important to wear comfortable shoes with laces so that they can expand with your feet. You should also wear loose socks – or compression socks as advised by the airline or your doctor. If you take your shoes off, put them back on a few hours before landing so that your feet have a chance to get used to them. Drink lots of water during the flight, and take no alcohol, since it has a dramatic dehydrating effect.

foot exercises in transit

Keeping the feet moving during a long air, bus or train journey minimizes swelling and helps to reduce the risk of deep-vein thrombosis (DVT), a potentially life-threatening condition. You should also do any exercises that are recommended by the airline. You will need an inflatable travel neck cushion to do the following routine.

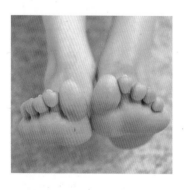

△ **1** Take off your shoes (and socks if you wish). Press the heels into the floor and lift your toes. Pull your toes towards your shins as far as you can; feel the stretch in the front of the lower leg. Then stretch them the opposite way, by pressing the toes into the floor.

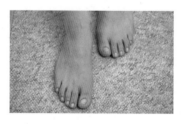

△ **2** Slide one foot forwards, then slide it back as you slide the other one forwards. Repeat this alternate action many times, starting off slowly and increasing the speed. If doing the exercise in bare feet, do not press too hard or you will get carpet burns.

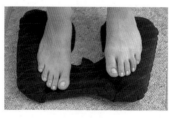

△ **3** Inflate a neck cushion to about three-quarters capacity. Place under the feet, then press alternate feet down as though you are walking. Push down hard enough to move the air from side to side.

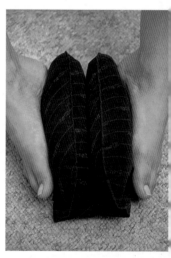

△ **4** Now fold the cushion in two and place it between the soles of your feet. Keeping the cushion in position, try to push your feet together. The partially inflated cushion provides resistance, giving a good workout for the thigh and buttock muscles. You will also feel the stretch in the abdomen. Relax, then push again a few times. Do the whole routine at regular intervals – twice an hour – during the flight.

jetlag routine

These steps will specifically help to relieve the symptoms of jetlag. They are an excellent way of keeping yourself going so that you can go to bed at the correct time.

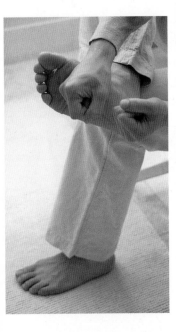

△ **1** Curl your hands into loose fists. Use the flat edge on the little finger side to strike the sole of the foot. Strike all over, working from toe to heel, then back to the heel.

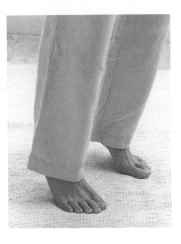

△ **2** Stand up. Stand on the balls of your feet to the count of ten – hold on to a chair or wall if you feel at all unsteady. Relax, then repeat.

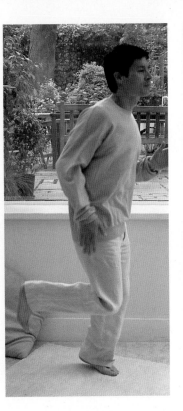

△ **3** Run on the spot to a count of 30. Relax for a count of 10, then run again. Do this about five times, depending on your fitness level.

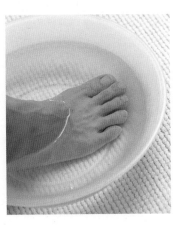

△ **4** Fill a large bowl with cool water (not too hot or cold), or run a very shallow, cool bath. Now place your feet in the bowl or bath. Lift up the toes, then the heels a few times. Rotate your right foot from the ankle, ten times clockwise, ten times anticlockwise. Do the same with the left foot. Repeat the rotation on both feet.

△ **5** Dry your feet. If you like, apply a tonic spray or some talcum powder, or stroke some revitalizing oil into your feet: rosemary is a good uplifting oil to use. Stroke the foot gently to warm up the muscles again.

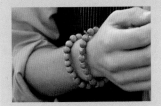

Circulation booster for the later years

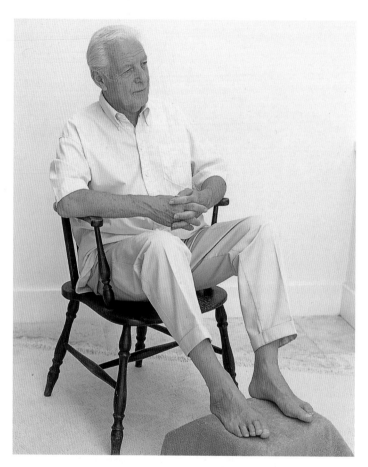

self-treatment routine

You need a towelling strap with loops for this routine, or you can improvise with a long folded towel, as shown. You also need some empty cotton reels threaded through some strong cord. At the start of the routine, it is good to use a light spray on the feet. You can make your own (plenty of light carrier oil, a little rosewater and glycerine and some of the essential oils listed below). Otherwise, use a ready-made spray.

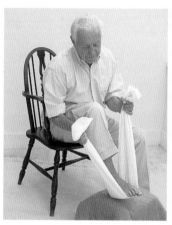

△ **1** Rest your feet on a footrest, covered with a towel. If using a spray, turn the right foot on to its edge to spray the sole, then straighten it up to spray the top. Drop a tissue on to the foot and rub with your left foot to blot excess spray. Now rub your soles over the towel on the footrest until they feel warm. Put the strap under your right foot and pull from side to side. Work all over the sole, from toe to heel, three times.

Everyone can benefit from foot massage. Older people, in particular, will benefit from the increase in blood flow that massage brings. We tend to become less active as we age, with the result that our circulation becomes less efficient. Self-treatment once a day will help to keep the feet healthy, bringing oxygen and nutrients to the area and boosting the circulation throughout the body. It will also help to keep the ankles and toes as mobile as possible.

The skin often becomes dehydrated when we are older; using a massage cream in this routine will help keep it moisturized.

△ **Self-massaging the feet once a day will help keep your circulation flowing. Always sit down to treat yourself. Rest your feet on a low stool so that you do not have to bend as far to reach them. Cover the stool with a towel to protect it from any foot spray or oil.**

safe for all

This treatment is very safe; it is fine to do if you have varicose veins, arthritis or other age-related complaints. The routine featured here is designed for self-treatment, but it can also be given by another person if you find that easier.

good oils for older skin

Try using one of these oils in a foot spray, or add a few drops to a carrier and smooth into the skin.
- Sandalwood, which is relaxing
- Cypress, which is stimulating
- Clary sage, which has pain-relieving properties

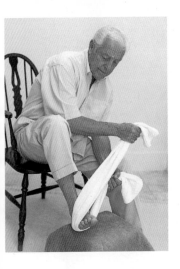

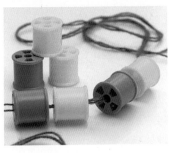

△ This routine involves using a home-made massage aid consisting of several cotton reels threaded on to a strong piece of cord or string. The string should be roughly the length of your leg. Devices such as these can be very helpful if you have difficulty bending down, or if it feels uncomfortable to rest your foot on your knee.

△ **2** Now turn the foot back on to its outside edge. Holding the strap out to one side, pull it back and forth so that you are gently rubbing the top of the foot as you did the sole. Again, work over the area three times, from toe to heel.

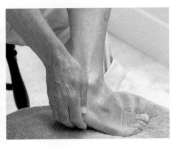

△ **3** Place the middle fingers of your right hand at the base of your heel. Draw them slowly up the back of the heel, using as firm a pressure as you can comfortably tolerate.

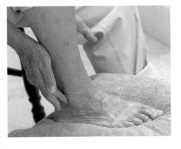

△ **4** Use the fingers of both hands to circle round the inner and outer ankle at the same time. Do steps 3 and 4 once again.

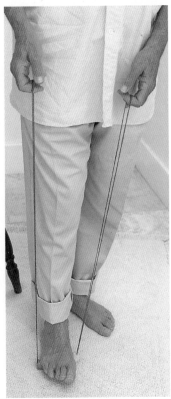

△ **5** Stand up (stay seated if you are unsteady). Place the threaded cotton reels under your right foot and hold the ends of the cord. Roll your foot backwards and forwards on the reels from heel to toe. Do five complete rolls in each direction.

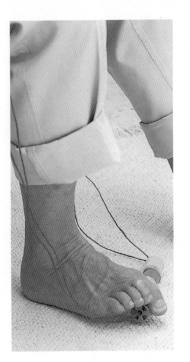

△ **6** Sit back down again, keeping the cotton reels under your right foot. Now try to pick up one or two of the reels with your toes. Practise this lifting exercise five times, making sure that you get all of your toes working.

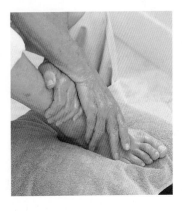

△ **7** Place a little nourishing oil in your hands and rub the palms together to distribute evenly. Using alternate hands, stroke over the top, then the sole, of the right foot. Continue stroking until there is no oil residue left on the top or bottom of your foot. Now repeat the whole routine on your left foot. Make sure there is no oil on the soles of your feet before you get up, so that you don't slip.

Getting closer

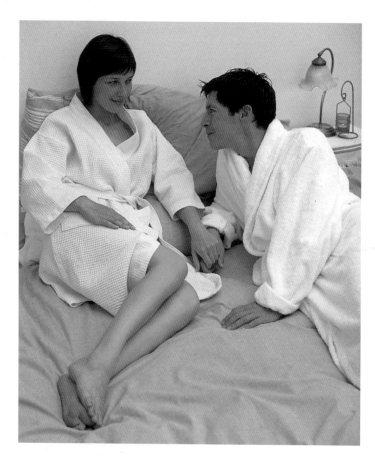

◁ This is a lovely massage to do in the bedroom, perhaps after a warm, relaxing bath or shower. Arrange plenty of cushions or pillows at the head of the bed, so that your partner can lean back and enjoy the massage.

aphrodisiac bath oil

The warm and spicy aroma of this sensual bath oil blend will linger seductively on the skin for some time after your bath – the perfect prelude to an intimate foot massage.

ingredients

- 100ml (3½fl oz) almond oil
- 20ml (4 tsp) wheatgerm oil
- 15 drops rose essential oil
- 10 drops sandalwood essential oil

Pour the almond and wheatgerm oils into a bottle with a screwtop or tight stopper, then add the essential oils. Shake well.

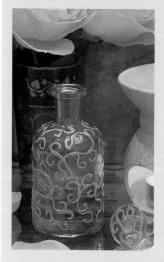

△ Storing oils in pretty bottles helps set the mood, but bottles like this are not ideal. Choose dark glass to keep the oils' aroma for as long as possible.

Sometimes, our days seem to be so filled with work and other commitments that it can be hard to make space for our most important relationship. Massage gives you an opportunity to spend some quiet time with your partner, without the TV, radio or other distractions.

A foot massage is a wonderful way of treating your partner, and for him or her to treat you. It allows you to touch each other in a loving, gentle way that is not necessarily always sexual. As well as soothing and calming the body, foot massage offers a quick route to reconnecting with each other, and re-establishing intimacy.

creating the right mood

When sharing massage with your partner, take a few moments to create an ambience of warmth and intimacy. Make sure that your bedroom is tidy, and that any clutter is cleared away. Have plenty of cushions on the bed so that you can lie back and relax. Use soft lighting – turn off overhead lights and use lamps or candles instead.

You might like to have music playing while you massage. Use the aroma of intoxicatingly-scented essential oils to add sensuality to the experience if you wish. Sandalwood is a warm, heady oil that is said to have genuine aphrodisiac qualities.

sensual foot massage

Try this routine with a relaxing or sensual essential oil, such as geranium or sandalwood, diluted in almond or another carrier oil. Place a towel over the bedcover to protect it from the oil.

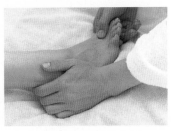

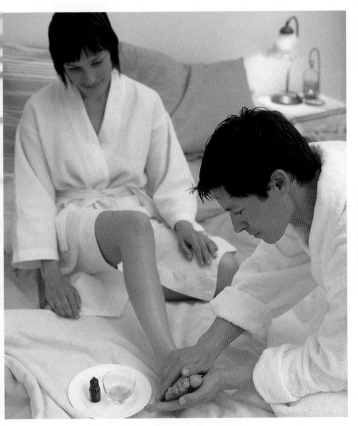

△ **1** Put three or four drops of massage oil in your hand, then lightly rub the palms together to spread it evenly. Take the right foot in a sandwich hold, with one hand across the top of the foot and the other across the sole. Hold for a minute or two, breathing quietly as you maintain contact.

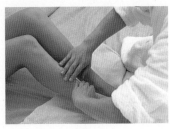

△ **4** Now support the inside edge of the foot, by holding your partner's toes quite firmly. Use the other hand to stroke down the outside edge of the foot, from the little toe to the base of the heel. Stroke back down to the little toe, working slowly and smoothly. Repeat this action two more times.

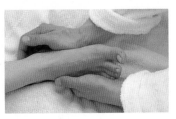

△ **5** Ask your partner to bend his or her knee, so that the foot rests flat on the bed. Apply a little more oil to your hands, then place both hands on the top of the foot – one slightly higher than the other. Stroke down the foot from the toes, and continue to stroke up the leg to the knee, using light pressure. Slide back down to the toes, using no pressure. Repeat twice more.

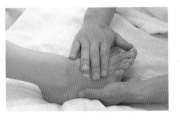

△ **2** Keeping the same hand position as Step 1, stroke the hands down the foot, towards the ankle, then slide back to the toes. The pressure should be firm, but pleasurable. Do this movement three times.

△ **3** Support the outside edge of the foot, so that the toes rest on the heel of your hand. Use the heel of the other hand to stroke down the inside edge of the foot from the big toe to the base of the heel. Work slowly and smoothly. Return the hand to the toe, and fan the inside edge in the same way twice more.

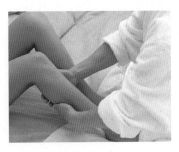

△ **6** Cup both hands around the heel, so that they point in opposite directions and one is higher than the other. Slide the hands up the lower leg to the knee: this helps release stored tension, so keep the pressure reasonably heavy. Slide down to the heel area, using no pressure, and repeat twice more. To finish, use alternate hands to stroke over the top and sole of the foot. Repeat the sequence on the left foot.

Therapeutic Foot Treatments

Most of us experience minor ailments from time to time, and many people suffer recurrent symptoms. In this section you will find some quick footwork that you can use to alleviate

tension headaches, menstrual pain and insomnia.

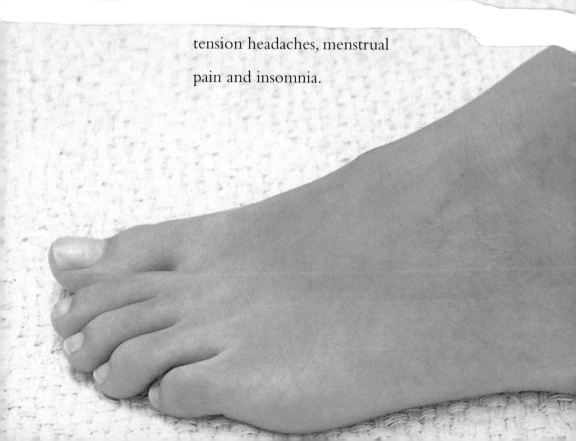

Reproductive problems

Reflexology is an excellent way of helping to maintain a healthy reproductive system, but surprisingly, it is far too often ignored when treating reproductive disorders. This is despite the fact that there are simple but highly effective techniques that will help to deal with a wide range of problems, including menstrual cramps, painful breasts, and even attacks of nausea. Note that all these reflexology movements concentrate on the feet, particularly on the area around the ankle, where the reproductive reflexes are located.

the reproductive system

You can use steps 1 to 3 on both men and women (note that the reflexes for the reproductive system are in the same places for both the sexes). Step 4 to 8 are designed specifically for women.

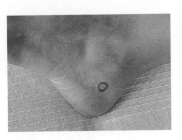

△ **1** Work the reflex for the ovaries or testes, located on the outside of the feet.

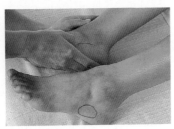

△ **4** Ease menstrual cramps by working the lower spine for nerves to the uterus.

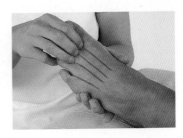

△ **7** Ease painful breasts by fingerwalking up the chest area on top of the foot with three fingers together.

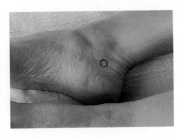

△ **2** Work the reflex for the uterus or prostate gland, which is on the inside of the feet.

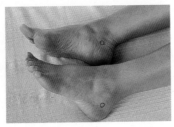

△ **5** Work the uterus reflex area on the inside of the feet using thumb circling.

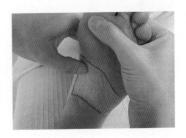

△ **8** Relieve nausea by working the whole abdomen, especially where it seems tender. Use very gentle pressure on painful spots.

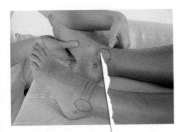

△ **3** Work the fallopian tubes or va deferens across the top of the ankle.

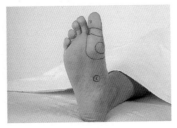

△ **6** Work the glands on both feet, on the areas marked above.

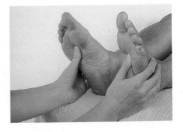

△ **9** Do the solar plexus breathing exercise: press on the in breath, and release on the out.

Boost your immune system

The immune system is a collection of defences that the body uses to fight infection and disease. Organs such as the liver and kidneys contribute to the immune system, as do whole body systems such as the lymph network. Many illnesses can result from a poorly functioning immune system.

Your body's defences can be depleted by lack of sleep, stress or poor diet. This is why you are more likely to fall ill when you are tired or anxious: your ability to fight infection and to recover from illness is reduced. You can help to keep your immune system functioning efficiently by making sure that you get enough sleep, and that you follow a healthy balanced diet. This should include at least five helpings of fresh fruit and vegetables each day.

Exercising regularly will also help to boost the immune system, because physical exertion helps the circulation. You should also avoid drinking excessively and smoking. Alcoholic drinks and cigarettes introduce toxins into the body and put pressure on the organs that deal with waste.

Complementary therapies such as massage, reflexology and acupressure can all help the immune system. Like exercise, they aid the circulation and they also encourage relaxation, which in turn helps all the organs of the body to function well. Regular treatments are the best way to maintain good health, but you can also use reflexology and acupressure as quick fixes. These are particularly good to do if you feel depleted or as if you are catching a cold.

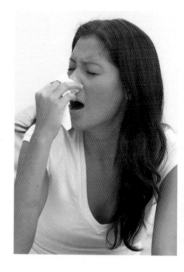

useful essentials

Essential oils can enhance the effects of an immune-strengthening treatment. Eucalyptus oil is a good oil to use here. It has antibiotic qualities, and can be added to a steam inhalation to clear a cough or cold, as well as being used in a footbath or in massage. The oil is very strong, so use it sparingly – one drop per 10ml (2 tsp) carrier.

Uplifting frankincense is another good oil for the immune system. It has anti-inflammatory properties, so it can help with chest infections, and it is also an antiseptic. If you do not want to use these oils in the foot treatments, try putting them in a vaporizer instead.

△ Try the quick immune-boosting acupressure treatments on these pages whenever you feel that you are succumbing to a cold due to stress or overtiredness. They may help to stave it off, or reduce the severity of your symptoms. It can also be helpful to use these routines on a preventive basis, especially if you know you have had a number of late nights or are under a lot of pressure at work.

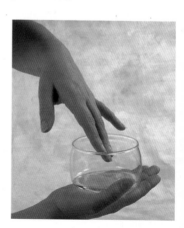

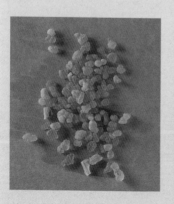

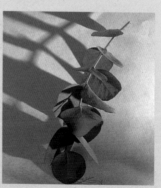

△ Frankincense oil smells warm and spicy.

△ Eucalyptus oil has a strong, lemony aroma.

△ Massaging essential oil into the feet enhances the effects of acupressure. Let the oil sink in.

getting a good night's sleep

The following steps may help to ensure a sleep-filled night.

- Establish a regular sleep routine: go to bed and get up at the same time each day. Avoid afternoon napping.
- Don't work late into the evening.
- Spend the last hour or two before bedtime calmly and quietly. In particular, do not do any vigorous exercise, watch TV or have difficult discussions during this time.
- Make sure that your bedroom is clear of anything to do with work, exercise or other activities – keep it for sleeping.
- Open the window a little, to get fresh air circulating.
- Have a warm bath and a hot milky drink before you go to bed.
- Make sure that you have enough bedcovers to keep you warm, but not so many that you become overheated.
- If you do not get to sleep within 20 minutes of turning out the light, get up and go into another room. Return to bed when you feel sleepy.
- Essential oils can assist sleep: add a few drops of chamomile or lavender into a night-time bath, or drop them on to a cotton-wool ball and slip this between the pillow and pillow cover.
- Try meditation or visualization: a short routine will help to ease you into a relaxed sleeping mode.

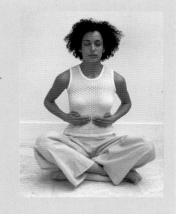

△ Meditating before you retire will help you to unwind and sleep more peacefully.

easing anxiety

This is a good routine to do before an important event. It uses two important acupressure points, which are calming and balancing. Working on the feet is an excellent way of combating anxiety because it has a grounding effect on you. Breathing deeply as you work will also be very helpful. Do each point on both feet.

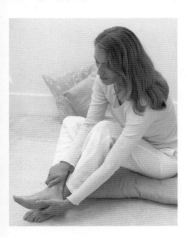

◁ **1** Put the thumb of your left hand on the inner side of the right foot, about one thumb-width below the ball. Press and hold for 30 seconds, breathing deeply. Release the point slowly, breathe for a count of 20, then press again for another 30 seconds. Do the left foot in the same way. This point is Spleen 4, which calms and balances.

▷ **2** Place the two middle fingers of your right hand on the outside of the right lower leg. The fingers should be four finger-widths down from the kneecap and one finger-width towards the outside of the shinbone. This is Stomach 36, which is a good balancing point. Rub up and down briskly to the count of 50, breathing as you work. Rest for one minute, then repeat. Do the same points on the left leg.

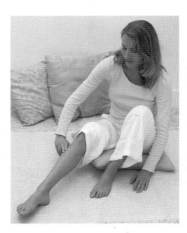

aromatic assistance

Essential oils can be useful addition to the anxiety treatment above. Many oils have a calming, soothing effect. You may like to try chamomile and lavender, diluted in a grapeseed or almond oil carrier. Basil is a good nerve tonic and its aroma combines well with neroli. Clary sage is a good oil to use if you feel very stressed, and sandalwood and rose are other useful oils for anxiety. Massage the oil blend into the ankles, using a circular motion, and allow it to disappear into the skin before working on the acupressure points.

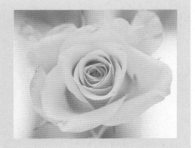

▷ **Rose essential oil is a most effective calmer. It is also very soothing if you are distressed.**

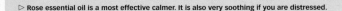

Colds, throats and sinuses

It is virtually impossible to avoid minor colds and the whole battery of side effects that go with them. Especially during the winter months, you can find yourself laid low at any time, by relentless outbreaks of sneezing, followed by sore throats and sinus problems. Fortunately, you do not have to grin and bear it. There are some excellent reflexology techniques that can help you overcome all the nasty extras that come with a cold. This sequence could soon have you back on the road to recovery.

clearing the system

Although the effects of a cold seem to concentrate in the head and upper body, in fact systems all over the body are involved. By working the reflexes to specific areas you can help relieve the symptoms quickly and effectively. Try always to work the reflexes in the same way as outlined here. This will bring the greatest relief.

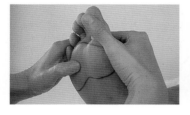

△ **1** Ease colds by working the chest area fully to encourage clear breathing.

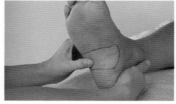

△ **4** Work the small intestines to aid elimination of toxins and uptake of nutrients. Then work on the colon to aid elimination.

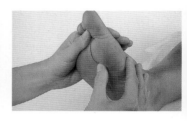

△ **7** Work the trachea and the larynx to stimulate them. Work the thyroid in the area of the chest under the big toe.

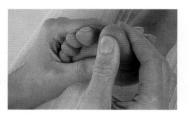

△ **2** Begin with the big toe and work the toe tops to clear the sinuses. Pinpoint the pituitary gland in the centre of the big toes for the endocrine system.

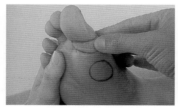

△ **5** Help sore throats by working the upper lymph system, the throat by working the neck, and the thymus gland for the immune system.

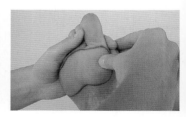

△ **8** Ease sinus problems by returning to work the whole chest area in order to aid good respiration.

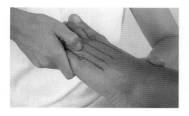

△ **3** Work the upper lymph system to stimulate the immune system.

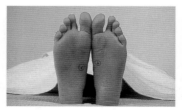

△ **6** Locate the adrenal reflex and rotate it in the direction of the arrow.

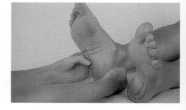

△ **9** Pinpoint the ileo-caecal valve to balance mucus levels. Then work the whole chest area and rotate the adrenal reflex again.

Improving the digestion

The digestive system is all too frequently overlooked, yet it is vital that it is operating in a smooth and efficient way. When we have digestive problems, they can leave us feeling sluggish and lethargic. To avoid any irritating problems, try carrying out the following quick and easy routine, and make it part of your daily or weekly reflexology session. One of the extra benefits of this sequence is that it will help fine-tune the rest of you, leaving you feeling wonderfully calm, refreshed and invigorated.

the digestive system

This sequence focuses on the abdomen area. Don't be surprised if your stomach starts gurgling – this is a good sign, showing that your digestive system has been stimulated to function more efficiently. Some reflex points are worked more than once in a sequence. This is a deliberate policy and should be followed through exactly as shown below.

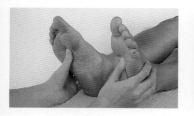

△ **1** Aid any indigestion by working the solar plexus to relax the nerves to the stomach area.

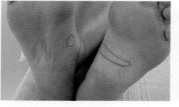

△ **4** Work the pancreas which regulates the blood sugar levels and also helps aid digestion.

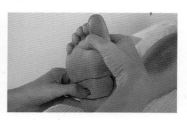

△ **7** Return to the liver and gall bladder: the liver reflex is shown above. Work this area, with the thumb rotating on the gall bladder.

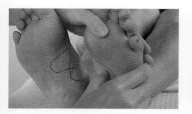

△ **2** Work the stomach, where digestion really begins. Then work the duodenum, the first section of the small intestines.

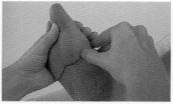

△ **5** Ease constipation by working the diaphragm area in order to relax the abdomen.

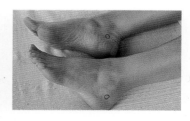

△ **8** Work the lower spine and its helper areas for the crucial nerve supply to the colon.

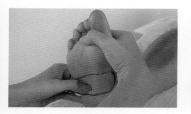

△ **3** Work the liver and the gall bladder: the liver area is shown above, with the thumb rotating on the gall bladder reflex. These deal with digestion of fats.

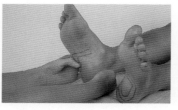

△ **6** Pinpoint the ileo-caecal valve, which links small and large intestines. Work the colon or large intestine.

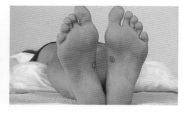

△ **9** Work the adrenals for muscle tone. Rotate the reflex with your thumb in the direction of the arrows.

Feet treat for mothers-to-be

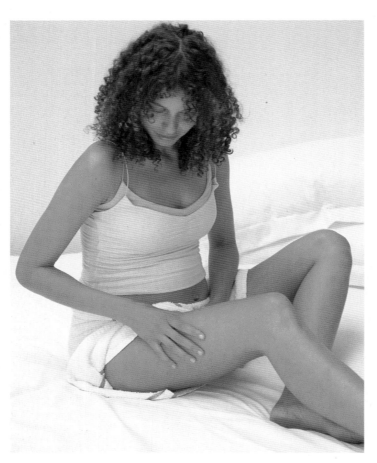

△ In early pregnancy, it is easy to self-massage your legs and feet, and it is extremely helpful for the circulation. However as your pregnancy advances, and the baby grows larger, you are likely to need props, such as marbles in a bowl, or a long-handled brush.

soothing pregnancy routine

This is a gentle and calming routine for pregnant women, which can be adapted for self-treatment (see box). Let the feet soak in the aromatic water for at least five minutes. It's a good idea to put your feet up for 15 minutes after receiving this treatment; enjoy a cup of herbal tea at the same time.

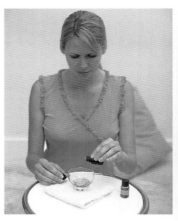

△ **1** Mix 2 drops of essential oil such as mandarin in 20ml/4 tsp of carrier oil – you need a lighter dilution than normal when treating in pregnancy.

safe oils in pregnancy

You should be careful about the essential oils that you use in pregnancy; many are not suitable because they may have an adverse effect. It is best not to use any essential oils other than citrus oils such as mandarin and tangerine during the first three months of pregnancy. Thereafter, always check that any oil is safe for use during pregnancy: camomile, geranium, lavender and sandalwood are good oils for most women, but should only be used well-diluted.

Some women sail through pregnancy with ease, but most will experience minor discomforts of one kind or another. Almost all women feel uncomfortable in the weeks before the birth, and may need some extra support at this time.

Massage has a feel-good factor, which may be particularly welcome in late pregnancy when the woman is likely to feel heavy and tired. Massage is also a good way of oiling of the skin, which can get very dry in pregnancy. Working on the feet and lower legs will also help to shift the fluid that tends

to collect in these areas during pregnancy. In addition, putting your feet up above heart level regularly will encourage fluid to drain out of the legs, which may prevent varicose veins and reduce feelings of heaviness and aching in the area.

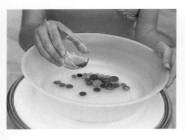

△ **2** Half-fill a foot bowl with warm water, then add a layer of marbles of different sizes. Pour in 5ml/1 tsp of the blended oil.

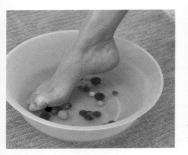

△ **3** Place the feet in the bowl, and push them backwards and forwards over the marbles: this gives a massage-like effect. Move the toes between the marbles. Stretch the feet by lifting up the heels and then placing them flat on the base of the bowl. Now raise up the toes. All these movements will help to open up the feet and to stimulate the circulation in the feet and lower legs. Remove the feet from the bowl and dry thoroughly.

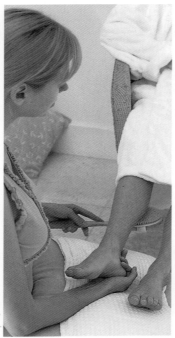

△ **4** Dampen a soft-bristled brush with warm water. Then pour about 5ml (1 tsp) of the oil over the bristles. Rub the brush over the top of the foot, using upward strokes. Cover the area three times, adding more oil if necessary. Rub up the heel and around the ankle area, followed by the front, and then the back, of the lower leg, using upward strokes. Again, cover the area three times. This helps to remove dead skin cells and will also stimulate the circulation.

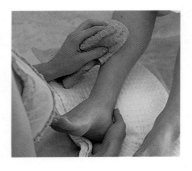

△ **5** Wipe off any excess oil with a cloth. Then use the cloth to stroke gently all over the top of the foot and the front of the lower leg. Once this area feels dry and comfortable, wipe the back of the leg.

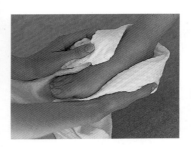

△ **6** Take a small hand towel and fold into a long strip. Holding either end, pass the towel backwards and forwards across the back of the leg. Start just above the ankle and work up the leg to just below the knee. As in step 4, this helps to activate the circulatory system. Now repeat steps 4 to 6 on the left foot and leg.

adapting the routine

Ideally, you should receive this treatment from someone else. However, if this is not possible, the routine works almost as well as a self-treatment. First of all, enjoy soaking your feet, rolling them backwards and forwards on the marbles and lifting the toes up and down – you may wish to spend longer than five minutes doing this. If so, have a kettle filled with boiled water nearby, so that you can top up the footbath when it starts to cool (take care near hot kettles).

It should be easy to apply the oil to your feet using a long-handled brush, as in step 4. To wipe off the excess oil (step 5), simply wrap a soft flannel around the brush, tucking in the edges at the top. Using this means that you do not have to bend down, which can be very uncomfortable in pregnancy. You can try step 6 using a longer towel. However, if this is too difficult for you to manage, simply skip this step. After the massage, make sure that you put your feet up and enjoy at least 15 minutes of peaceful and enjoyable relaxation.

▷ **If you are treating yourself, wrap the head of the brush in a flannel or small towel so that you can remove oil from your feet easily.**

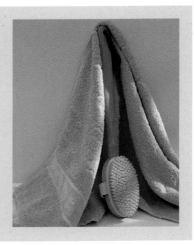

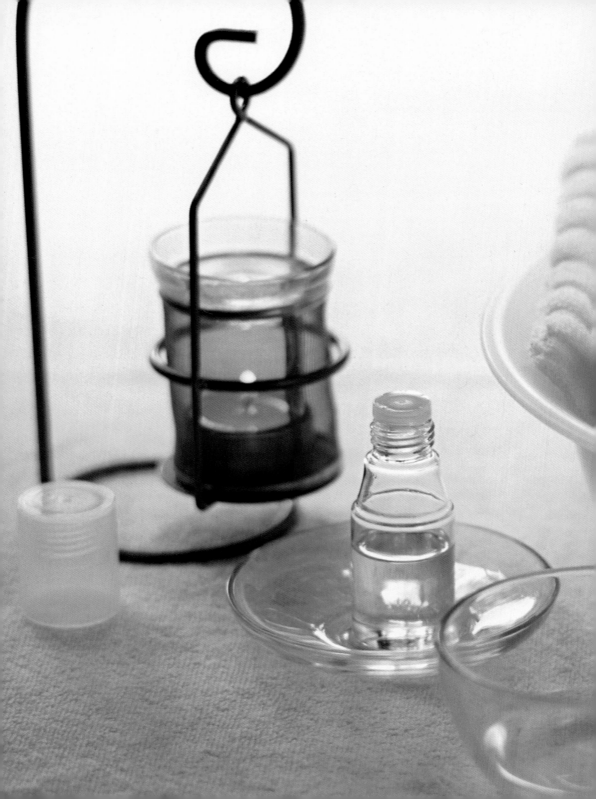

Aromatherapy Principles

Aromatherapy works on every level to cleanse the body and balance the mind. This chapter introduces aromatic essential oils: what they are, how they work, and which oils and blends can be used to target specific problems and restore the mind–body harmony that is needed for good health and improved vitality.

An ancient art

The value of natural plant oils has been recognized for more than 6,000 years, for their healing, cleansing, preservative and mood-enhancing properties, as well as for the sheer pleasure of their fragrances. Today, these properties are being rediscovered as we look to the wisdom of past eras and civilizations to restore the balance that has been lost in modern-day life. Stress, pollution, unhealthy diets, hectic but sedentary lifestyles – all these factors have adverse effects on our bodies and spirits. The art of aromatherapy harnesses the potent pure essences of aromatic plants, flowers and resins, to work on the most powerful of senses – smell and touch – to restore the harmony of body and mind.

secrets of the oils discovered

The origins of aromatherapy can be traced through the religious, medical and social practices of all the major civilizations. It is likely that the Chinese were the first to discover the remarkable medicinal powers of plants around 4500BC. However, it is the Egyptians who must take the credit for recognizing and fully exploiting the physical and spiritual properties of aromatic essences. From hieroglyphs and paintings we know that aromatic preparations were used as offerings to the gods. Furthermore the natural antiseptic and antibacterial properties of essential oils and resins, particularly cedarwood and frankincense, made them ideal for the purpose of preserving corpses in preparation for the next world. The discovery of remarkably well-preserved mummies up to 5,000 years after their preparation is a tribute to the embalmer's art.

By around 3000BC priests who had been using the oils in religious ceremonies and embalming rites became aware of the usefulness of their properties for the living, too. Closely guarding their secrets, they became the healers of their time, mixing and prescribing "magic" medicinal potions. Use of essential oils gradually permeated all levels of society as cosmetics and perfumes became widespread.

From Hippocrates we know the Greeks had some awareness of the therapeutic properties of the oils and their value as sedatives and stimulants was certainly recognized. The Greeks and Romans used aromatics widely in rituals and ceremonies and the oils played an important role in the rise in popularity of baths and massage, and body-culture generally. However, with the fall of the Roman Empire the use of essential oils died out in Europe.

The art of aromatherapy flourished elsewhere, though, particularly in Arabia, where Avicenna was the first to distil rose essence around AD1000. Arabia became the world's centre for production of perfume, importing raw materials from Egypt, India, Tibet and China, and trading their products internationally.

With the Crusaders the art of perfumery was reintroduced to Europe around the twelfth century. Records show that aromatics were used as protection against the plague and the lower incidence of death among perfumiers suggests they were to some degree effective. The fifteenth century saw the rise of the great European perfumiers, and their wares were widely used to disguise body smells and ward off sickness. By the seventeenth century the aphrodisiac properties were certainly well recognized, and with the work of the great herbalists, such as Culpeper, the therapeutic properties also started to be recorded, laying the foundation for modern-day aromatherapy.

the modern renaissance

The term "Aromathérapie" was first used in 1928 by a French chemist, René-Maurice Gattefossé, to describe the therapeutic action of aromatic plant essences. His work was taken up by Dr Jean Valnet who found the essences' remarkable regenerative and antiseptic properties effective for healing the wounds of World War II soldiers.

The application of aromatherapy to beauty therapy and healthcare was pioneered by Marguerite Maury in her influential book, *The Secret of Life and Youth*. She also developed the method of applying the oils through massage.

Today there is a worldwide revival in the art of aromatherapy and contemporary research is beginning to understand the

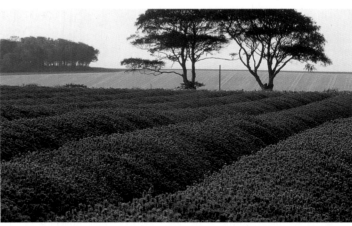

◁ **Lavender is one of the best-known essential oils**, evocative of a summer breeze over the lavender fields of Provence.

scientific foundations of the oils' properties and applications, discovered by trial and error over thousands of years.

essential oils

The vital element in any aromatherapy treatment is the pure essential oil. These oils are very different from the heavy oils we use for cooking; they are concentrated essences, much lighter than water and highly flammable. Their volatility means that they evaporate quickly, so they are usually mixed with other ingredients to preserve their effectiveness. Because they are so concentrated, essential oils are measured in drops.

essence

This is a natural living substance: the "living" element of a plant which is captured and capsuled. It is a delicate operation. For instance, certain petals and leaves must be picked at exactly the right moment, or the quality of the oil is affected. Only the purest essences are used in aromatherapy, so that the therapeutic properties are maximized and the effects are predictable.

Essential oils are extracted from an array of plant sources – petals, leaves, seeds, nut kernels, bark, stalks, flower heads and gums and resins from trees. Apart from their sensuous vapours, which provide the fragrance in many perfumes, they can be used in the bath, smoothed over the body, and used in the myriad ways described in this book.

Because of their small molecules, essential oils can penetrate the skin more effectively than vegetable oils, which only

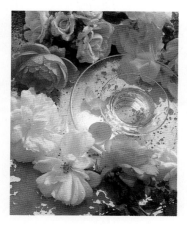

△ Rose oil is one of the more expensive oils as very large quantities of petals are needed in the extraction process.

lie on the surface. Used medicinally over the centuries, essential oils have now become an established complementary natural therapy which can assist in the treatment of almost every type of ache and pain, as well as smoothing away the stress and strains of modern life.

how they work

Essential oils are composed of tiny molecules which are easily dissolved in alcohol, emulsifiers and, particularly, fats. This allows them to penetrate the skin easily and work into the body by mixing with the fatty tissue.

As these highly volatile essences evaporate they are also inhaled, thus entering the body via the millions of sensitive cells that line the nasal passages. These send messages straight to the brain, and affect the emotions by working on the limbic system, which also controls the major functions of the body. Thus in an aromatherapy treatment the essential oils are able to enhance both your physical and psychological well-being at the same time.

Each oil has a distinct chemical composition which determines its fragrance, colour, volatility and, of course, the ways in which it affects the system, giving each oil a unique set of beneficial properties.

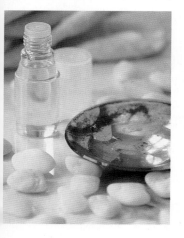

◁ Store essential oils in small bottles with dropper tops to prevent children swallowing them, as oils should never be taken internally.

methods of extraction

distillation

The Egyptians stored their raw materials in large clay or alabaster pots. Water was added and the pots heated so that steam rose and was pushed through a cotton cloth in the neck of the jar. This soaked up the essential oil which was then squeezed and pressed out into a collection vessel. The same principle remains in use today as high-pressure steam is passed over the leaves or flowers in a sophisticated still, often using a vacuum, so that the essential oils within them vaporize. When the steam carrying the essential oil passes through a cooling system, the oil condenses and can be separated easily from the water.

maceration

Flowers are soaked in hot oil to break down the cells, releasing their fragrance into the oil which is then purified and the aromatics extracted.

enfleurage

This is the method by which flower essences, such as jasmine, neroli and rose, which are more delicate and difficult to obtain, were once extracted. Flowers or petals are crushed between wooden-framed, glass trays smeared with an odourless fat until the fat is saturated with their perfume.

pressing

This simple method literally squeezes essential oils out of the rinds and peel of ripe fruit, usually citrus fruits, into a sponge.

quality control

Once the flowers and plants are harvested they are usually processed and stored quickly to preserve the freshness. Climate, soil and altitude can all affect the character of an oil. French lavender, for example, is famous for its rich aroma but, like wine, the quality can vary from year to year.

Always buy pure and natural essential oils as synthetic clones or adulterated oils do not act on the body in the same way and many of the beneficial properties are lost. The best-quality oils may be expensive but they are always worth the extra cost.

Using essential oils

You can soak and splash in them, feed your skin, sensually smooth them all over, or simply breathe in their wonderful aromas. The pleasure and versatility of aromatic oils make them one of nature's kindest gifts. Essential oils contain the active ingredients of a plant in a highly concentrated and potent form. They therefore need to be treated with care and should never be applied directly to the skin undiluted. However, there are many ways of dispersing their fragrance and utilizing their therapeutic properties, and most do not require any special equipment.

inhalation

Steam inhalation is an excellent method for treating respiratory problems, colds and so forth, but should not be used by asthmatics. Add 6–12 drops to a bowl of hot but not boiling water. Place a towel over your head and breathe deeply. This is also a great way of deep-cleansing the face.

therapeutic massage

This is the classic aromatherapy treatment, triggering the body's natural healing processes by using lymphatic massage and essential oils to stimulate the flow of blood and lymph fluid. The aromas also act upon the emotional centre in the brain (the "limbic" system) which governs the way we feel.

For massage use a 1–3 per cent solution of essential oil to base oil.

fragrancers

These attractive pots, also known as diffusers or vaporizers, are simple to use. Fill the top china bowl with water and add a few drops of essential oil. The candle in the pot underneath heats the water, slowly releasing the oil's natural fragrance into the room.

Stand the burner on a plate or tile, not on plastic surfaces. Depending on the size of the room, 3–6 drops of essential oil are sufficient. It is also possible to buy battery-

driven fan vaporizers – these blow air through oil-impregnated pads, which can be changed to suit the mood.

baths

Run hand-hot water and then add 5–10 drops of the essential oil to suit your mood. Close the door to keep in the vapours, and soak for 15 minutes. For sensitive skin it is better to dilute the oil in a base oil first, such as sweet almond, apricot or peach kernel. Essential oils can mark plastic baths if they are not dispersed thoroughly. Wipe the bath straight after use.

foot bath

Refresh tired feet by adding 4–5 drops of peppermint, rosemary and thyme to a large bowl of hot water. Soothe with lavender.

hand bath

Soothe chapped skin by soaking in a bowl of warm water (not hot) with 3–4 drops of patchouli or comfrey before a manicure.

shower

After soaping or gelling, rinse well. Dip a wet sponge in an oil mix of your choice, squeeze and rub over your whole body while under a warm jet spray.

sauna

Add two drops of eucalyptus or pine oil per 330ml (½ pint) of water and throw over the coals to evaporate. These are great cleansers and detoxifiers.

jacuzzi or hot tub

Relax by adding 10–15 drops of sandalwood, geranium or ylang ylang, or simply bubble over with the stimulating effects of pine, rosemary and neroli.

room sprays

To make a room spray blend 10 drops of essential oil in 100ml (7 tbsp) of water. 15ml (1 tbsp) of vodka or pure alcohol added to

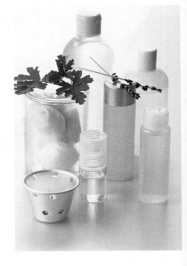

△ Aromatherapy bath products can be bought ready-made, or mix them yourself using non-scented base products.

the solution will act as a preservative, but this is optional. Shake well before filling the sprayer.

pillow talk

Perfume your pillow with 2–3 drops of oil. Choose a relaxing oil to unwind or one for insomnia if you have sleep problems. For a different mood, try an aphrodisiac like ylang ylang or be extravagant and use rose or jasmine, two of the most expensive oils.

perfumes

The finest perfumes are traditionally blended from pure essential oils, particularly the flower extracts, though these days synthetic aromas tend to be used, particularly for cheaper perfumes. The art of the perfumier is subtle and skilled, and difficult to emulate at home as it is hard to find a medium to use as a substitute for alcohol. If you have a favourite oil or blend of essences you can use it all over in a body oil (three per cent

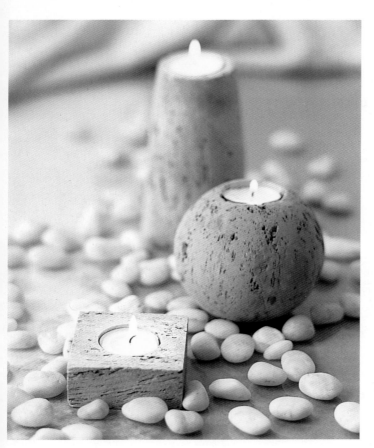

◁ **Aromatherapy candles are now widely available in a range of different scents, and are often intended to enhance certain moods.**

wood fires

Sprinkle drops of cypress, cedarwood, pine or sandalwood over the logs to be used about an hour before lighting the fire and then burn them to release your favourite aroma.

scented candles

Wax candles can be bought ready-impregnated with essential oils and are a delightful way of fragrancing a room. Or you can add a few drops of essential oil to an oil lamp for the same effect.

compresses

Soak a clean cotton cloth (such as a face flannel, handkerchief or small towel) in 160ml (¼ pint) warm water with 5–10 drops of essential oil. Squeeze out and lay across the area to be treated. Cover and leave until cold. A useful method for sprains, bruising, headaches (place the compress across the forehead) and hot flushes.

body and facial oils

These can be used daily to nourish the skin. Use a one per cent blend of essential oil to carrier oil for the face, and a three per cent blend for the body.

solution), or make a very concentrated blend (25 per cent) to dab behind your ears and knees, and on your wrists and temples.

pomanders

Hang porous corked bottles in the wardrobe. The essential oil is absorbed by the clay and released slowly. Fill with the fragrance of your choice: try melissa or bergamot, or cedarwood to keep away moths.

pot pourri

Add a few drops of an appropriate flowery or spicy essential oil to refresh tired pot pourri, or make your own.

handkerchief

The most portable way of using essential oils. Add 3–4 drops to a handkerchief and inhale when you have a cold or headache, or for clearing your head at work.

shoe rack

Freshen the shoe cupboard with lemongrass oil. Deodorize your shoes with two drops of pine or parsley oil, dropped directly on to the insole.

humidifiers

You can add your favourite oil to the water of a humidifier or improvize by adding five drops of essential oil to a small bowl of water placed on top of a radiator. This will have the same effect as using a fragrancer.

ring burners

Use the heat generated by light bulbs to release perfumed oils. Small ring burners, usually made of porcelain or aluminium, sit over the top of the bulb and are perfectly safe to use. Add a few drops of essential oil, and the heat from the bulb will gently distribute the aroma.

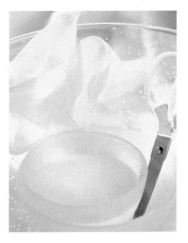

△ **You don't need to buy expensive equipment to use essential oils in the home. The simplest methods can be very effective.**

Preparing oils for application

Essential oils can be added to a range of carrier bases: vegetable oils, unscented lotion or cream. The choice of base depends on how the mixture is to be used, and is also a matter of personal preference.

types of carrier oil

There are many suitable vegetable oils, each with its own benefit. Unrefined, cold-pressed oils are the best for aromatherapy. The basic oils are widely available, while special and macerated oils are available from suppliers. As a guide, use 15–20 drops of essential oil in 50ml (2fl oz) of the base oil for mixtures to be applied to the skin. Use only 5 drops for preparations to be used on the face.

basic oils
Sunflower *Helianthus annuus*

This oil is taken from the seeds of the giant yellow sunflower. It can relieve eczema and dermatitis, lower blood cholesterol, soothe rheumatism, and ease leg ulcers, sprains and bruises. It may also have diuretic properties.

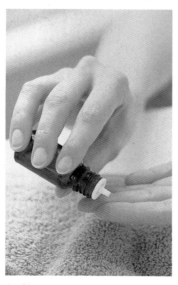

△ Apply one or two drops of neat essential oil direct to the skin to soothe cuts, bites and stings.

Sweet almond *Prunus dulcis*

Almond oil is taken from the kernel of the almond nut, but it is difficult to obtain cold-pressed almond oil. This oil alleviates inflammation and irritation of the skin, helps to relieve constipation, lowers blood cholesterol, and is good for eczema, psoriasis and dry skin.

special oils

These can all be used alone or as 25 per cent of a basic carrier oil.

Evening primrose *Oenothera biennis*

Yellow evening primrose flowers open at dusk, one circle of flowers at a time. The flowers open so quickly that the buds can be watched as they open. The flowers' seeds are cold-pressed when the stem has finished flowering. Evening primrose oil will relieve arthritis, lower blood cholesterol, help PMS, and soothe wounds. It is excellent for eczema, psoriasis and dry skin, and is said to have a beneficial effect on wrinkles.

Hazelnut *Corylus avellana*

Cold-pressed hazelnuts yield an amber coloured oil. Hazelnut oil has astringent properties and can be used to relieve acne, stimulate circulation and protect against the harmful effects of the sun.

Jojoba *Simmondsia chinensis*

Jojoba is not an oil but a liquid wax, which gives it excellent keeping qualities. Jojoba is an analgesic with anti-inflammatory properties, and it will soothe arthritis and rheumatism, acne, eczema, psoriasis, dry skin and sunburn. Jojoba is good for the scalp, and is a useful addition to shampoo.

Rose hip *Rosa canina*

These small berries produce a syrup, a rich source of Vitamin C, and a golden-red oil. Rose hip oil is anti-aging and will help to regenerate tissue. It softens mature skin, and is good to use for burns, scars and eczema.

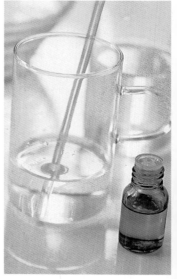

△ Essential oils can be added to cold spring water to make your own customized skin toner. Choose the right oils for your skin type.

macerated oils

The process of macerating (soaking) plants in olive or sunflower oil enhances base oils with the plants' therapeutic properties. These macerated carrier oils can be added to a base vegetable oil, lotion or cream to enrich it. Macerated melissa and lime oils can also be used to enrich base oils.

Calendula *Calendula officinalis*

Often referred to as marigold (although it is not related to French marigold, *Tagetes patula*), Calendula has anti-inflammatory and astringent properties, and can relieve broken and varicose veins. Apply directly in undiluted form to ease sprains and bruises.

St John's wort *Hypericum perforatum*

With its analgesic and anti-inflammatory properties, St John's wort will help to relieve haemorrhoids, sprains, bruises and arthritis, and can heal burns, sunburn and wounds.

carrier lotion and cream

Unperfumed lotion, which is made from emulsified oil and water, can be used instead of vegetable oil as a carrier base. Lotion is particularly good for all self-application techniques as it is non-greasy. Use a cream if a base richer than a lotion is needed.

To prepare a blend for use on the body, mix 15–20 drops of essential oil with 50ml (2fl oz) of lotion or cream. For a blend to be used on the face, mix 5 drops of essential oil per 50ml (2fl oz) lotion or cream. For a foot reflex treatment (*see* page 252) add 50 drops of oil to 50ml (2fl oz) of cream.

safety note

Except for a cream blend to be used in a reflex treatment, use only half the specified quantity of essential oils in any base carrier – vegetable oil, lotion or cream – if the mixture is to be used on children and the elderly.

Preparing a blend for the body using vegetable oil

Vegetable oils are excellent carriers for massage. The essential oils readily dissolve in them, and they allow the hands to move continuously on the skin without dragging or slipping. Mineral oil, such as baby oil, is from a mineral, not a vegetable source. It aims to protects the skin by keeping moisture out and will not allow essential oils to penetrate: it is not suitable as a base oil.

ingredients
- essential oils
- vegetable carrier oil

equipment
- screw-top bottle
- label and marker pen

tips

Care should be taken not to use too much of the mixed oil as it can stain sheets and clothes. To stop too much oil coming out at a time, place your fingers over the top of the bottle, tipping it against them. Apply the fingers to the area to be treated, repeating only if you need more oil.

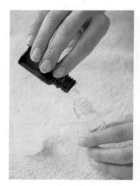

△ **1** Pour 15–20 drops of your chosen essential oil or oils into a 50ml (2fl oz) screw-top bottle.

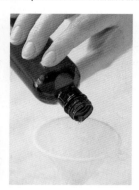

△ **2** Fill the bottle to within 2cm (¾in) of the top with your chosen vegetable carrier oil. Use a funnel, if preferred, to avoid any unnecessary spillage.

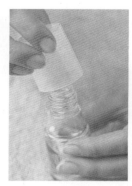

△ **3** Screw on the top and label the bottle with the quantity of each oil used, what the mixture is to be used for, your name and the date.

Preparing a blend for the body using lotion

A bland, non-greasy lotion is preferable to oil as it is less messy and is absorbed quickly by the skin. A lotion base is better for self-application techniques, as a vegetable oil bottle will become greasy and can easily slip through your fingers.

ingredients
- bland white lotion
- vegetable oil (optional)
- essential oils

equipment
- screw-top jar or bottle
- label and marker pen

tips

Prepare a blend with a cream base in the same way. For a preparation to use on the face, mix 50ml (2fl oz) of the base lotion or cream with only 5 drops of your chosen essential oil.

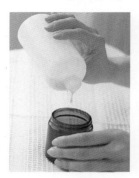

△ **1** For a lotion to use on the body, fill a 50ml (2fl oz) jar or bottle three-quarters full with an unperfumed white lotion, or a lotion mixed with a little vegetable oil, if preferred.

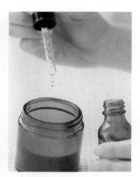

△ **2** Add 15–20 drops of the chosen essential oil or oil blend. Screw on the top and shake thoroughly. Add the rest of the lotion but do not fill right to the top, to allow room for reshaking.

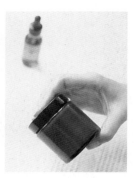

△ **3** Screw the top on firmly and shake again. Label with the contents, use, your name and the date. For a facial lotion, mix 50ml (2fl oz) of the base lotion with 5 drops of essential oil.

The essential oils

Essential oils are powerful agents and all of them – even those nominated as safe – must be used in the correct amounts and for the conditions to which they are best suited. One or two pure essential oils, and most synthetic and adulterated ones, may cause irritation and skin sensitivity. The botanical varieties chosen for this book have been carefully selected from those which do not present this problem. However, these varieties are not always commonly available in the shops and appropriate cautions are included here for the sake of safety.

Except in emergencies, as in cases of burns, stings or wounds, essential oils should not be applied undiluted to the skin, but should be mixed first in a base carrier oil. Citrus oils are photosensitive and should not be used before sunbathing. If you are unsure about the suitability of an oil, always seek the advice of a qualified aromatherapist.

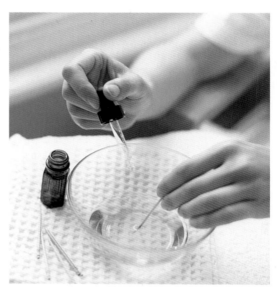

◁ Prepare a compress for treatment at home by blending your favourite essential oils and adding them to water.

▽ Setting the scene at home will contribute to the benefits of aromatherapy. Choose a quiet part of the house and light candles to help you relax.

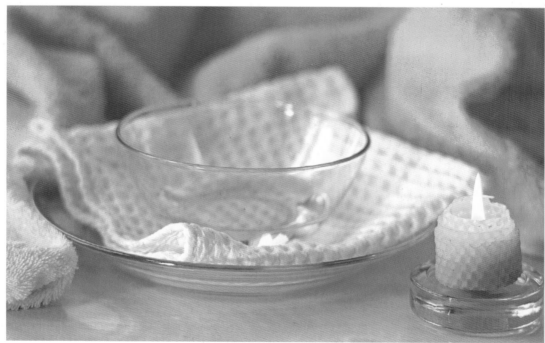

Boswellia carteri – frankincense
family *Burseraceae*

properties
analgesic, anti-infectious, antioxidant, anticatarrhal, antidepressive, anti-inflammatory, cicatrizant, energizing, expectorant, immunostimulant

These small trees, also known as olibanum, grow in north-east Africa and south-east Arabia. Cuts are made in the tree bark from which a white serum exudes, solidifying into "tear drops". When distilled, these produce a pale amber-green essential oil. Frankincense, an ancient aromatic product once considered as precious as gold, has been burnt in temples and used in religious ceremonies since Biblical times.

Frankincense is a gentle oil which is particularly useful for emotional problems, where it allays anger and irritability and soothes grief.

safety
• No known contraindications in normal aromatherapy use.

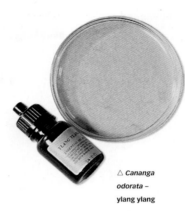

△ **Cananga odorata – ylang ylang**

Cananga odorata – ylang ylang
family *Annonaceae*

properties
antidiabetic, antiseptic, antispasmodic, aphrodisiac, calming and sedative, hypotensive, general tonic, reproductive tonic

Ylang ylang trees, with their long, fluttering yellow-green flowers, are native to tropical Asia: ylang ylang is a Malay word meaning "flower of flowers". The blooms are picked early in the morning and steam-distilled to yield an oil with an exotic and heady aroma.

Widely reputed for its aphrodisiac qualities, ylang ylang is said to counter impotence and frigidity. It can help emotional problems such as irritability and fear; and is effective against introversion and shyness. Ylang ylang also helps to regulate cardiac and respiratory rhythm.

safety
• No known contraindications in normal aromatherapy use.
• Use in moderation. Excess can lead to nausea and headaches.

Cedrus atlantica – cedarwood
family *Pinaceae*

properties
antibacterial, antiseptic, cicatrizant, lipolytic, lymph tonic, mucolytic, stimulant

There are 20 or more species of the trees which yield an oil of cedar. This particular tree, the Atlas cedarwood, grows in the Atlas mountains of north Africa. The first oil extracted was used by the Egyptians for embalming. Most of the oil was taken from wood chippings left from making boxes and furniture (King Solomon used cedarwood extensively when building the temple at Jerusalem). Cedarwood oil is now obtained by steam distillation. It has a pleasant, sweet, woody aroma and can be used in a variety of ways.

Cedarwood is effective for oily skin and scalp disorders, and its antiseptic properties and cleansing aroma are beneficial to bronchial problems.

safety
• Unsuitable for pregnant women and small children.
• Should not be taken internally.

▽ **Cedrus atlantica – cedarwood**

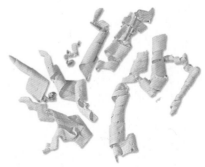

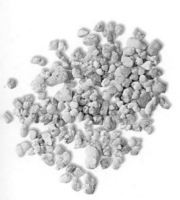

△ **Boswellia carteri – frankincense**

Chamaemelum nobile – chamomile (Roman)
family *Asteraceae*

properties
antianaemic, anti-inflammatory, antineuralgic, antiparasitic, antispasmodic, calming and sedative, carminative, cicatrizant, digestive, emmenagogic, menstrual, vulnerary, stimulant, sudorific

Roman chamomile is native to the British Isles and is a small perennial with feathery leaves and daisy-like flowers. The essential oil is a pale blue-green colour because of the chamazulene content (see *Matricaria recutica* – German chamomile).

The oil is gentle, soothing and calming. It is suitable for children and babies for irritability, inability to sleep, hyperactivity and tantrums. Roman chamomile is also useful for a range of adult complaints, including rheumatic inflammation, indigestion and headaches.

safety
• No known contraindications in normal aromatherapy use.

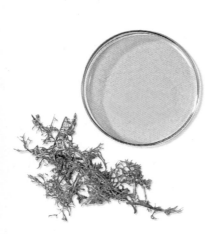

△ *Chamaemelum nobile* –
Roman chamomile

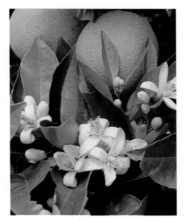

△ *Citrus aurantium* var. *amara* – neroli

Citrus aurantium var. amara – neroli
family *Rutaceae*

properties
antidepressant, aphrodisiac, sedative, uplifting

Neroli oil is the distilled oil from the blossoms of the bitter orange tree. It has a soft, floral fragrance, and is the most costly of the orange oils.

Neroli is beneficial for the skin and helps improve its elasticity. It is good for scars, thread veins and the stretch marks of pregnancy, and has a sedative and calming effect on the emotions.

safety
• No known contraindications in normal aromatherapy use.

Citrus aurantium var. amara – orange (bitter)
family *Rutaceae*

properties
anti-inflammatory, anticoagulant, calming, digestive, sedative, tonic

Oranges have a long tradition in both therapeutic and culinary use. A variety of essential oils are obtained from the fruit, flowers and leaves of both bitter (Seville) and sweet orange trees: neroli oil from the flowers, petitgrain from the leaves, and orange oil from the peel. Bitter orange is expressed from the peel of Seville oranges (most orange marmalades are also made from the peel of Seville oranges).

Bitter orange can be helpful for poor circulation, digestive problems and constipation. It has antidepressant qualities, and will promote positive thinking and cheerful feelings.

safety
• Photosensitizer. Do not expose the skin to sunlight or a sunbed for at least two hours after use.
• No known contraindications in normal aromatherapy use.

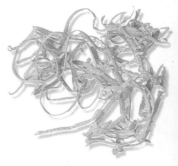

△ *Citrus aurantium* var. *amara* –
bitter orange

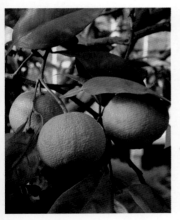

△ *Citrus aurantium var. amara* – petitgrain

Citrus aurantium var. *amara* – petitgrain
family *Rutaceae*

properties
antibacterial, anti-infectious, anti-inflammatory, antispasmodic, calming and energizing

Taken from the leaves of the bitter orange tree, petitgrain's aroma is a cross between the delicate fragrance of neroli oil and the fresh aroma of bitter orange peel. A good petitgrain oil, distilled with some of the blossoms also, is often referred to as the "poor man's neroli" because of its enhanced aroma. Unlike the oil from the fruit, which is expressed, petitgrain oil is obtained by distillation.

Petitgrain is balancing to the nervous system and is recommended for infected skin problems. Emotionally, it can help with anger and panic.

safety
• No known contraindications in normal aromatherapy use.

Citrus bergamia – bergamot
family *Rutaceae*

properties
antibacterial, anti-infectious, antiseptic, antispasmodic, antiviral, calming and sedative, cicatrizant, tonic, stomachic

The main area of bergamot production is southern Italy, although it is also grown on the Ivory Coast. The greenish essential oil is expressed from the peel of this bitter, inedible citrus fruit, which in Cyprus is often crystallized and eaten with a cup of tea. Traditionally, bergamot is a principal ingredient in eau-de-cologne because of its refreshing aroma, and is famous for its use as the flavouring in Earl Grey tea.

Bergamot is useful both in the treatment of digestive problems, such as colic, spasm and sluggish digestion, and for calming emotional states, such as agitation and severe mood swings. It is effective on cold sores but use with extreme caution if in strong sunlight.

safety
• Photosensitizer. Do not expose the skin to sunlight or a sunbed until at least two hours after using.
• Bergapten-free bergamot is an adulterated oil and should not be substituted for the whole essential oil. If not going into the sun, bergamot can be used in the same way as any other oil without risk.

▷ *Citrus bergamia* – bergamot

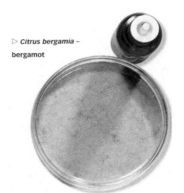

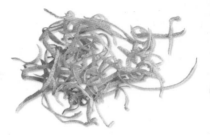

△ *Citrus limon* – lemon

Citrus limon – lemon
family *Rutaceae*

properties
antianaemic, antibacterial, anticoagulant, antifungal, anti-infectious, anti-inflammatory, antisclerotic, antiseptic, antispasmodic, antiviral, calming, carminative, digestive, diuretic, expectorant, immunostimulant, litholytic, phlebotonic, stomachic

Lemon juice and peel are widely used in cooking, and the essential oil is expressed from the peel of fruit not sprayed with harmful chemicals. Natural waxes in the oil may appear if it is kept at too low a temperature, but this does not detract from its quality or effectiveness.

Oil of lemon is an underestimated and extremely useful oil. It has an anti-infectious and expectorant effect on the respiratory airways and can help to eliminate the toxins which cause arthritic pain. It is also good for greasy skin. The clean, lively scent can lift the spirits, dispel sluggishness and indecision and relieve depression. Oil of lemon can also help to dispel fear and apathy.

safety
• Photosensitizer. Do not expose the skin to sunlight or a sunbed for two hours after using.

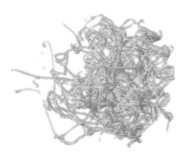

△ *Citrus paradis* –
grapefruit

Citrus paradis – grapefruit
family *Rutaceae*

properties
antiseptic, aperitif, digestive, diuretic

Originating in tropical Asia and the West Indies, the grapefruit tree is now cultivated mainly in North and South America. The yellow oil, produced mainly in California, is obtained by expression of the peel and has a sweet, citrus aroma.

It is effective in caring for oily skin and acne, and regular use twice daily is helpful for cellulite, water retention and obesity. Its antiseptic property is particularly useful in a vapourizer to disinfect the air of a sickroom. It is useful to add a little (4 drops per litre) to spring water when travelling to help prevent digestive problems.

safety
• No known contraindications in normal aromatherapy use.

Citrus reticulata – mandarin
family *Rutaceae*

properties
antifungal, antispasmodic, calming, digestive

The mandarin orange tree originates in China, and its fruit was named after the Chinese Mandarins. The fruit of the mandarin tree is very similar to the tangerine and oils from both fruits may be sold as mandarin. The essential oil is expressed from the peel.

Mandarin oil has digestive properties, and is excellent for treating both adults and children with indigestion, stomach pains and constipation. It can be very useful for over-excitement, stress and insomnia. It is often popular with children because of its gentle action and familiar orangey aroma.

safety
• No known contraindications in normal aromatherapy use.

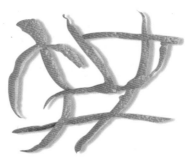

△ *Citrus reticulata* –
mandarin

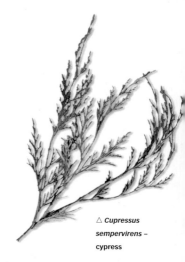

△ *Cupressus*
sempervirens –
cypress

Cupressus sempervirens – cypress
family *Cupressaceae*

properties
antibacterial, anti-infectious, antispasmodic, antisudorific, antitussive, astringent, calming, deodorant, diuretic, hormone-like, neurotonic, phlebotonic, styptic

Cypress oil is distilled from the leaves, cones and twigs of the cypress tree. *Sempervirens* is Latin for evergreen, and the resinous wood of this ancient tree has long been used as an aromatic.

The astringent action of cypress oil helps to regulate the production of sebum, reduce perspiration (even of the feet) and to staunch bleeding. It is reputed to help calm the mind where grief is present, and to induce sleep.

safety
• No known contraindications in normal aromatherapy use.

Eucalyptus smithii – eucalyptus
family *Myrtaceae*

properties

analgesic, anticatarrhal, anti-infectious, antiviral, balancing, decongestant, digestive stimulant, expectorant, prophylactic

Known as gully gum, this tree is native to Australia. The oil distilled from its leaves is equally beneficial to, and much gentler than, the more common *Eucalyptus globulus*, or blue gum, which needs care in use. Because of its gentle action, gully gum eucalyptus is ideal for children; its aroma is also not as piercing as blue gum eucalyptus, which is usually rectified to increase its cineole content.

Eucalyptus is good for muscular pain and is effective against coughs and colds, both as a preventive and as a remedy. *E. smithii* oil has great synergistic power.

safety

• No known contraindications in normal aromatherapy use.
• Keep to the recommended dilution when using as an inhalant for children.

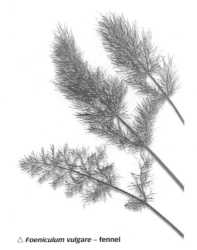

△ **Foeniculum vulgare – fennel**

Foeniculum vulgare – fennel
family *Apiaceae* (or *Umbelliferae*)

properties

analgesic, antibacterial, antifungal, anti-inflammatory, antiseptic, antispasmodic, cardiotonic, carminative, decongestant, digestive, diuretic, emmenagogic, lactogenic, laxative, litholytic, oestrogen-like, respiratory tonic

Fennel is widely grown in the Mediterranean area and the essential oil is distilled from its seeds. The delicate flower heads of all this family resemble umbrellas, as indicated by the original family name, *Umbelliferae*.

Fennel is recommended for lack of breast milk and because it is oestrogen-like, it can be valuable for PMS, the menopause and ovary problems. It will also work efficiently as a diuretic.

safety

• Safe in normal aromatherapy amounts.
• Should not be used during pregnancy before the seventh month.

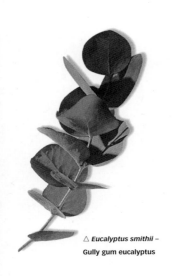

△ **Eucalyptus smithii –
Gully gum eucalyptus**

Juniperus communis – juniper
family *Cupressaceae*

properties

analgesic, antidiabetic, antiseptic, depurative, digestive tonic, diuretic, litholytic, sleep-inducing

The juniper tree is a small evergreen from the same family as cypress. The essential oil, distilled from the dried ripe berries (and sometimes the twigs and leaves), has a sweet fragrant aroma. Take care when buying juniper oil, as the berries are used to flavour gin and the residue is often distilled to produce a poor quality essential oil. Even genuine juniper oil can be frequently adulterated.

Juniper oil has a strong diuretic action which is useful for treating cystitis, water retention and cellulite. It has a cleansing, detoxifying action on the skin, and is useful for oily skin problems, such as acne. It is especially good for feelings of guilt and jealousy, and for giving strength when feeling emotionally drained.

safety

• No known contraindications in normal aromatherapy use.
• May be neurotoxic if used without due care and attention.

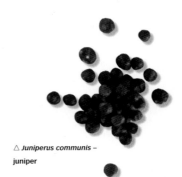

△ **Juniperus communis –
juniper**

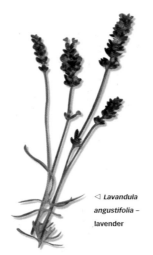

◁ *Lavandula*
angustifolia –
lavender

Lavandula angustifolia – lavender
family *Lamiaceae*

properties
analgesic, antibacterial, antifungal, anti-inflammatory, antiseptic, antispasmodic, calming and sedative, cardiotonic, carminative, cicatrizant, emmenagogic, hypotensive, tonic

Lavender is the most widely used aromatherapy oil. It is obtained from the plant's flowering tops, and grows wild throughout the Mediterranean region, although it is now cultivated worldwide. In spite of this, it is not easy to find a quality oil. Lavandin, a cheaper oil from a hybrid plant, is often substituted for true lavender.

Lavender is a skin rejuvenator, and helps to normalize both dry and greasy skins. It works in combination with other oils to alleviate arthritis and rheumatism, psoriasis and eczema. It aids sleep, relieves tension headaches, and is good for calming nerves, lifting depression, relieving anger, and soothing fear and grief.

safety
• No known contraindications in normal aromatherapy use.

Matricaria recutica – chamomile, German
family *Asteraceae*

properties
antiallergic, antifungal, anti-inflammatory, antispasmodic, cicatrizant, decongestant, digestive tonic, hormone-like

German chamomile, an annual herb, grows naturally in Europe and its small white flowers are widely used in teas and infusions to aid relaxation and induce sleep. When the flowers are distilled a deep blue oil is produced. The blue colour is produced by the presence of chamazulene, a chemical not present in the plant but formed during the distillation process.

Chamazulene, in synergy with the other components of the oil, is a strong anti-inflammatory agent, which is especially useful for skin problems (particularly irritated skin) and rheumatism, when a compress is most effective. The oil is recommended for premenstrual syndrome, and for calming anger and agitated emotional states.

safety
• No known contraindications in normal aromatherapy use.

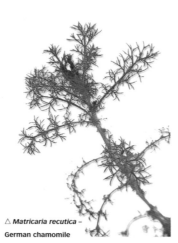

△ *Matricaria recutica –*
German chamomile

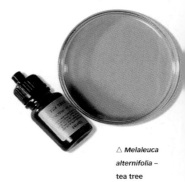

△ *Melaleuca*
alternifolia –
tea tree

Melaleuca alternifolia – tea tree
family *Myrtaceae*

properties
analgesic, antibacterial, antifungal, anti-infectious, anti-inflammatory, antiparasitic, antiviral, immunostimulant, neurotonic, phlebotonic

The tea tree plant is native to Australia. Traditionally, a type of herbal tea is prepared from its leaves, and the oil has long been recognized by the Australian Aborigines for its powerful medicinal properties.

Essential oil of tea tree has strong antiseptic properties with a matching aroma, and has excellent antimicrobial and antifungal action. It is a powerful stimulant to the immune system. The unadulterated essential oil has been found to be non-toxic and non-irritating to the skin, and is one of the few essential oils that can be applied directly and undiluted on the skin and all mucous surfaces. The antifungal activity of tea tree oil is much used against *Candida albicans*. It is also effective against some viruses, such as enteritis.

safety
• No known contraindications in normal aromatherapy use.

Melaleuca viridiflora – niaouli
family *Myrtaceae*

properties

analgesic, antibacterial, anticatarrhal, anti-infectious, anti-inflammatory, antiparasitic, antipruritic, antirheumatic, antiseptic, antiviral, digestive, expectorant, febrifuge, hormone-like, hypotensive, immunostimulant, litholytic, phlebotonic, skin tonic

Niaouli trees originate from the region of Gomene in the South Pacific island of New Caledonia, hence "gomenol" became an alternative name. The trees are large with a bushy foliage and yellow flowers. The steam-distilled leaves and young stems yield an essential oil, which has a eucalyptus-type aroma. The majority of the oil is produced in Australia and Tasmania and very little is exported, making the genuine oil hard to find.

Niaouli is useful for a range of problems experienced by women. It is also a powerful antiseptic and anti-inflammatory agent, and is effective for respiratory problems, such as bronchitis and colds. Its properties suggest it will help against grief and anger.

safety

• No known contraindications, but pregnant women and children should use with care.

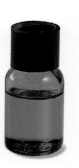

◁ *Melaleuca viridiflora –* niaouli

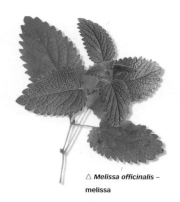

△ *Melissa officinalis –* melissa

Melissa officinalis – melissa
family *Lamiaceae*

properties

anti-inflammatory, antispasmodic, antiviral, calming and sedative, choleretic, digestive, hypotensive, sedative, capillary dilator

Melissa, also known as lemon balm, is a small herb with tiny, white flowers originating from southern Europe. A daily drink of tea prepared from the fresh leaves is supposed to encourage longevity. The distilled yield from the leaves is tiny, making it a very expensive oil. Much of the melissa oil sold commercially is blended with cheaper essential oils and achieves a similar aroma.

Melissa's sedative action relieves headaches and insomnia and is particularly beneficial for a problematic menstrual cycle. It is also a tonic for the heart, calming the turbulent emotions of grief and anger and helping to relieve fear.

safety

• Photosensitizer. Do not expose the skin to sunlight or a sunbed for two hours after using.
• It is difficult to obtain pure melissa oil, and many fakes contain skin irritants.
• No known contraindications in normal aromatherapy use.

Mentha piperita – peppermint
family *Lamiaceae*

properties

analgesic, antibacterial, antifungal, anti-inflammatory, antimigraine, antilactogenic, antipyretic, antispasmodic, antiviral, carminative, decongestant, digestive, expectorant, liver stimulant, hormone-like, hypotensive, insect repellent, mucolytic, neurotonic, reproductive stimulant, soothing, uterotonic

The peppermint plant has dark green leaves from which its essential oil is distilled. The oil has a strong, refreshing aroma and is used extensively in the food and pharmaceutical industries, particularly for toothpaste, chewing gum and drinks.

Peppermint is renowned not only for its beneficial effect with digestive problems, such as indigestion, nausea, travel sickness and diarrhoea, but also for respiratory problems. It can help to clear congestion or catarrh and is useful for bronchitis, bronchial asthma, sinusitis and colds. It helps to clear the mind, and will aid concentration and overcome mental fatigue and depression. It is also useful against anger, guilt and apathy. This is a good essential oil to keep to hand in the first aid cabinet.

safety

• Use sparingly and keep to recommended dilution.
• May counteract homeopathic remedies.

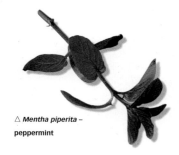

△ *Mentha piperita –* peppermint

Ocimum basilicum var. album – basil
family Lamiaceae

properties
analgesic, antibacterial, antifungal, anti-inflammatory, antiseptic, antispasmodic, antiviral, cardiotonic, carminative, digestive tonic, nervous system regulator, neurotonic, reproductive decongestant

Basil oil has a distinctive aroma and is distilled from the whole plant. Several varieties of basil, with different chemical composition, grow in warm Mediterranean climes (especially France and Italy), with leaves that vary in both size and colour, from green to a deep purplish red. The preferred variety for aromatherapy is *album*, as it is not likely to have a neurotoxic effect.

    Basil is known mainly for its effect on the nervous system. It is a good tonic and stimulant and is helpful in coping with unwanted emotions, such as fear and jealousy. Its analgesic property makes it useful in cases of arthritis. It is also good for muscle cramp. Basil is an effective insect repellent, particularly against house flies and mosquitoes.

safety
• No known contraindications in normal aromatherapy use.
• May be neurotoxic if used without due care and attention.

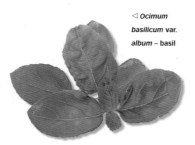

◁ **Ocimum basilicum var. album** – basil

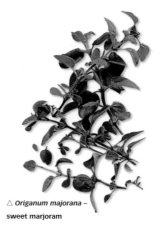

△ **Origanum majorana** – sweet marjoram

Origanum majorana – sweet marjoram
family Lamiaceae

properties
analgesic, antibacterial, anti-infectious, antispasmodic, calming, digestive stimulant, diuretic, expectorant, hormone-like, hypotensive, neurotonic, respiratory tonic, stomachic, vasodilator

Sweet marjoram is a popular culinary herb and has a reputation for promoting long life. The plant grows in the Mediterranean regions and has tiny, white or pink flowers: the oil is distilled from the plant's leaves and flowers. Sweet marjoram should not be confused with the sharp-smelling Spanish marjoram (*Thymus mastichina*), which is a species of thyme.

    Sweet marjoram has been shown to be antiviral and is useful for cold sores. It can ease tension and irritability, lift headaches (especially those connected with menstruation) and promote sleep. It is useful for grief and anger, and its ability to calm and uplift makes it useful to combat moodiness.

safety
• No known contraindications in normal aromatherapy use.

Pelargonium graveolens – geranium
family Geraniaceae

properties
analgesic, antibacterial, antidiabetic, antifungal, anti-infectious, anti-inflammatory, antiseptic, antispasmodic, astringent, cicatrizant, decongestant, digestive stimulant, haemostatic, styptic, insect repellent, phlebotonic, relaxant

The geranium plant is cultivated in Egypt, Morocco, the Reunion Islands and China. The oil is distilled from the aromatic leaves, the aroma of which depends on the variety of the plant and where it is grown. Some geranium oils have a definite rose-like smell and are often referred to as rose geranium. More correctly, rose geranium is when a tiny percentage of rose otto is added to the geranium oil.

    Geranium will reduce inflammation and is good for acne, herpes, diarrhoea and varicose veins. It is also a relaxant, and will help grief and anger. It is useful for general moodiness and to balance the mood swings associated with PMS.

safety
• No known contraindications in normal aromatherapy use.

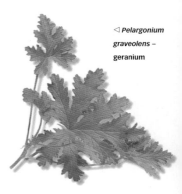

◁ **Pelargonium graveolens** – geranium

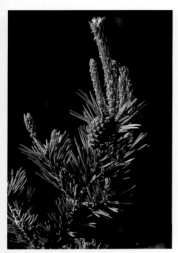

△ *Pinus sylvestris* – pine

Pinus sylvestris – pine
family *Pinaceae*

properties
analgesic, antibacterial, antifungal, anti-infectious, anti-inflammatory, antisudorific, balsamic, decongestant, expectorant, hormone-like, hypotensive, litholytic, neurotonic, rubefacient

Pine-needle essential oil has a warm, resin-like aroma and is distilled from the Scots-pine tree, which grows widely throughout Europe and Russia.

Pine is an excellent disinfectant and air-freshener: when dispersed in the air, its antiseptic qualities help to prevent the spread of infections. It is recommended for respiratory tract infections and hay fever, while its anti-inflammatory action makes it useful for cystitis and rheumatism. Pine is an excellent pick-me-up for general debility and lack of energy, and is said to dispel melancholy and pessimism.

safety
• No known contraindications in normal aromatherapy use.

Pogostemon patchouli – patchouli
family *Lamiaceae*

properties
antifungal, anti-infectious, anti-inflammatory, aphrodisiac, cicatrizant, decongestant, immunostimulant, insect repellent, phlebotonic

The plant grows mainly in East Asia and its essential oil has a soft, balsamic aroma. The leaves are cut every few months as the newest ones yield the most oil. Patchouli oil improves with age and has a musty, exotic aroma that is very penetrating.

Patchouli is particularly valuable for broken, chapped and cracked skin, as well as inflamed skin, eczema and acne. It promotes the growth of new skin cells, which makes it helpful in reducing scar tissue. It is beneficial against haemorrhoids and varicose veins. It has a sedative effect on the emotions; its anti-inflammatory property helps calm anger and its antifungal property is useful for jealousy. It is said to help soothe an overactive mind.

safety
• No known contraindications in normal aromatherapy use.

▷ *Pogostemon patchouli* – patchouli

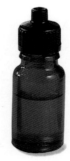

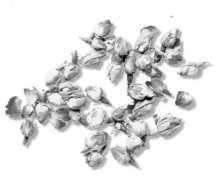

△ *Rosa damascena* – rose otto

Rosa damascena – rose otto
family *Rosaceae*

properties
antibacterial, anti-infectious, anti-inflammatory, astringent, cicatrizant, neurotonic, sexual tonic, styptic

The much-prized rose otto, also known as attar of roses, is distilled from the deep pink rose petals of this flowering shrub. The genuine, pure oil is extremely expensive as the petals contain very little oil. Roses for distillation are cultivated chiefly in Bulgaria, Turkey and Morocco. Rose absolute is extracted from the petals by a different process, and is a cheaper oil.

Rose otto has been favoured by women through the ages for its gentle action and fragrant aroma. It is said that rose otto balances the hormones and that it is helpful for irregular periods. Rose soothes the skin, lifts depression, and calms inflamed emotions, promoting feelings of happiness and well-being.

safety
• No known contraindications in normal aromatherapy use.

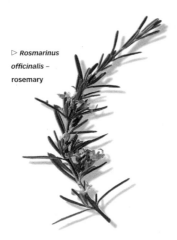

▷ *Rosmarinus officinalis* – rosemary

Rosmarinus officinalis – rosemary
family *Lamiaceae*

properties

analgesic, antibacterial, antifungal, anti-infectious, anti-inflammatory, antispasmodic, antitussive, antiviral, cardiotonic, carminative, choleretic, cicatrizant, venous decongestant, detoxicant, digestive, diuretic, emmenagogic, hyperglycaemic, blood pressure regulator, litholytic, cholesterol-reducing, mucolytic, neuromuscular effect, neurotonic, sexual tonic, stimulant

Native to the Mediterranean region, rosemary has a long history of culinary and medicinal use. This oil, with an impressive list of helpful properties, is obtained from the pale-blue flowers of the aromatic plant.

Rosemary is helpful for respiratory problems, arthritis, congestive headaches and constipation. It is also a tonic for the liver. This oil stimulates both body and mind. It lifts depression, clears the mind, and is an excellent memory aid.

safety
No known contraindications in normal aromatherapy use.

Salvia sclarea – clary sage
family *Lamiaceae*

properties
antifungal, anti-infectious, antispasmodic, antisudorific, decongestant, detoxicant, oestrogen-like, neurotonic, phlebotonic, regenerative

The strong smelling essential oil of clary sage is distilled from the dried clary sage plant and is used in eau-de-cologne, lavender water, muscatel wines and vermouth. It should not be confused with sage oil and is not a substitute for it.

Clary sage is excellent for all menstrual complications; its oestrogen-like qualities make it good for hormonal problems. It encourages menstruation and is useful for the hot flushes of the menopause. Clary sage is helpful for depression and fear, and during general convalescence.

Safety
• No known contraindications in normal aromatherapy use.
• Prolonged inhalation may cause drowsiness.
• Avoid alcohol consumption for a few hours before or after use.

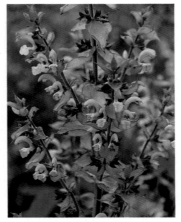

△ *Salvia sclarea* – clary sage

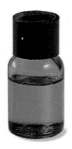

▷ *Santalum album* – sandalwood

Santalum album – sandalwood
family *Santalaceae*

properties
anti-infectious, astringent, cardiotonic, decongestant, diuretic, moisturizing, nerve relaxant, sedative, tonic

The sandalwood tree is native to India, and its cultivation is controlled by the government of that country – for each tree felled, another is planted. The offcuts and wood chips from the sandalwood furniture industry in India, together with the tree roots, are distilled to obtain the essential oil. The sweet, woody aroma of the oil has a soft and therapeutic effect.

Sandalwood, although a gentle oil, is important in the treatment of genito-urinary infections, especially cystisis. It is used for its effect on the digestive system, relieving heartburn and nausea, including morning sickness. It has been found to benefit both acne and dry skin (including dry eczema), as well as being useful for haemorrhoids and varicose veins. Its tonic properties are thought to be helpful in cases of impotence. Sandalwood can also be useful against fear.

Safety
• No known contraindications in normal aromatherapy use.

Thymus vulgaris – thyme, sweet
family *Lamiaceae*

properties
antifungal, anti-infectious, anti-inflammatory, antiseptic, antispasmodic, antiviral, diuretic, immunostimulant, neurotonic, sexual tonic, uterotonic

Thyme is native to the Mediterranean region and is a well-known culinary herb. The essential oil is distilled from its leaves and tiny purplish flowers. There are many different varieties of thyme oil, some of which need careful handling. The alcohol chemotypes of thyme (linalool and geraniol) are the safest for general use.

Sweet thyme is useful for respiratory problems, infections, and digestive complaints. It is especially helpful for insomnia of nervous origin. Sweet thyme is a safe, uterotonic oil to use towards the end of pregnancy and during labour, and it is known to facilitate delivery.

safety
• No known contraindications in normal aromatherapy use.

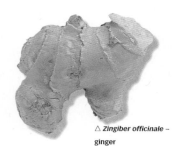
△ *Zingiber officinale* – ginger

Zingiber officinale – ginger
family *Zingiberaceae*

properties
analgesic, anticatarrhal, carminative, digestive stimulant, expectorant, general tonic, sexual tonic, stomachic

This perennial herb is native to the tropical parts of Asia. The root, which is used in cooking, is renowned for its heat and for its digestive properties. Its yellow oil is distilled from the roots and, although it has a spicy aroma, the heat does not come through into the essential oil during distillation.

Ginger essential oil has properties which alleviate most digestive problems, including flatulence, constipation, nausea and loss of appetite. Its ability to dull pain is beneficial to muscular pain and sciatica, while its tonic properties are useful for emotions like fear and apathy, and will also help to draw out a reticent, withdrawn personality.

safety
• No known contraindications in normal aromatherapy use.

Special essential oils

Myristica fragrans – nutmeg
Pimpinella anisum – aniseed
Salvia officinalis – sage
Syzygium aromaticum – clove bud

There are some highly beneficial, but very powerful oils which are recommended in this book for special use only. These are used in pregnancy to facilitate delivery. However, their use is not advised without training in aromatherapy or aromatic medicine.

safety
• These oils must only be used in the manner and amounts advised.
• Always seek advice from a qualified aromatherapist before home use.

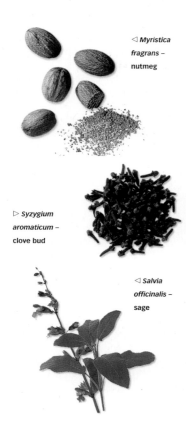
◁ *Myristica fragrans* – nutmeg

▷ *Syzygium aromaticum* – clove bud

◁ *Salvia officinalis* – sage

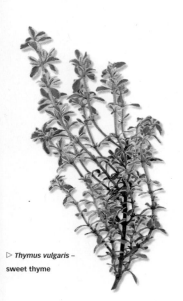
▷ *Thymus vulgaris* – sweet thyme

Using inhalations and baths

Essential oils are rarely used in their original, concentrated form but are always taken into the body via a carrier substance. This can be anything which takes the oils into the body: air, water, vegetable oils, lotions and creams are all carriers.

inhalation

When we breathe in the fragrance of an essential oil, some of its molecules travel to the lungs, pass through the lining and into the bloodstream, where they travel around the body. Other molecules take an upward route to the brain, which receives a healing message – to relax or energize, for example – and transmits the appropriate signal along the nerve channels of the body.

Inhalation is the quickest way for oils to enter the body, and is the most effective way to deal with fragile emotions, and negative states of mind such as stress and depression. It is very useful for respiratory conditions, especially those that may present an emergency situation, such as bronchitis or asthma. Although essential oils may be inhaled directly from the bottle, other methods are preferred.

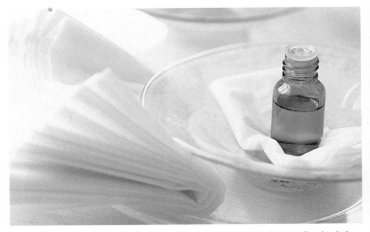

△ A few drops of lavender oil, added to a tissue and sniffed throughout the day, can relieve headaches.

the hands

This method is useful for emergencies. Put one drop of essential oil into your palm and rub your hands briefly together. Now cup your hands over your nose, avoiding the eye area, and take a deep breath.

a tissue

Place a few drops of essential oil on to a tissue and take three deep breaths. The tissue can then be placed on your pillow or inside your shirt, so that you will continue to benefit from the oil's aroma.

steam inhalation

Fill a basin with hot water and add no more than 2–3 drops (use 1–2 drops for children and the elderly) of essential oil. Keeping your eyes closed to protect them from the powerful vapours, lower your head over the bowl and breathe in deeply.

a vaporizer

This is one of the most popular methods of all for oil inhalation. Electric vaporizers are available, and are the safest types to use. Night-light vaporizers (or oil burners) are inexpensive and readily available in different sizes and designs. The basic model involves a night-light candle standing under a tiny

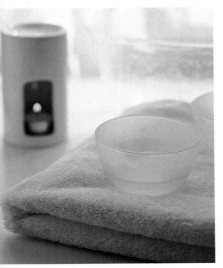

◁ Using an oil burner is a popular way of vaporizing essential oils. Keep enough water in the top to stop it drying out.

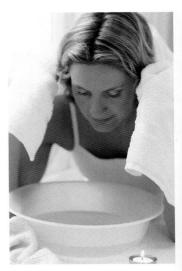

▷ A steam inhalation using eucalyptus oil can help to relieve head colds and sinus congestion.

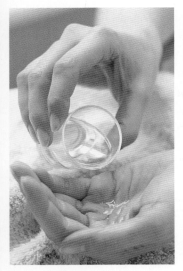

△ **Dry skin will benefit from an essential oil mix: it is best massaged on to your body after a bath.**

cup filled with water, to which a few drops of oil are added. Keep the vaporizer out of the reach of children and pets. Top up the water and add more oils as necessary.

Use a vaporizer to keep infections at bay, to relax after a stressful day, or to set the mood for a party or a romantic evening. The number of oil drops is not critical and really depends on the size of the room.

safety

• The quantities of essential oils given above for inhalations are suitable for children and the elderly unless otherwise stated.

bathing

Essential oils do not dissolve well in water, and it is important that the molecules are evenly distributed. Bathing can enhance the effects of essential oils: the oils are not only absorbed through the skin but their aroma is also inhaled. There are several ways to enjoy bathing with essential oils.

bath

Run the water in the bath to a comfortable temperature. Next, add 6–8 drops of oil, then swish the water thoroughly to disperse

▷ **Pamper yourself and unwind with a relaxing aromatherapy bath at the end of a tiring day.**

the oil. Sit in the bath, and for maximum benefit, stay in the water for at least ten minutes to allow the oil to penetrate your skin and to enjoy the benefits of its aroma.

If you prefer, the oils can be mixed with 15ml (1 tbsp) dairy cream or honey before being added to the bath. This will help to disperse the oils. Alternatively, you can mix the oils into powdered milk, adding water to make a paste, before adding the mixture to the bath water. Bath oil prepared from vegetable oil and mixed with essential oils is fine for dry skin, but will feel greasy on normal skins.

foot and hand bath

For sprains, localized swelling, bruising, or similar general discomforts, ten minutes in a foot or hand bath containing 6–8 drops of your chosen oils will bring welcome relief. Remember to keep a kettle of warm water nearby to add to the water in the bowl before it cools too much for comfort.

sitz–bath

For vaginal thrush, a sitz–bath with essential oils is an effective treatment. Fill a large bowl one-third full with warm water and add 3–4 drops of your chosen oil. Sit in the bath for ten minutes.

showers

It is not as easy to benefit from essential oils in the shower. However, you can add some oils to your shower gel or put some on to a sponge. Rub this over your body in the shower, or before you get into it. Make the most of the aroma, breathing deeply and rubbing with your sponge or hands while slowly rinsing. If you wash off the oils too quickly, you won't feel the benefit. Finish with a body lotion mixed with an oil.

safety

• For children and the elderly the essential oil quantities should be halved.

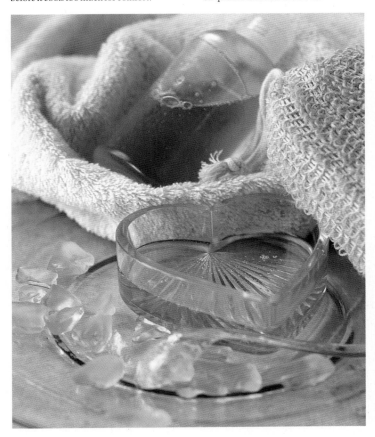

Using compresses, gargles and drinks

Further effective ways of carrying essential oils into the body, using water as the carrier, are with compresses, gargles, mouthwashes and drinks. For the latter, it is important that the essential oils used, and the number of drops, are exactly as recommended.

compresses

A compress brings effective relief in cases such as insect bites, arthritic joints, period or stomach pain, headache, sprains and varicose veins. Use a cold compress if there is inflammation and/or heat, and a warm compress if there is pain or a dull ache.

To make the compress, you need a piece of clean material and a container of water. Soft cotton or linen are the best materials to

▽ A compress is a simple way to use essential oils, and the result can be very soothing.

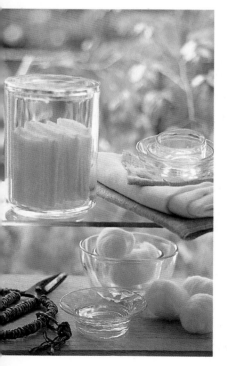

use. The container should be big enough to hold just enough water to soak into the compress: for example, an egg cup will be big enough for a finger compress, and a small bowl is suitable for an abdomen compress. Add your chosen essential oils to the water: 2 drops of oil is enough for a finger compress, and up to 8 drops of oil is enough for larger body compresses.

Stir the water in the container to disperse the essential oils, then gently lower the compress material on top to allow it to absorb the oils. When the material is wet, squeeze it lightly, position it on the area to be treated, and cover with clear film (plastic wrap) to hold it firmly in place.

For a cold compress, place a sealed, plastic bag of frozen peas or crushed ice cubes over the treatment area and hold in place. For a warm compress, wrap a strip of material such as a scarf, thermal garment or a small towel around the cling film. To keep a compress in place on an arm or leg, an old sock or pair of tights is ideal. Leave the compress in place for at least an hour, or overnight for a septic wound.

gargles and mouthwashes

For sore throats, voice loss and colds which may go on to the chest, gargling with one or more essential oils can be very helpful. Put 2–3 drops of antibacterial essential oils into a glass and half-fill with water. A drop of a soothing oil can also be added. Stir well, take a mouthful, gargle and spit out. Stir again and repeat. It is important to stir the mixture before each mouthful so as to redisperse the oils. Gargling should be done twice a day for best results.

The procedure for mouthwashes is the same as for gargling, except that the liquid is swished around inside the mouth (rather than at the back of the throat) for 30 seconds before spitting out.

▷ Adding a few drops of an antibacterial oil to a glass of water makes an effective gargle mix.

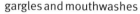

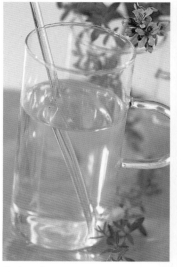

△ When using a mouthwash, make sure the oils are well stirred in the water before each sip.

safety
• For children and the elderly the essential oil quantities should be halved.

drinks

To use essential oils in drinks, the oils must be organic and mixed in a suitable carrier.

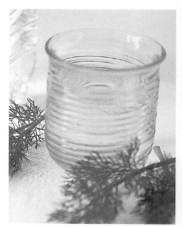

> Organic plants are grown without the use of chemicals. When taking oils internally, it is important to use only those of therapeutic and certified organic quality.

You are advised first to consult a qualified aromatologist or an aromatherapist working alongside a medical doctor. If you wish to use essential oils in water or tea at home without taking professional advice, it is imperative that the essential oils, and the dosage and time scales recommended in this book are strictly adhered to.

water

Drinking plenty of water is good for us. If you are not fond of water as a drink, put 2 drops of an essential oil such as lemon or orange into 1 litre (1¾ pints) of water in a bottle and shake well. For a healthy digestive system, use 1 drop each of peppermint and fennel oil and mix as before. Shake the bottle before drinking. In conjunction with healthy eating habits, 1 drop each of grapefruit and/or cypress, used as before, can help weight loss as part of a slimming and exercise programme.

teas

Only aromatologists are able to prescribe essential oils for internal, medicinal use. Tea is not a medicine, however, but a pleasant drink. If the tea tastes too strong when the oils are added, dilute it with more water.

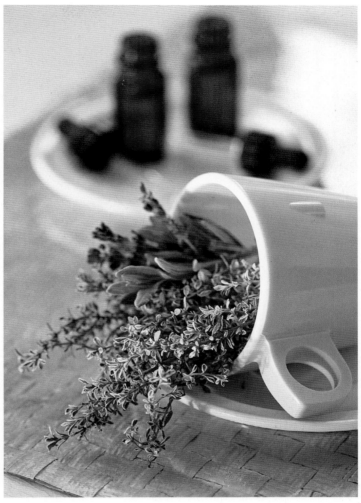

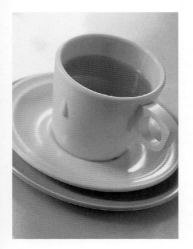

Tannin-free china tea or rooibos (red bush) tea make the best bases. Put 2–3 drops of essential oil on to the tea leaves or tea bag, add 1 litre (1¾ pints) of hot water, stir well, then remove the tea leaves or bag. The tea will taste better without milk. Never pour essential oil directly into tea: it will be too strong, and the oils will not disperse. Any tea not drunk immediately can be stored in the fridge and reheated as necessary.

For digestive disorders, a cup of tea drunk two or three times a day is a very gentle and effective remedy. Common

◁ Teas made with essential oils can be a pleasant way of enjoying the healing properties of plants.

urinary tract problems, such as cystitis, respond well, as do insomnia and pain from arthritic joints.

safety

• Use only organic essential oils of therapeutic quality for adding to drinks.
• Absolutes or resins should never be ingested.
• These methods should not be used on children, but are suitable for the elderly.
• Never put essential oils directly into a cup of tea or glass of water. Otherwise, the drink will taste far too strong and will be very unpleasant. The oils should be used only by the methods stated.

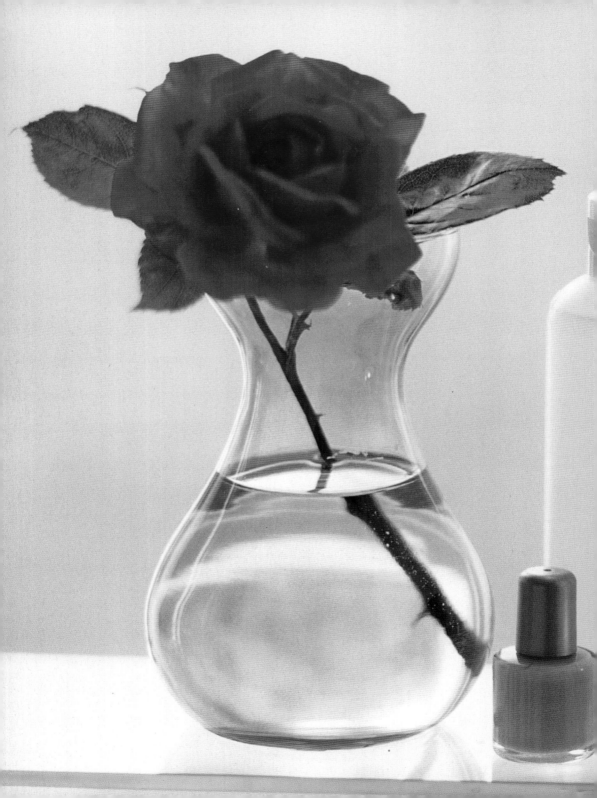

Aromatherapy Routines

Aromatherapy can be used in a wide range of gentle, simple applications – from drinks, gargles, baths and compresses to inhalation and massage. Essential oils are perfect for many beauty treatments for the face, body, hair and nails, and suitable oils can be found for all skin types and conditions. Within this chapter there are also special routines for using aromatherapy during pregnancy.

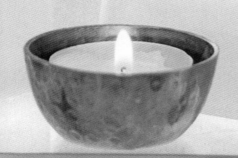

Daily skincare

The sooner a woman begins a good skincare routine, the more she will reap the benefits as she gets older. A good moisturizer is arguably the most important item in a woman's wardrobe – you can replace your clothes, but not your skin. It is well worth investing in an efficient, quality moisturizer that you like to use.

There is a vast array of commercial products available, designed for every skin permutation imaginable: teenage, normal, dry, oily, mature, sensitive, and allergy-prone skins. Although well-formulated cosmetics without essential oils may benefit the skin, a natural, quality range with added essential oils will increase the benefits.

choosing products

With aromatherapy, you should only have to choose between two basic product types because all essential oils are normalizing,

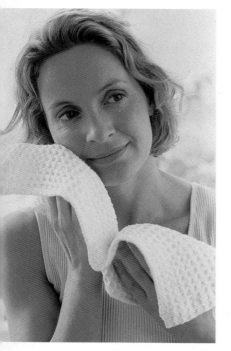

giving exceptional care to the skin. If the skin is normal to oily, then look for a cleansing milk and moisturizing *lotion*. Choose cleansing and moisturizing *creams* when the skin is more dry and in need of nourishment. Look for products which have good quality bases and which don't contain alcohol, lanolin or other animal products. Night creams containing lanolin make your skin greasy, as the molecules are actually too big to penetrate the skin, and the cream will "sit" on top of your face all night, rubbing off on the pillow. Prepare your products with well chosen essential oils in a concentration of 0.5 per cent.

tips for healthy skin

If you wear make-up, it is important to cleanse your skin thoroughly before bed. In the morning, toner on cotton wool (cotton ball) is usually sufficient. Give yourself a treatment mask once a week. After a mask, you should moisturize twice, as masks draw out moisture as well as toxins. If you don't wear any make-up, a mask once a fortnight is usually sufficient.

If you don't wear make-up, use a mild toner only at night-time after cleansing. Moisturize first thing in the morning, after cleansing and toning.

creating your own products

To make your own skincare products, use unperfumed bases, adding the appropriate essential oils, 1 drop for each 10ml (2 tsp) of carrier. Cold spring water is an excellent basic toner.

oily skin or acne

daytime base lotion with 10 per cent spring water added slowly while stirring.
night-time base lotion with 10 per cent hazelnut oil added slowly while stirring.

◁ **Always pat your face dry with a soft towel after rinsing. The skin on the face needs careful handling, whatever our age.**

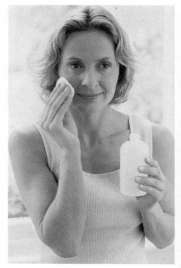

△ **Spring water can be used as a basic toner for all types of skin. Add your chosen essential oils.**

dry or mature skin

daytime base lotion with 25 per cent rose hip or jojoba oils added slowly while stirring.
night-time base cream with 50 per cent rose hip or jojoba, or the macerated oils of lime blossom or melissa added while stirring.

at the menopause

Try using hormone-like essential oils such as clary sage and niaouli which both have oestrogen-like properties.

skin disorders

A skin problem can arise from many causes, some of which may be more obvious than others. It may stem from an internal physical problem, such as poor digestion or painful periods, or from a mental problem, such as deep-rooted anxiety or grief. The effects of on-going mental and emotional stress can also cause skin problems, which in turn may aggravate the condition as we become worried, anxious and embarrassed about how others see us.

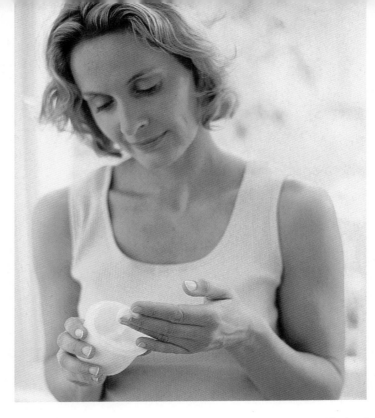

▷ Roman chamomile is excellent for soothing dry, irritable and inflamed skin. Try adding a few drops to your moisturizer and apply daily.

aromatherapy treatment

Aromatherapy can play an important part in the treatment of skin disorders. The oils are not only able to treat the physical symptoms but, through their aromas, can also affect the mental state of the sufferer. For example, many people suffering chronic, painful skin conditions, such as eczema and psoriasis, may have high stress levels because of the impact of the disease on their physical appearance.

Essential oils are able to break this cycle effectively, lightening the mind as well as tackling the physical symptoms. Where the skin is already being moisturized, whether on the face, hands and/or body, it is easy enough to combine appropriate essential oils with the existing treatment for a two-in-one effect. For example, arthritis oils added to a hand and body lotion base reduce pain and inflammation at the same time as making the skin less dry and scaly.

For severe eczema it is very beneficial to change your diet to one that is dairy-free, eliminating cow's milk and related products from what you eat. This is usually enough to cure the condition, although it can take a few months for the results to be evident. Meanwhile, correct use of the appropriate oils will bring relief from the symptoms.

Acne rosacea, a form of acne which usually attacks women over 30, has similar symptoms to *Acne vulgaris*. It seems to affect women who like highly seasoned foods and drink large amounts of tea and coffee. Dietary changes will be highly beneficial in all cases, while the use of aromatherapy treatments will improve the condition of the skin.

Blending essential oils with a moisturizer

For customized skincare, select the appropriate essential oils and add them to a good quality, bland base cream. Add a little rose hip carrier oil if your skin is particularly dry.

ingredients
• 40ml (8 tsp) unperfumed base cream
• rose hip oil (optional)
• blend of appropriate essential oils

equipment
• small jar
• swizzle stick or teaspoon
• spatula (optional)

tip

Always apply creams to the face with clean hands, and best of all using a spatula, to avoid transmitting germs from your fingernails to the cream, and possibly to your skin.

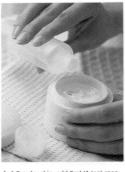

△ **1** For dry skin, add 5ml (1 tsp) rose hip oil to a jar containing 40ml (8 tsp) base moisturizing cream.

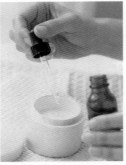

△ **2** After blending your own selection of appropriate essential oils, add 5 drops to the moisturizing cream.

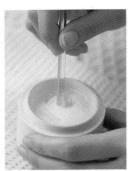

△ **3** Stir thoroughly with a swizzle stick or the handle of a clean teaspoon to blend the mixture.

Beauty basics

Looking good starts with great skin, and aromatherapy can help you achieve this in various ways: the remarkable penetrative properties of essential oils make them excellent moisturizers, and the wide range of their properties means there is always the right oil for the right condition. For instance, rosemary stimulates the circulation and thyme helps the cells to regenerate. As well as stimulating the lymphatic system, which helps cleanse the tissue that causes sluggish skin, essential oils can be used as part of your daily skincare routine and to treat specific problems such as acne.

feed your skin

Skin needs to be fed and nourished – inside and out. Healthy diets can keep the body in shape but to keep skin in peak condition it needs to have a ready supply of valuable vitamins and minerals. Many factors can drain the body of this valuable resource – canned and over-processed foods, caffeine, alcohol, nicotine, sunlight, central heating, carbon monoxide and habitual drug taking. The effects of these can build up and attack the skin so from time to time you need to give it a break.

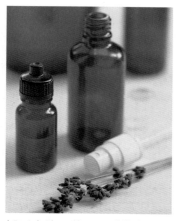

△ Empty bottles and jars are available from most aromatherapy suppliers.

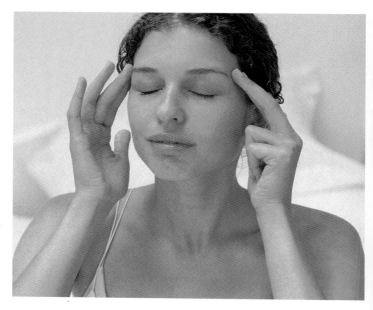

△ Combine your daily cleansing routine with a gentle face massage to stimulate the lymph flow and help remove toxins.

skin types

Choose the right oils for your skin type and use them to blend your own cleansers, toners, masks and moisturizing facial oils. Remember that skin types can vary: skin may be drier in winter or summer, or more prone to oiliness around the time of your period, and it can change several times between puberty and menopause. So review the oils you use to suit your skin now and vary them to meet the changing needs of your complexion.

Few people are blessed with normal skin and even those who are may tend towards dryness or oiliness at times. Letters in parentheses indicate what other skin types an oil is suitable for. D = dry, S = sensitive, O = oily, A = all skin types.

oils for normal skin

Chamomile (D, S) • Fennel (O) • Geranium (A) • Lavender (A) • Lemon (O) • Patchouli (D) • Rose (D, S) • Sandalwood (D, S)

oils for dry skin

Chamomile • Geranium • Hyssop • Lavender • Patchouli • Rose • Sandalwood •Ylang ylang

oils for sensitive skin

Chamomile • Lavender • Neroli • Rose • Sandalwood

oils for oily skin

Bergamot • Cedarwood • Cypress • Lavender • Lemon • Geranium • Juniper • Frankincense • Sage

combination skin has an oily T-zone panel from the forehead down to the nose and chin area, and may be normal or even dry elsewhere. Prepare your skin treatments accordingly, using oils for oily skin on the greasy patches and oils for normal or dry skin on the rest of the face area.

cleansers

Choose the correct essential oils for your skin type from the list above and blend them in with an ordinary unperfumed brand of cleanser, liquid soap, or tissue-off lotion/cream, and they will do nature's work of rebalancing the skin.

facial steam

Add five drops of chamomile for a soothing steam or try lavender, peppermint, thyme or rosemary to stimulate; comfrey or fennel for their healing properties.

toners

Essential oils are the gentlest way of toning up. Rose water for normal or dry/sensitive skin or witchhazel for oilier skins are ideal bases for fresheners. These can be applied with cotton wool or, for a more refreshing tone, sprayed on to the face.

Herbal tea infusions are also ideal toners. Boil a cup of water and infuse chamomile, marigold, rosehip or nettle teas (you can use herbal tea bags if you can't get hold of the herbs), add two drops of orange or lavender oil and leave to cool. Oily skin benefits from juniper or lemongrass, whereas drier skins would appreciate rose or sandalwood.

facial oils

Well-moisturized skin is soft and supple, reflects a healthy glow and ages less quickly. Younger skin only needs light conditioning, whereas older skin needs specific nourishing treatments. Most moisturizers soothe and sit on the surface of the skin, but essential oils, with their fine molecular structure, work their way through from the surface to the inner dermis (the skin's deeper regenerating

△ Caring for your skin becomes an enjoyable experience when you know that you are mixing exactly the right blend for your skin type.

layer). Mixed with the correct amount of base oil, these pure essentials do not clog up pores: they are light enough to be absorbed spontaneously by skin.

masks

Both clay and oatmeal are ideal ingredients for any face mask. A natural powdered clay is Fuller's earth, which can be mixed into a paste with hot water. Cool and then add yogurt for a smoother consistency. Similarly, finely ground oatmeal can be mixed into a paste and left to cool. Add 15 drops of essential oils to suit your skin type per cupful of paste. Smooth on to your face, leave to dry slightly and then sponge off. For particularly dry/sensitive skins add 15ml (1 tbsp) of evening primrose base oil to give a more moisturizing mask. When applying, avoid the eye area.

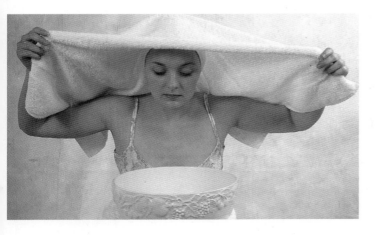

△ Steam inhalation has the benefit of treating a cold and your skin at the same time.

eye treats

While relaxing with a face mask on, close the eyes and cover with cotton pads soaked in rose water, or soothe with two slices of fresh cucumber.

acne

Because of their anti-bacterial, anti-inflammatory and rebalancing properties, essential oils are ideal skin treatments for acne sufferers.

It is often a mistake to scrub oily skin over-zealously: this only activates the sebaceous glands which in turn produce more sebum. If you suffer from pustular acne then avoid excessive facial steams which may spread the condition: use a mask instead. Often it is better to opt for a daily sensitive-skin type cleanser and moisturizer, adding

two drops of juniper, which is stimulating and antiseptic. Opt for a deeper clay-type mask treatment once a week, adding a couple of drops of juniper, which is healing, soothing and tightening, or eucalyptus which is anti-inflammatory, antiseptic and antibiotic. Increase your intake of vitamin E, which is a great skin healer.

broken veins

These small, red, spider-like thread veins often appear on the surface of skin around the cheek area. They are broken capillaries and seem to affect those with a delicate or fragile skin type. Hot and cold, along with stimulants such as alcohol and caffeine, can often trigger this condition. To treat it at home the secret is to protect the skin from losing excess moisture and to give it extra

essential oil treatments using parsley, geranium, chamomile, rosemary or cypress in a heavy base oil.

cold sores

Cold sores are small blisters on the lips or surrounding area. They are caused by the virus herpes simplex, which normally lies dormant but can surface following a cold or flu. Any lip sore that persists should be treated medically, but for the common cold sore a dab of undiluted tea tree oil will help.

odd spots

If prone to occasional spots then mix one drop each of neroli, lemon and lavender in 5ml (1 tsp) of base oil and treat just the affected area. For a single spot dab on one drop of undiluted sandalwood with a cotton bud.

facial massage

Massage helps the skin to absorb oils and creams easily. Give skin a clear start with this step-by-step facial.

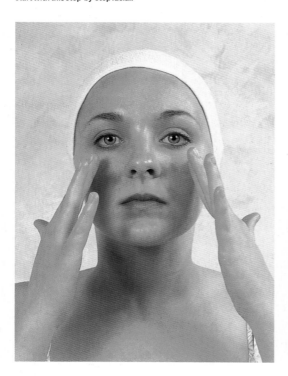

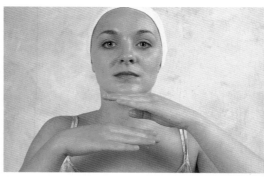

△ **2** With the back of your hands, gently tap the skin around the jawline and underneath the chin to stimulate the skin cells.

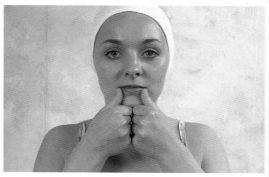

△ **1** Pour a small amount of blended oil into the palm of your hand and gently apply all over the face, avoiding the eyes.

△ **3** Apply small circular movements to the chin area using your thumbs, to tone, help circulation and eliminate toxins.

aromatherapy routines

346

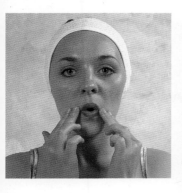

△ **4** Make an "oooh"-shaped mouth. Massage either side easing out fine lines.

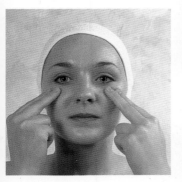

△ **5** With your fingertips, press along the top of the cheekbones and massage outward up to the temples to release toxins.

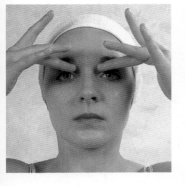

△ **6** With the middle fingers, apply pressure to points above the bridge of the nose and underneath the eyebrows. Hold for five seconds and smooth across from the inner to the outer corners of the eyebrows and continue up to the temples.

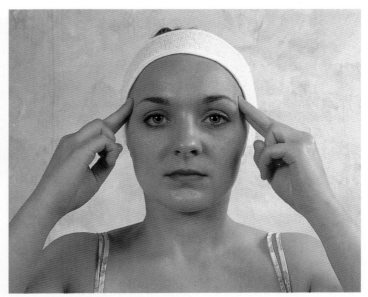

△ **7** To relieve tension, apply firm pressure at either side of the temples, and rotate backward.

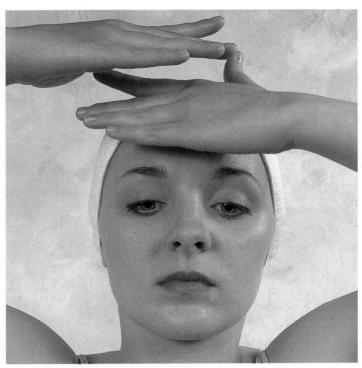

△ **8** Stroke up the forehead to the hairline with the palms of the hands, smoothing out fine lines.

Healthy hair

Hair can define your image and style but it is also a mirror of your health. Emotional or physical problems can soon result in a lack of bounce or shine. Keeping hair in peak condition is a combination of caring for it on the surface and nurturing it from inside with a well-balanced diet.

scalp massage oils

dry hair is rough to touch, thick in texture and dries out at the first sign of heated rollers or tongs. Avoid chemical colourants and perms and opt for shampoos and conditioners with jojoba and almond oils. Hot oil treatments allow essential oils to soak in easily and condition the hair. After massaging warm oil into the scalp, wrap the head in a warm towel and leave on for half an hour.

oils for dry hair
Rose • Sandalwood • Ylang ylang • Lavender • Geranium

greasy hair tends to look dull, lank, lacks body and won't hold a style. Central heating and environmental elements aggravate the condition but it can stem from a hormonal imbalance. Check your diet and avoid harsh degreasing shampoos. Clean your hairbrushes and combs weekly. Plastic brushes are better for brushing through as bristle continually stimulates the scalp. Choose light conditioning rinses to detangle, and try a scalp massage to regulate the oil-producing sebaceous glands.

oils for greasy hair
Basil • Eucalyptus • Cedarwood • Chamomile • Lemongrass • Cypress • Sage • Rosemary

normal hair is glossy with plenty of natural body and bounce. An occasional hot-oil scalp treatment will keep it looking good and growing healthily.

oils for normal hair
Geranium • Lavender • Lemongrass • Rosemary

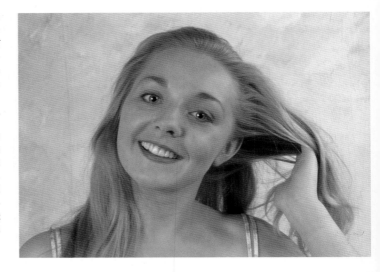

combination hair has ends that are dry or normal, and greasy roots. Avoid using hot appliances near the scalp and keep the ends regularly trimmed and conditioned. Use a scalp treatment with oils for greasy hair but don't comb through to the ends.

how to mix
base oils Choose from sweet almond, apricot kernel, avocado, jojoba, evening primrose and sunflower.

essential oils For one scalp treatment, choose up to three oils and use five drops of each for 30ml (2 tbsp) base oil (for very long hair you may need more oil). Warm the blended oils by placing the container in a bowl of boiling water, and then massage into the scalp. Wrap with a hot towel, leave for 15 minutes and then shampoo.

hair problems
dandruff
There are two types: dry and the more common oily. It's not catching! It can be caused by factors such as chemical body changes, stress, poor eating habits or wrong use of

△ **A combination of a healthy, balanced diet and regular use of essential oils will help you maintain a head of shiny, healthy hair.**

hair products. Both flaky and dry scalps can be treated with essential oils. Use special dandruff shampoos and conditioning rinses and treat the scalp by gently massaging with oils to suit. Use a base oil formula with patchouli and tea tree. For a dry, itchy scalp try cedarwood and lavender.

grey hair
Grey hair is more porous and needs extra conditioning, particularly if it is chemically treated or coloured. Use a scalp formula for dry hair adding essential oil enhancers, such as chamomile to lighten or sage to darken any discoloration.

hair loss
Hair coming out in handfuls is often due to a hormonal imbalance, stress or anxiety, so the first step is to learn to relax. Any unusual thinning patch should be looked at by a trichologist but, as a general remedy, use a scalp massage with lavender and rosemary oils.

scalp massage

This is a wonderful way to condition the hair, stimulate the scalp and relieve tension in the head. You can use these steps to treat your own hair but it's even more relaxing if you can persuade a friend to help, especially if you've got long hair. You can offer a treatment in exchange. Remember to wash the oil out of your hair at the end of the treatment.

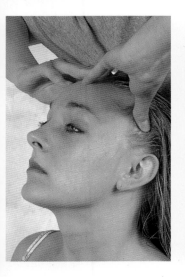

△ **1** Shampoo the hair and towel dry to absorb excess water. Comb through with a wide-tooth comb. Tilt your head back and pour some oil on to the hairline, massaging in with thumbs on the temple and fingers spread apart over the centre of the head.

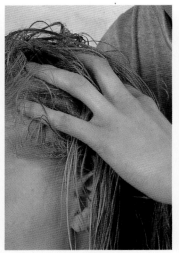

△ **3** Massage the head with kneading movements. Grip and push (with fingerpads, rather than fingernails) against the scalp. The scalp should gently rotate against the skull. Concentrate on one area at a time, with the hands positioned on either side of the scalp.

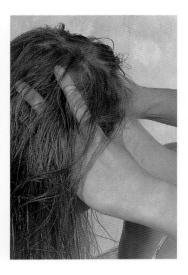

△ **4** At the base of the skull, press firmly and push the whole scalp up toward the crown to release tension. If the scalp feels particularly tight, then concentrate on areas where the scalp doesn't want to move.

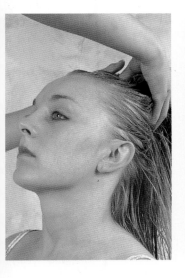

△ **2** Loosely run fingers and oil over the top of the scalp from front to back, lifting hair at the crown. Keep dipping your fingertips in the treatment oil to spread through the hair while massaging.

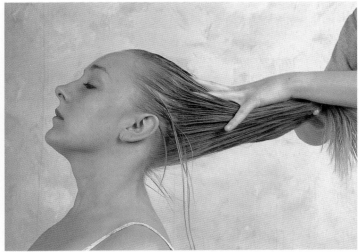

△ **5** Pull any extra oil through the hair, working out from the roots to the tips. Make sure all the hair is well oiled, and then leave towel-wrapped for at least 15 minutes before shampooing.

Daily hand, foot and nail care

Our hands are exposed daily to the elements and to household detergents, and our feet carry us wherever we want to go. Both deserve as much attention as the face, and will benefit greatly from aromatherapy.

hand care

It is said that there are two ways to tell a woman's age: by her neck and by her hands. Our hands, like our necks and faces, are always exposed to the air and are always on visible display. However, it is easy to neglect them when leading a busy life.

treatment

Essential oils can be added to a base lotion and used after each time you wash your hands. Patchouli is one of the best oils for cracked, dry skin, and clary sage helps delay cellular aging. If your hands are neglected and in need of a boost, try giving them an exfoliating "mask" treatment before going to bed. After using an exfoliating face mask on your hands, apply your hand lotion. Cover your hands with cling film (plastic wrap) and pull on a pair of cotton gloves, or cotton socks, over the cling film. Keep the mask in place for an hour before rinsing off.

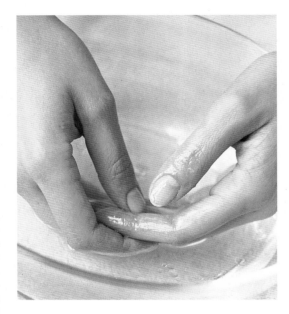

◁ Having well-cared for hands is a beauty asset. To give your hands a treat, prepare a mix using oils of geranium and rose otto and work well into the skin.

foot care

Think of the amount of work our feet have to do – we walk on them daily, often in inappropriate footwear, and yet we give them surprisingly little care and attention.

treatment

Spend some time each week giving your feet a treatment massage (see page 252), which benefits your feet and the rest of your body at the same time. Keep them as scrupulously clean as your face, regularly removing dead skin at the heels and drying properly between the toes. Watch for any broken skin between the toes as this may be a sign of athlete's foot – a fungal condition which can be difficult to treat once it takes hold. Plastic shoes are a common cause of athlete's foot as they create moisture and cause the feet to sweat,

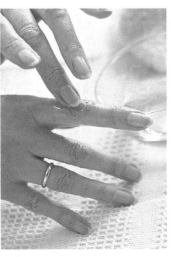

◁ For cracked knuckles, try patchouli oil mixed in a carrier cream or lotion base and applied to the affected area on clean, dry hands.

creating the ideal conditions for fungus to develop. Essential oils can be used to treat all fungus-type infections as well as viral ones, including warts and verrucas. You will also need to address the underlying causes. These may be related to stress and poor nutrition, and will be helped with relaxing essential oils.

nail care

Strong, well-manicured nails on the hands and feet play an important role in a woman's appearance. Brittle, damaged or weak nails can detract from this. Essential oils can be used to improve nail condition.

treatment

Essential oil of lavender is particularly good for strengthening nails. Each evening, put your finger on to the nozzle of a bottle of lavender oil, tip the bottle, and rub the oil into the cuticles. After two or three months you should see some improvement as the treated nail grows through.

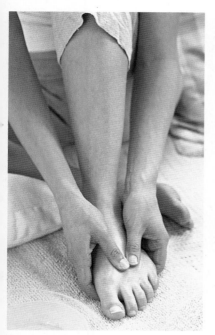

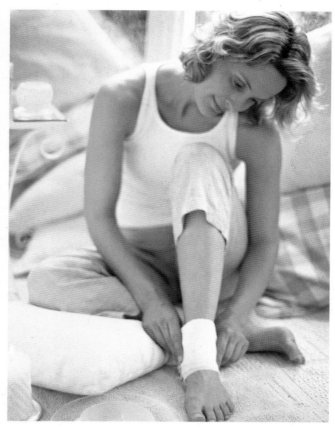

△ Giving yourself a foot massage not only feels good but also energizes the many reflex points on your feet, which in turn correspond to different parts of the body.

▷ For tired or swollen ankles, a cool compress soaked in Roman chamomile and lavender oil is both soothing and refreshing and can also alleviate any inflammation.

Nail treatment

Pampering your nails with this weekly treatment will keep them healthy and strong. If your nails are particularly weak and damaged, you may prefer to apply this quick treatment every evening. Because nail growth is a slow process, the results are not immediate – it will be a couple of months before you see any improvement, but it will be worth the wait.

ingredients
• warm water
• lavender essential oil
equipment
• bowl
• cuticle stick
• cotton bud (Q-tip)

tip
Sucking a jelly cube each day is said to stengthen the nails. If you often have white flecks across your nails, increasing the calcium in your diet could also help.

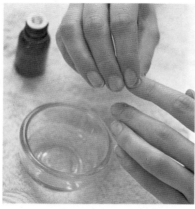

△ 1 Soak your fingertips in warm water before gently cleaning the surplus cuticle from the nails.

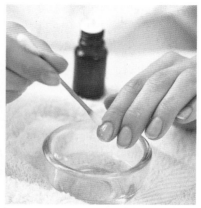

△ 2 Use a cotton bud (Q-tip) to apply neat lavender oil to each cuticle to strengthen them.

Daily bodycare

Our bodies are protected for much of the time with clothes, and because of this, the skin of our torso is usually in a better condition – softer and smoother – than that of our arms and legs, which are more frequently exposed to sunlight.

conditioning treatments

The arms and legs benefit hugely from the daily use of creams and lotions containing essential oils; improvements are particularly apparent when moisturizing bath or shower oils or gels have not been used as a matter of course. If your skin is dry or flaky, put your essential oils into a carrier oil to add a gleam to your skin. (*See* Preparing Oils for Application *to select the most beneficial oil for your skin type.*)

For a bath treatment for dry skin, grate 15g (½oz) unscented, non-alkaline soap into 120ml (½ cup) boiling water, and stir to dissolve the soap. When cool, add 8 drops of your favourite essential oil or oil mix. Hold your mixture under the running tap to dissolve in the bathwater and make some bubbles. If you prefer lots of bubbles, add essential oils to a non-drying bubble bath.

If you have normal to oily skin, which is not known to be sensitive, give yourself a body rinse before leaving the bath or

▷ Varicose veins can be painful and unsightly. A cool compress, made with cypress, clary sage or niaouli oil and applied to the affected area, can help.

shower. Dissolve your essential oil or oils into 15ml (1 tbsp) vodka, and mix with 1 litre (1¾ pints) spring water. Add 120ml (½ cup) white wine or cider vinegar to the spring water mixture for an extra zingy feel.

If you have a problem with body odour, use the vodka rinse above, but without the vinegar. Add 3 drops of nutmeg essential oil and 3 drops of cypress essential oil; both of these have deodorizing properties.

For hard, rough skin on elbows and heels, use a facial exfoliating mask, followed by a moisturizing body lotion or oil to which 2–3 drops of essential oil have been added.

Cellulite is caused by ineffective blood circulation, which leads to poor lymphatic drainage and fluid retention. Aromatherapy can help with a daily regime. Pummel the area vigorously before applying essential oils in a carrier lotion or oil.

Varicose vein treatment

Apply the essential oil blend or lotion mix to the whole leg before following the directions below. Upward strokes are important to help the blood move towards the heart. Ensure an even pressure when stroking the legs and take care when moving over any tender areas. Use phlebotonic oils such as clary sage, cypress and niaouli.

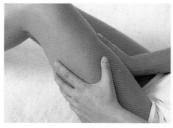

△ **1** Massage the upper half of the leg first with upward movements. This clears the valves to allow the blood to pass more easily from the lower leg.

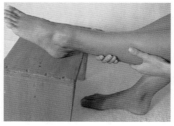

△ **2** Massage in an upward direction only, using the palms of both hands. Make long, firm strokes alternately with each hand up the calf muscle.

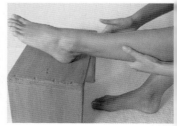

△ **3** Take the fingers of both hands alternately up the calf muscle. Complete the sequence by repeating step 2.

Anti-cellulite treatment

Cellulite is recognized by its resemblance to orange or grapefruit peel. A daily aromatherapy treatment, along with an improved diet and a thorough exercise plan, will boost the circulation and improve lymphatic drainage, helping to disperse the cellulite. Try this exercise immediately after a bath or shower and practise daily for the best results.

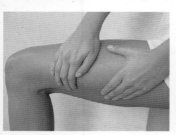

△ **1** After firmly rubbing in your prepared oil mix or lotion, take both hands alternately up the outside of the leg. Use a loofah or bristle brush if preferred.

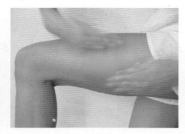

△ **2** Use the heel of your hands to pummel the cellulite vigorously. This stimulates the circulation and allows quicker penetration of the essential oils.

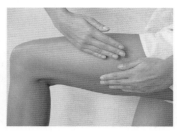

△ **3** Continue to work over the cellulite area using the heels of both hands alternately. Maintaining the firmness of the strokes, repeat step 1.

Useful essential oils

essential oil	treatment
skin types	
DRY SKIN	
Chamomile (Roman) *Chamaemelum nobile*	anti-inflammatory (irritable skin)
Geranium *Pelargonium graveolens*	anti-infectious, cicatrizant
Lavender *Lavandula angustifolia*	antiseptic, anti-inflammatory, cicatrizant (healing)
Patchouli *Pogostemon patchouli*	anti-inflammatory, cicatrizant
Rose otto *Rosa damascena*	anti-inflammatory (blotchy skin), cicatrizant
OILY SKIN	
Cedarwood *Cedrus atlantica*	antiseptic, antibacterial, cicatrizant.
Lemon *Citrus limon*	astringent, antibacterial, anti-inflammatory
Ylang ylang *Cananga odorata*	tonic, balancing, calming, hypotensive
MATURE SKIN	
Clary sage *Salvia sclarea*	regenerative (cellular aging)
Frankincense *Boswellia carteri*	antioxidant (combats aging process), cicatrizant
anti-aging	
Clary sage *Salvia sclarea*	oestrogen-like, regenerative (counteracts cellular aging)
Frankincense *Boswellia carteri*	antioxidant (combats aging process)
Lemon *Citrus limon*	antisclerotic (combats aging process)

essential oil	treatment
skin conditions	
PSORIASIS (INCLUDING NAILS)	
Bergamot *Citrus bergamia*	cicatrizant
Lavender *Lavandula angustifolia*	cicatrizant
ECZEMA	
Bergamot *Citrus bergamia*	anti-infectious (weeping eczema), cicatrizant
Geranium *Pelargonium graveolens*	analgesic, anti-infectious, anti-inflammatory, cicatrizant
ACNE ROSACEA	
Chamomile (German) *Matricaria recutica*	anti-inflammatory, cicatrizant
Chamomile (Roman) *Chamaemelum nobile*	anti-inflammatory, cicatrizant
Frankincense *Boswellia carteri*	analgesic, cicatrizant
ATHLETE'S FOOT AND NAIL FUNGI	
Clary sage *Salvia sclarea*	antifungal (skin conditions)
Geranium *Pelargonium graveolens*	antifungal, anti-infectious
Lavender *Lavandula angustifolia*	antifungal, antiseptic
CELLULITE	
Cypress *Cupressus sempervirens*	diuretic
Fennel *Foeniculum vulgare*	diuretic, circulatory stimulant
Juniper *Juniperus communis*	diuretic, lypolytic

The aromatic bath

The relaxing and remedial properties of water and of massaging oils into the body were recognized in ancient Greek and Roman cultures, when bathing first became a daily ritual.

A bath with essential oils is one of the simplest and most effective aromatherapy treatments. It can be stimulating or relaxing, depending on the temperature of the water and whether you choose oils with uplifting or calming properties. In the bath, the therapeutic action of the oils is two-fold: they are absorbed through the skin, moisturizing the dermis and entering the circulatory system, and at the same time their aromas are inhaled, stimulating the brain and increasing your sense of well-being. An aromatic bath can detoxify the body, help problems like cellulite, joint stiffness, general aches and pains, colds and headaches, tone and condition skin, and relieve anxiety and tension.

running the bath

Bath temperature and the time spent in the tub are important. A cooler bath is more stimulating and warmer water relaxes. Very hot water is damaging, however: it causes blood vessels and capillaries to expand and increases the heartrate. You should particularly avoid hot water if you have varicose veins, haemorrhoids, high blood pressure or are pregnant. A 15–20 minute

therapeutic baths
Oils for dermatitis
Chamomile • Hyssop • Lavender
Oils for eczema
Chamomile • Geranium • Hyssop • Juniper • Rosemary • Myrrh
Oils for psoriasis
Bergamot • Chamomile • Lavender
Oils for arthritis/rheumatism
Chamomile • Eucalyptus • Juniper • Lavender • Rosemary • Thyme

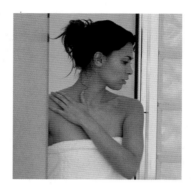

△ **Neroli, lavender and rose oils make a lovely, relaxing bath blend, or choose basil, sage and sandalwood for a man.**

soak is long enough before skin cells over-hydrate and swell with water. Wait until the bath is almost full before adding the oils, as they evaporate so quickly.

oils for the bath

Essential oils are the best way of making a bath both aromatic and therapeutic. They sink into the skin easily and at the same time impart their lovely herbal or floral fragrances. You can add drops of oil directly to the bath and they will float on the surface in a fine film and evaporate, giving you the full benefit of their aromas. Or if you want to absorb them more you can disperse them through the water by mixing with a base carrier oil such as sweet almond, apricot kernel, jojoba or evening primrose (these rich base oils all nourish and rejuvenate the skin in their own right).

Mix a bath oil with a combination of up to three essential oils, five drops from each, in 15ml (1 tbsp) of skin-softening base oil. Choose oils with complementary effects so they do not override one another.

▷ **If you have time to soak in a bath, use relaxing aromatherapy oils to soothe or stimulating oils to invigorate.**

the relaxing bath

To calm yourself after a fraught day or to prepare yourself for a peaceful night's sleep, turn your bathroom into a private sanctuary. Keep the light as soft as possible, using aromatic candles if the light is harsh, or you could use an eye mask. Introducing plants into the bathroom will help create an oxygenated atmosphere. Once in the bath, support your head with a bath pillow, close your eyes and inhale deeply. Concentrate on your breathing, empty your mind and let the oils soothe away the stresses and strains. After a 15–20 minute soak, get out and wrap yourself in a large, warm towel and rest quietly for a few moments.

oils for relaxation

Basil • Bergamot • Cedarwood • Chamomile • Frankincense • Hyssop • Juniper • Lavender • Marjoram • Melissa • Neroli • Patchouli • Rose • Sage • Sandalwood • Ylang ylang

Although these oils have predominantly calming effects, some can also be used to stimulate the circulation and lymphatic system, in particular lavender oil and also bergamot.

the stimulating bath

Best for the morning to get you started or to revive you before an evening out. Keep the water fairly cool and use an invigorating

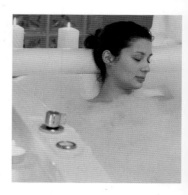

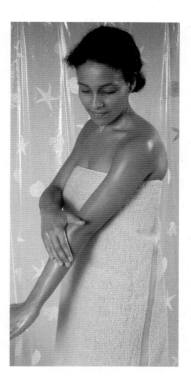

body-oil formula
Essential oils sink beautifully into warm damp skin. For a lasting effect, mix the three chosen bath essential oils, five drops of each, in 30ml (2 tbsp) base oil. If you want to make up a larger quantity of body oil, use a concentration of three per cent essential oil in base oil.

bath mitt to rub down and stimulate the circulation. When you've soaked, rinse yourself with water as cold as you can bear, either by splashing directly from the tap (faucet) or shower, or by adding more cold water to cool down your bath.

As you get out, either slap yourself dry to make the skin tingle or rub yourself vigorously with a towel.

oils for stimulation
Cypress • Eucalyptus • Fennel • Geranium • Juniper • Lavender • Lemon • Lemongrass • Peppermint • Pine • Rosemary • Thyme

showers and cold rinses
Invigorating jets of water are ideal for getting the blood pumping and there's no need to forego the benefits of aromatic oils. Skin tends to be sluggish in the cold winter months but sloughing off dead top layers can help regenerate cells and allow moisturizers to be absorbed more easily. Showers are ideal for smoothing skin with exfoliating rubs using wet salt, a loofah or a mitt to slough off the top surface of dead skin cells. A dry friction glove or loofah is too harsh for most skins so soften first in warm water. Soft bristle brushes can also help to get the circulation going with gentle massage on problem areas like hips and thighs. To keep friction brushes and mitts fresh always rinse and hang up to dry.

Essential oils can be used under the shower: try a base oil mixed with invigorating essences poured on to a clean face-cloth or sponge and rubbed all over the body. To clear the sinuses and help coughs, sponge the chest with a mix of eucalyptus and peppermint oils. A cold shower after cleansing improves the circulation and tightens skin pores.

after-bath body treatments
Moisturizing oils and lotions applied after the bath or shower help to nourish the skin, keeping it soft and supple. As we get older our skin dehydrates since the oil glands do not produce as much oil as in youth. Apply a body oil all over, starting from the feet and working right up to the neck and the tips of the ears. Avoid talcum powders as they clog the pores and tend to have a drying effect.

problem zones
Hands and nails take some rough treatment with everyday chores. The ideal time for a manicure or pedicure is after soaking in a bath when nails and skin are softened, making it easy to clean around the nail bed and to clip uneven nails without snagging. Fragile or flaky nails benefit from a rich, nourishing treatment: rub them with apricot kernel, wheatgerm or jojoba oil. Restore hands with a soothing, moisturizing mix of 15ml (1 tbsp) sweet almond oil and five drops each of patchouli, lavender and lemon.

Feet are often neglected until they hurt. Polish hard skin around heels and soles with a handful of damp salt or use a pumice stone. While in the bath, bend one knee, grip the toes and then work with the fingers massaging in an upward direction, from the toes to the heels and up the calves, in order to stimulate blood flow and relax tired feet. Massage a body oil into the feet after a bath, shower or pedicure.

For a deodorizing and soothing footbath add three drops each of cypress and lavender to a basin full of water. Chilblains can be treated with a massage blend of three drops

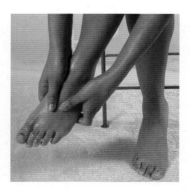

△ Apply body oil to the arms with smooth upward strokes to boost circulation, concentrating on the elbows and upper arms where the skin is often rougher and drier.

of geranium and a drop each of lavender and rosemary in 15ml (1 tbsp) sweet almond base oil.

Elbows can soon build up hard protective layers of grey, unsightly skin. A good softener for tough elbows is a sweet almond oil and oatmeal scrub. Mix 45ml (3 tbsp) sweet almond oil with 45ml (3 tbsp) fine oatmeal and mix to a paste with fresh milk or yogurt. Smooth and rub over the elbows and any grey, goosey areas of skin around upper arms. Add six drops of fennel if arms are flabby. Another great elbow booster is the traditional recipe of cutting a lemon in half, squeezing out the juice and rubbing the elbows in the hollow of the lemon.

◁ Soften the feet after a bath by massaging between the toes and then working around the tougher skin and heel areas. Finish with sweeping movements all over to stimulate the circulation.

Sensual aromas

The power of perfume to inspire romance has been known since the Babylonians, and today perfume and flowers are still the favourite gifts of lovers. Cleopatra's seduction of Mark Antony was carefully staged with a carpet of rose petals and rare and exotic scents in every conceivable form – even the sails of her barge were drenched in perfume to catch the breeze and announce her arrival to the object of her desire.

The sense of smell is fundamental to our sensuality. Pheromones, chemicals secreted in human sweat, act as the most basic trigger to sexual attraction. The smells of flowers and plants are the plant equivalent of pheromones, irresistible to birds and bees and just as attractive to humans. We can use natural aromatic plant oils to relax, heighten our awareness, excite the senses and create a mood for love.

setting the scene

Create a calming and sensual atmosphere with scented candles placed safely around the room or a few drops of essential oil evaporated in a fragrancer or light-bulb ring. Dim the lights and turn up the heat.

Scent your lingerie or bedlinen by adding three drops of your favourite oil to the final

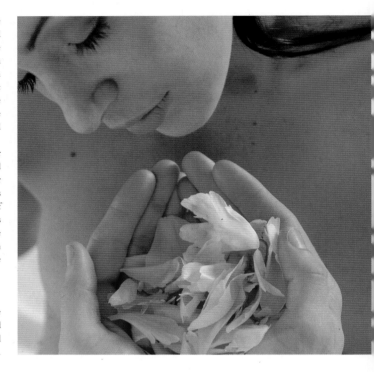

rinse, or store them in drawers with aromatic bags or scented balls. Sprinkle drops of rose or jasmine on the pillows.

preparing your body

Luxuriate in an aromatic bath or hot tub, or better still, share it with your partner. After soaking, perfume your whole body with a rich body oil or use a strong concentration to dab pulse points such as wrists, temples and behind the ears and knees, and wait for your partner to discover these secret scented areas.

partner massage

We are all sensual beings and yet at times we may need help to switch off from

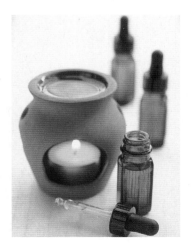

◁ **Create a romantic mood with a blend of oils from the list opposite, vaporized in an oil burner.**

△ **The sense of smell is one of the most powerfully evocative of the human senses and essential oils can be used to speak volumes.**

everyday concerns and tune in to our senses. The loving touch of partner massage is always enjoyable; it is relaxing and yet sensually stimulating – a total physical experience.

You can adapt the basic essential massage, using plenty of effleurage all over, deeper kneading for tense areas and light feather strokes with the fingertips to excite the surface of the skin. Avoid the lymph drainage movements as these are distinctly unerotic! Discover your partner's erogenous zones – explore the ears and feet and the inside of the forearms and thighs. Find some more. Be tender and loving, playful and creative – let your imagination guide you.

oils for seduction

Most of the aphrodisiac oils combine well with each other, but be careful not to use too many together or they may clash and work against each other. Subtlety is the key to the art of seduction.

- **clary sage** – sweet, sensuous and slightly intoxicating, but be careful – if used in very high doses its sedative effect will inhibit sex drive.
- **geranium** – a strong floral oil that both relaxes and uplifts.
- **jasmine** – the heady floral fragrance boosts confidence and creates a luxurious atmosphere.
- **neroli** – fresh and sweet, its fortifying effect helps overcome shyness and inhibitions.
- **patchouli** – heavy and exotic, it is stimulating in small doses, and heightens the senses.
- **rose** – the quintessential oil for lovers. Rare and powerful.
- **sandalwood** – woody, sweet and exotic with spicy undertones. It blends with many oils as it is mild and mellow.
- **ylang ylang** – the long-lasting floral scent gives a feeling of relaxed well-being, helpful for impotence or fridigity. Use in small doses as the scent is very heady.

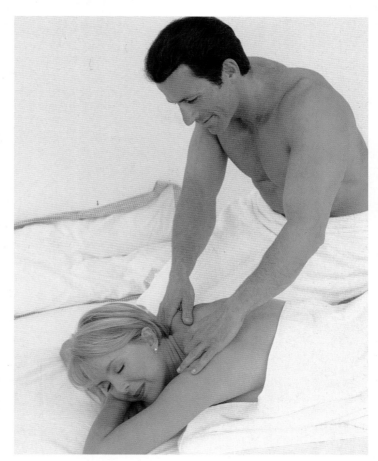

△ With a massage oil blended from floral and spicy aphrodisiac essences you can arouse the intimate senses of touch and smell simultaneously as you explore the skin and curves of your partner's body with strong smoothing strokes. Let the heady scents work their spell on the senses and emotions.

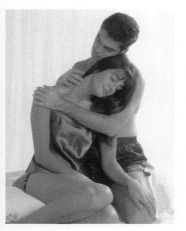

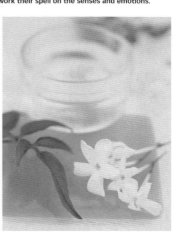

You can also try the warm, spicy exotics such as black pepper, ginger, cardamom, cinnamon and cedarwood, but be sparing with these as they can easily overpower.

Layer the scents by choosing just three or four and using them in different strengths and combinations for the room fragrance, bath, body oil and massage blend.

◁ Combine the use of essential oils with a sensual massage to relax your partner's body and stimulate their senses.

▷ Sesame or almond oil, infused with jasmine, makes a soothing massage oil and will create a sensual, relaxing atmosphere.

Ambient aromatics

A lingering smell, whether pleasant or foul, is usually the first thing we notice when we enter a room, and it can strongly affect the way we feel. Fragrancing the home to cover unpleasant smells and delight the senses is an old tradition. For centuries the Chinese have suspended balls of jasmine flowers over the bed to clear the air and promote pleasant dreams, while posies of jasmine were handed to guests to refresh them on leaving banquets or dances. Lavender sachets placed in drawers and bowls of pot pourri used to scent a room were particular favourites during the Victorian era.

studies and offices

Work-places are often stuffy and full of unpleasant smells, but if you work in an open-plan space fragrancing the whole area may not be a viable option. Inhaling a few drops of oil from a handkerchief is the most personal way of using a fragrance, or you

▽ A bowl of pot pourri can greatly enhance the atmosphere and mood of a room. Don't forget to refresh the mixture regularly.

can spray your immediate environment with a room spray, or add a couple of drops of oil to a cup of hot water on your desk.

Useful oils for the work-place are basil, rosemary, bergamot, lemon and melissa. Bergamot and lemon are particularly antiseptic, and lemon has the added advantage of helping efficiency. Basil stimulates a tired brain and rosemary is a great aid to concentration. Rosemary is also helpful in relieving headaches. If you are feeling overwrought try clary sage or juniper, but watch the dosage as too much will cause sleepiness.

living rooms

The methods for fragrancing a room are many and diverse. Those that involve evaporating the oils, such as fragrancers/diffusers, water bowls, light-bulb rings and room sprays, are best for preventing ill-health, balancing the emotions and disguising unpleasant smells such as cigarette smoke or cooking odours. All these methods disperse the fragrance through a large space extremely quickly and effectively. For more

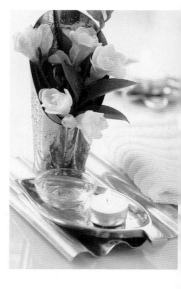

△ Use flower oils, such as rose, geranium, jasmine, neroli or lavender, to create the same effect as a vase of freshly cut flowers.

lingering and subtle scents, blend your own pot pourri or, alternatively, use pomanders. Rose, geranium, orange and lavender are uplifting scents for a room, used individually or blended together. For an exotic, intimate atmosphere use sandalwood or patchouli, or to unwind in the evening try geranium, lavender, sandalwood or ylang ylang.

perfumes for parties

Clary sage or jasmine will create a heady, "feel-good" atmosphere for a party, or use orange, lemongrass or neroli for a lighter, fresher touch.

For a festive blend choose from the spicier oils such as frankincense, cedarwood, sandalwood, cinnamon and orange.

bedrooms

Whether to ensure a restful night's sleep or to turn your bedroom into a place of passion, fragrancing the bedroom just before

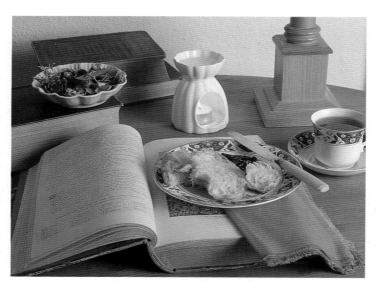

retiring will create an appropriate atmosphere. Rose, neroli and lavender are delightful all-purpose oils for the bedroom. Use lavender to freshen a musty spare room to make it welcoming for guests.

insect repellent

Use tea tree, eucalyptus, melissa, lemongrass or the closely related citronella in a diffuser to keep insects at bay.

disinfecting

Vaporized molecules of any essential oil will neutralize airborne bacteria, but some – such as tea tree, bergamot, lemon, pine and lavender – are particularly antiseptic. Use these in a fragrancer or room spray. A few drops of pine, lemon and tea tree can be used on a damp cloth to disinfect surfaces in the kitchen or bathroom. Clear the atmosphere of a sickroom with bergamot, eucalyptus and juniper.

pot pourri

To make your own pot pourri assemble fully-dried flowers, petals, herbs, leaves and other plant materials. Using completely dry ingredients prevents the potpourri from going off. There are no hard and fast rules about quantities and proportions, but an allowance of two or three tablespoons ground spices, two tablespoons orris-root powder, two teaspoons dried lemon, orange or lime peel, and six drops of essential oil to every four cups of dried plant material makes a pleasant well-balanced mixture.

If your pot pourri loses a little of its aroma over a period of time, it can be revived. Simply stir in another two or three drops of essential oil. And if the mixture loses its colour sharpness just stir in a few dried flowers such as miniature rosebuds, santolina flowers or tansy clusters.

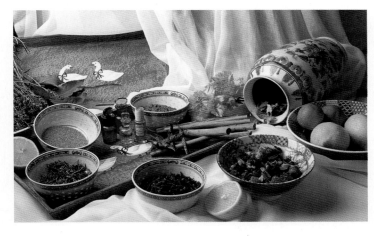

△ **Ingredients which can be used to make pot pourri. From the left: dried lavender, bay leaves, dried ground orris-root powder, dried rosemary leaves, a selection of essential oils, ground cinnamon, dried chillies and cinnamon sticks, whole cloves, a blend of dried flowers, limes and lemons. The dried peel of citrus fruit is finely grated or chopped for use in the spice mixture.**

cottage garden mix

115g (4oz) dried lavender flowers
225g (8oz) dried rose petals
225g (8oz) dried pinks (*Dianthus*)
115g (4oz) dried scented geranium leaves
15ml (1 tbsp) ground cinnamon
10ml (2 tsp) ground allspice
5ml (1 tsp) dried grated lemon peel
30ml (2 tbsp) orris-root powder
3 drops rose oil
3 drops geranium oil
Mix ingredients together in a covered container, and set aside for six weeks. Stir daily to distribute the fragrances.

woodland mix

25g (1oz) lime seedpods, or "keys"
50g (2oz/1 cup) cedar bark shavings
50g (2oz/1 cup) sandalwood shavings
115g (4oz) small cones
15ml (1 tbsp) whole cloves
15ml (1 tbsp) star anise
1 cinnamon stick, crushed
30ml (2 tbsp) orris-root powder
4 drops sandalwood oil
2 drops cinnamon oil
Mix ingredients together in a covered container, and set aside for six weeks. Stir daily and refresh as necessary.

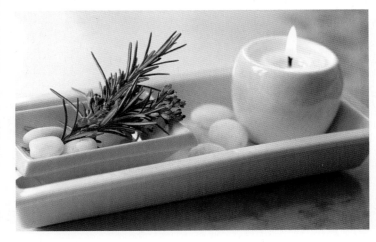

▷ **Candles scented with essential oils can fragrance a whole room. Use a safe container and never leave candles burning unattended.**

Pregnancy treatments

Pregnancy can be one of the most exciting and fulfilling times of a woman's life. The joy of bringing another human being into the world creates a tremendous feeling of contentment and anticipation, but it is also a time of great physical and emotional upheaval. Together with the ever-important trio of exercise, good diet and rest, essential oils can play an important role in helping a woman cope with the stresses of nine months of pregnancy, the pain of labour and post-natal recovery.

common ailments

Surging hormone levels and changes in your swelling body can bring a host of discomforts, many of which can be alleviated by aromatherapy treatments and other simple steps.

backache

The lower back region takes a lot of strain during pregnancy, and will benefit from a firm massage with four drops each of lavender and sandalwood in 30ml (2 tbsp)

base oil. Six drops of lavender in the bath will help to soothe away the aches.

morning sickness

Eat little and often during the day, avoiding junk food and heavy meals late at night. Choose fresh foods which are free from preservatives or chemicals. Try herbal tea infusions such as chamomile, peppermint or orange blossom, which are good for the digestion.

heartburn

Avoid heavy meals and particularly rich, spicy foods. Peppermint tea infusions help, and you can rub the solar plexus with a blend of two drops each of lemon and peppermint essential oils in 15ml (1 tbsp) base oil.

sore breasts

These need extra care and attention during pregnancy as they expand. Use a gentle massage oil with rose and orange, three drops of each in 15ml (1 tbsp) sweet almond

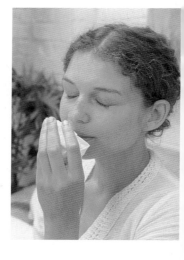

△ Spoil yourself with the luxurious and relaxing scent of rose for body and facial oils, to keep your spirits up during pregnancy.

oil; or if breasts are very swollen and sore, make a cool compress using rosewater and place over the breasts while having an afternoon rest. Sweet almond oil on its own is very good for sore, cracked nipples during breast-feeding. Never use pure essential oils on the breasts during this period as they can easily be transferred to the baby while feeding.

constipation

Make sure your diet contains plenty of fresh and high-fibre foods and drink plenty of still water. Tension can also be a contributory factor, so try a relaxing bath with three drops of lavender and four drops of rose. Carefully massage your abdomen and the small of the back with a blend of four drops of chamomile or orange in 15ml (1 tbsp) base oil.

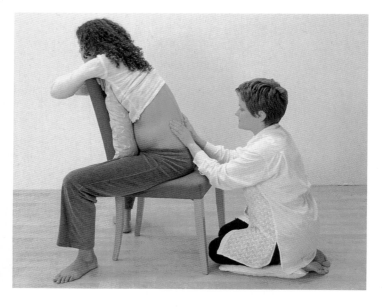

◁ A back massage is lovely during pregnancy. In the later stages, sitting up will be more comfortable than lying on your front.

cautions

The following oils should be avoided during pregnancy (particularly the first five months) because of their strong diuretic properties or tendency to induce menstruation:

Bay • Basil • Clary Sage • Comfrey • Fennel • Hyssop • Juniper • Marjoram • Melissa • Myrrh • Rosemary • Sage • Thyme

Use essential oils in half the usual quantity during pregnancy and take extra care when handling them. Make sure you only use pure essential oils, as adulterated blends or synthetic oils can have less predictable results.

Chamomile and lavender are extremely safe oils and excellent for pregnancy, but if you have a history of miscarriage, all oils should be avoided for the first few months.

Because of their potentially toxic nature and strong abortive qualities, the following oils should never be used except by a qualified aromatherapist, and must be avoided during pregnancy:

Oreganum • Pennyroyal • St John's Wort • Tansy • Wormwood

sleep problems

In the last few months of pregnancy, with the baby kicking and other discomforts, it is often difficult to get a good night's sleep. A relaxing bath with neroli and rose is soothing, and you can add ylang ylang for its calming, sedative effect – a maximum of eight drops in total. Two drops of rose or lavender on the edge of the pillowcase will help induce sleep.

stretch marks

When the stretched skin returns to the body's normal shape it can leave tiny jagged scars. A daily massage around the hips and expanding tummy, using five drops of lavender in 15ml (1 tbsp) jojoba, wheatgerm or evening primrose oil, will help keep

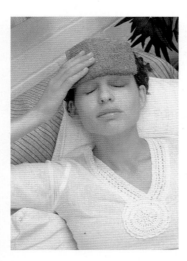

skin smooth and supple. Start around the fifth month of pregnancy and continue after the birth until you return to your normal weight.

swollen ankles

These can be reduced with a cool to warm footbath of benzoin, rose and orange. Add two drops of each directly to the bowl or mix with 15ml (1 tbsp) base carrier oil such as sesame seed. Rest with feet raised on cushions or pillows.

varicose veins

During pregnancy the blood flow to the legs is often slowed down, causing the veins to dilate. Two drops each of cypress, lemongrass and lavender, mixed with 30ml (2 tbsp) apricot kernel base oil, can be smoothed gently over the legs for relief. One of the best oils for the circulation is geranium, though this should always be very dilute for use in pregnancy. Add four drops to the bath or to 15ml (1 tbsp) carrier oil to massage the leg with upward movements. Do not work directly on the veins or apply too much pressure to the leg.

labour

To create a relaxing atmosphere in the labour room, use a few drops of lavender in a fragrancer, or try rose, neroli or ylang ylang

▷ **This is a time to pamper yourself – use soft, warm towels for any treatment.**

◁ **When you're feeling hot and bothered, use a cool and soothing compress of lavender and chamomile, both extremely safe oils.**

to fortify you as the labour progresses. Any of these oils can be used in a massage blend for the lower back to help with contractions. If labour is progressing slowly, try marjoram as a massage oil or compress across the abdomen to stimulate contractions.

after the birth

The "baby blues" often occur around the third or fourth day after childbirth, though some women can suffer a more severe form of post-natal depression for up to a year. A bath of jasmine and ylang ylang will lift your spirits and help you feel better, or use a body oil of chamomile, geranium and orange (5 drops to 30ml (2 tbsp) sweet almond oil), which is a good mix for hormonal imbalance.

To ease any perineal pains, a bath with a few drops of lavender is very soothing. Tea tree can also be added, since this is a powerful antiseptic and helps heal internal wounds and stitches.

recommended oils for pregnancy

Chamomile • Geranium (in low doses) • Lavender • Lemon • Neroli • Orange • Rose • Sandalwood

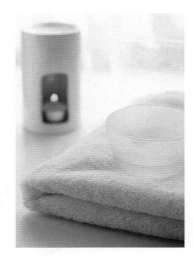

Pregnancy massage

These simple touch massage movements can help to relieve many of the stresses and discomforts of pregnancy, and the back massage is particularly welcome during labour. The basic essential oil massage is modified in various ways to take account of the pregnant condition.

Check the box on the previous page to find which oils are suitable and which are to be avoided.

Use a lower concentration of essential oil to base oil; ½–1 per cent is ideal.

Keep strokes lighter than usual.

In addition to the routine suggested on the following pages, you can incorporate a facial and gentle breast massage.

It is particularly important to observe the rest period after the massage and to help your partner get up gently.

The positions you work in need to be adapted for a pregnant woman, as she cannot lie out straight on her front or back and needs to be well supported.

the back

After about the fourth month, it becomes awkward and uncomfortable for a pregnant woman to lie on her stomach, so work with your partner sitting up with a towel-wrapped pillow or back of a chair to lean over for support.

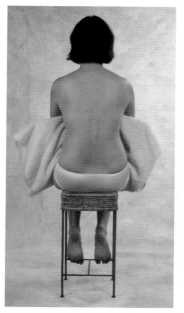

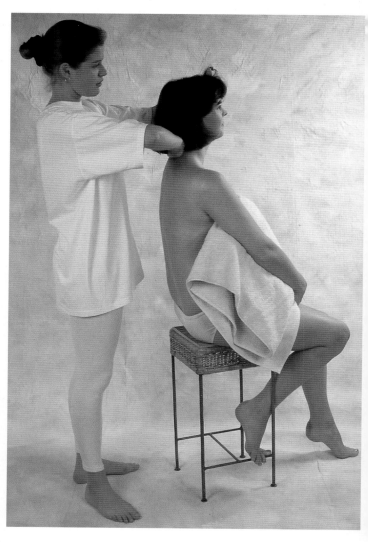

△ **1** Make sure your partner is comfortable and place your left hand over the forehead and the palm of your right hand across the back of the neck. Hold for a few moments and then release.

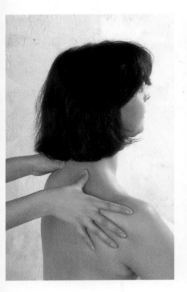

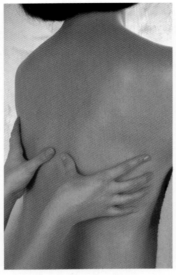

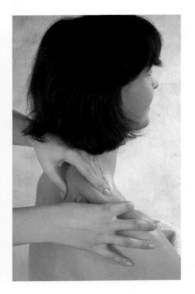

△ **2** Apply a little oil to your fingers and using a slight but gentle pressure, softly massage each side of your partner's neck and shoulders, kneading mainly with the thumbs. This will help to relieve the tension often caused by the weight of enlarged breasts.

△ **4** Using the thumbs, work upward on each side of the spinal column from the lower back to the neck to help release congestion along the spinal nerves. Repeat four times. Clear the movement by sweeping up the back using the calming effleurage stroke.

△ **6** Using a double-handed movement, press down and then gently lift the muscles to the side of the neck, rolling with the thumb, and then release. Work out from the neck across the shoulder, and then repeat across the other shoulder. Performed slowly with rhythmic movements this is very relaxing and will alleviate stiffness.

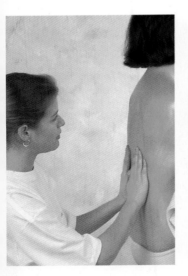

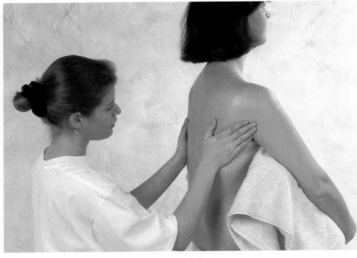

△ **3** Stroke the oil evenly over the back and begin an effleurage movement (a soothing, stroking motion with two hands, moving up the sides of the spine and out over the shoulders). Repeat several times to establish a rhythm and relax your partner.

△ **5** Starting from the centre of the back, begin working up and outward across the width of the back with superficial effleurage movements. Repeat the movements several times until your partner is relaxed. This will help to stimulate the circulation and has a soothing effect on the nerve endings.

the abdomen

For a pregnant woman, the weight of the baby in her uterus can constrict important blood vessels if she lies down flat on her back, so provide plenty of pillows, cushions, bolsters or rolled towels to support your partner behind the back, under the neck and knees and anywhere else she needs it to feel comfortable.

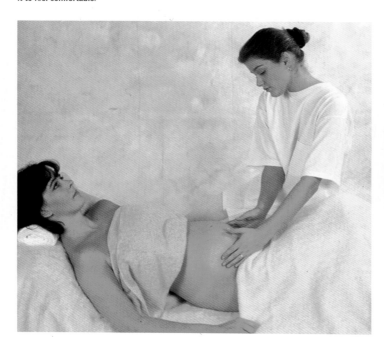

△ **1** It may seem alarming to massage the abdomen during pregnancy but, providing the strokes are light and careful, it is safe and relaxing for mother and baby. Gentle massage all over the abdominal area can be very soothing and is beneficial for relieving the stretched feeling often experienced during pregnancy. Apply oil evenly over the area to help feed the tissues and lessen the possibility of stretch marks.

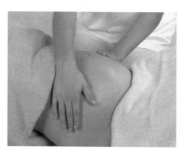

△ **2** Using the flat of your hands, carefully glide them up from either side of the waist with a pulling motion, lifting your hands off as they reach the navel, and then start again. Continue to stroke the area with a light, soft touch, working over the whole of the abdomen to soothe and calm.

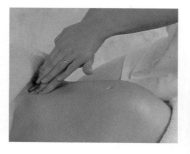

△ **3** After a minute of gentle circular movements, place the fingertips of your left hand on the higher section of the solar plexus region and cover with your right hand. Rest both hands for a moment and then release to help alleviate stress.

the legs

Make sure your partner is comfortable, with the knees supported by cushions.

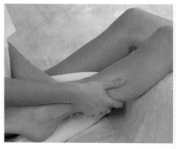

△ **1** Begin gently stroking the leg with an effleurage from the ankle to the knee, smoothing up the shin, and then glide around the calf.

Massage can help to relieve the swelling, varicose veins or cramp which afflict many pregnant women. Do not use any heavy strokes to the legs and avoid any reflexology movements to the feet, though gentle stroking around the ankles may well be appreciated.

to finish

With both hands positioned at the back of the neck, apply light circular pressures to the cranium (skull) with your fingertips working in an upward direction to help release tension.

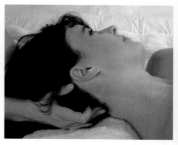

△ **1** End the massage by smoothing the hair away from the neck and forehead, releasing all the negative energy. Allow your partner to rest for 15 minutes and then help her to get up very gently.

self-massage on tired legs

Self-massage can be very soothing and beneficial – and you can do it whenever you like. You can use it to energize yourself before an appointment during the day or to unwind in the evening before going to bed. Massaging the legs is especially good if your legs ache after standing. It stimulates the circulation and soothes tiredness or swelling. Do not apply heavy pressure, and use very light movements on the inner leg.

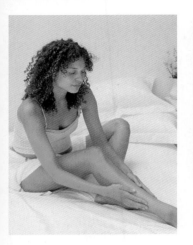

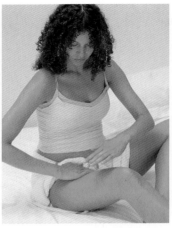

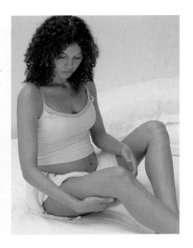

△ **1** Rest the foot of the leg you are working on flat, and bend the knee slightly so you can reach the lower leg. Stroke the whole leg with alternate hands, one on each side of the leg. Work up from the foot to the top of the thigh. Repeat five or six times, then work on the other leg.

△ **3** Stroke the thigh, working up from the knee and using both hands, with one hand following the other. You will enjoy the smooth, flowing strokes as a contrast to the more energetic kneading. Now repeat on the other leg.

△ **5** Using the tips of your fingers, stroke the area around the kneecap. Hold the thigh steady with your other hand. Now stroke gently behind the knee, then continue the action up your thigh. Repeat this step on the knee and thigh of the other leg.

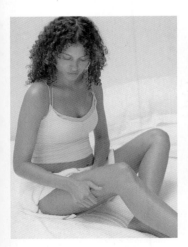

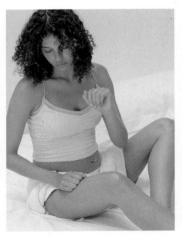

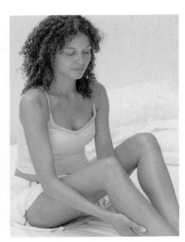

△ **2** Now use alternate hands to knead the thigh. Squeeze and release the flesh, working in a rhythmic fashion from just above the knee to the top of the thigh. Repeat this two or three times, and then work on the thigh of the other leg.

△ **4** Make loose fists and lightly pummel the front and outside of the thigh. This movement will help to relieve any stiffness. Pummel up the thigh a few times, and then repeat on the other thigh.

△ **6** Knead the calf muscle using both hands, alternately squeezing it and releasing it. Then stroke the area gently, with each hand following the other one up the back of the leg. Repeat on the other leg.

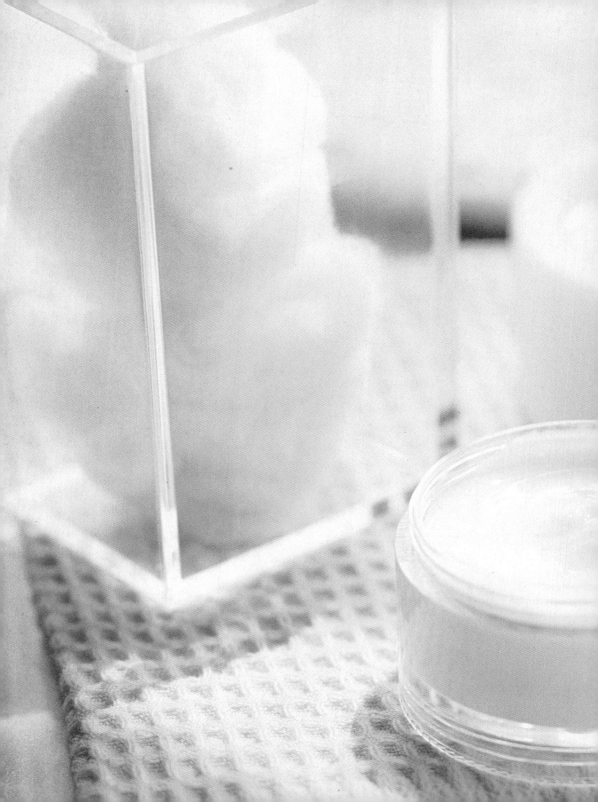

Therapeutic Aromatherapy Treatments

Therapeutic treatments using aromatic essential oils are both pleasurable and effective. The oils draw on the healing properties of plants, and with regular use they can stimulate the immune system to strengthen the body against disease. Within this chapter you will find treatments to alleviate common health conditions including headaches, mood swings, stress, pre-menstrual syndrome and the symptoms of the menopause.

Stress soothers

Sadly, stress is now playing far too large a part in all our lives, and while we cannot always avoid the causes, we can at least dispel its effects on us. All you need to do is set aside just a few minutes at the end of the day when you can be quiet and relax. Then, using a variety of soothing, relaxing therapeutic measures, such as a marvellous, long, slow rhythmic massage, you will end up feeling totally invigorated and refreshed.

stress relievers

Stress, or rather our inability to cope with too much of it, is one of the biggest health problems today. Lifestyles seem to include so many varied and often conflicting demands that it is not surprising that most of us feel stressed at times, sometimes constantly. We all react to excess stress in different ways, perhaps through anxiety, depression or exhaustion, but we can all certainly benefit from the wonderfully balancing and calming effects provided by aromatic oils.

Our bodies are geared to cope with a stressful situation by producing various hormones that trigger a series of physiological actions in the body; they are known collectively as the "fight or flight" response,

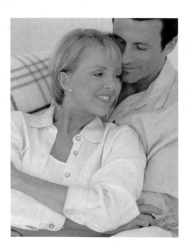

◁ **Aromatherapy can help reduce your levels of stress enabling you to lead a happier and more fulfilled life.**

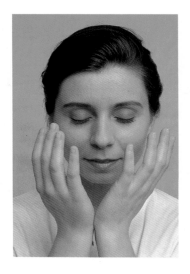

△ **Experimenting with the calming oils will help you to discover which particular essential oils work best for you as an individual.**

and serve to place the body in a state of alert in a potentially dangerous situation. Extra blood is shunted to the muscles, and the heart rate speeds up while the digestion slows down. These responses are appropriate when we are faced with a physical threat, but can nowadays be triggered by quite different kinds of stress and end up placing a strain on our bodies without fulfilling any useful need.

In order to help reduce the impact of stress on the whole system, it is necessary to find ways both to avoid getting overstressed in the first instance, and to let go of the changes that occur internally when under stress. Aromatherapy can be a great help in each case, especially during and immediately after a long relaxing massage, because the oils will help to keep you calm.

anxiety calmers

When people are described as being "uptight", that is often exactly what they are: tense muscles in the face and neck are a sure sign of anxiety. You can release that tension with a face massage, using gentle, soothing strokes on the temples and forehead especially. This is very good as an evening treat, calming away the day's cares and worries.

Use just a few drops of oil because most people do not like having a greasy feeling on the face, and avoid getting oil in the hair. Make up a blend of 4 drops lavender and 2 drops ylang ylang in a light oil such as sweet almond.

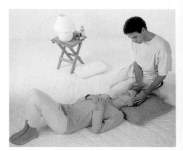

△ **1** Ideally have the person lying down with the head in your lap or on a cushion. With your fingertips, gently begin smoothing the essential oil into the face.

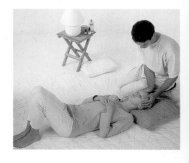

△ **2** Using your thumbs, one after the other, stroke tension gently and carefully away from the centre of the forehead.

blood pressure

It should be emphasized that anyone with very high blood pressure should first seek expert medical (or professional) treatment. You should not even think about trying to tackle such a condition yourself without accurate guidance. However, in much milder, far less dangerous or acute cases, which are almost entirely related to anxiety and tension, you can help get temporary relief by using essential oils.

▽ **1** Begin by giving yourself or your partner a soothing footbath. For such a bath you should fill a large bowl three-quarters full with hot water. Then carefully add 2 drops rose, 2 drops ylang ylang and 3 drops lavender. Using a clean, new wooden kitchen spoon specially reserved for the job, mix everything in, and let stand for a couple of minutes. Then place the feet into the water and soak for at least five relaxing minutes.

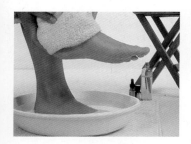

muscular aches

When you are under any kind of stress for any length of time, your body promptly reacts by becoming and staying permanently tense. Clearly this is not good for your body or your emotional state. It can make quite specific muscles, or indeed all of your muscles, ache and feel overwhelmingly tired and sluggish, leaden and heavy.

▽ **1** In order to relieve this all-too-familiar list of thoroughly unwanted symptoms, and also to start releasing the underlying tension, use essential oils in what is called a massage blend. As the massage movements begin to work on the aching muscles at surface and deeper levels, the oils begin to be absorbed. In time they too get to work and start tackling the inner tension.

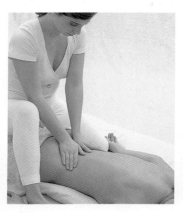

△ **1** Rest your hands on the lower back to either side of the spine. Lean your weight into your hands and stroke up the back towards the head. Mould your hands to the body as they glide firmly along.

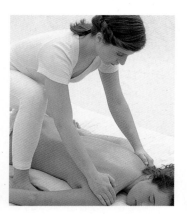

△ **2** As your hands reach the top of the back, fan them out towards the shoulders in a long, smooth, flowing, ceaseless motion.

colic

Colic is the term that is used to describe spasmodic bouts of cramping pain, building up in intensity until it finally reaches a peak, before abating and returning a short while later. The causes can range from an obstructing stone, for which professional medical treatment is required, to intestinal gas. The latter is extremely common in babies, and it may strike adults as a result of high tension levels. Fortunately, you can easily aid the adult condition by having a short gentle massage that will also leave you feeling calm and gently relaxed. It only takes about ten minutes.

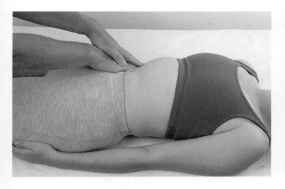

△ **1** Starting in the lower right-hand corner, steadily and firmly press in using both your hands, but taking care not to cause any discomfort.

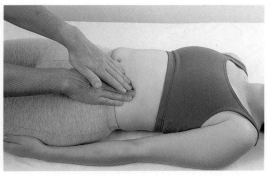

△ **2** Slowly move the hands in a clockwise direction around the abdomen. Keep making continuous small circles to massage the colon.

anxiety

Whether it's a temporary bout of nerves caused by something like an impending examination or interview, or an ongoing response to a persistent problem, anxiety can be a debilitating response to stress. It prevents you from dealing effectively with a problem, and makes you feel tense. Essential oils, when inhaled, stimulate the limbic portion of the brain which is responsible for all our feelings of well-being and discontent. They can balance the senses before deep depression sets into a more serious state. Temporary anxiety can also trigger skin eruptions so watch your diet and boost levels of vitamins C and E and B-complex.

Anxiety can be alleviated with a combination of uplifting and calming oils. You can use the following oils individually or mix them in a blend, using two relaxing oils to one uplifting oil:

Basil (uplifting) • *Bergamot (uplifting)* • *Geranium (relaxing)* • *Lavender (soothing)* • *Neroli (sedative)* • *Sandalwood (calming)*

▽ **Taking time for yourself is an important ingredient in easing anxiety and depression.**

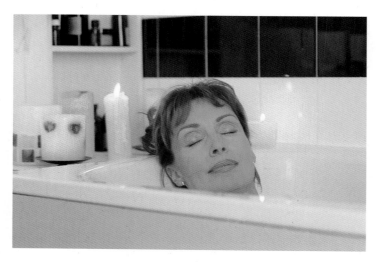

A good combination for an anxiety-reducing blend is basil, neroli and lavender. Stick to the same blend and proportions for bath and body, mixing five drops of each of the three oils in 15ml (1 tbsp) base oil for the bath and 30ml (2 tbsp) for the body. All of the oils can be used individually in ring burners or fragrancers.

mild shock

This is a temporary form of stress, but the impact on the system can nonetheless be very strong, so a fast-acting remedy is needed.

Chamomile (calming) • *Melissa (anti-depressant)* • *Neroli (relieves anxiety)* • *Peppermint (invigorating pain-reliever)* • *Rosemary (stimulating)*

Use only two essential oils: both chamomile and melissa work well individually with neroli, and peppermint has an affinity with melissa. Use a total of six drops in 25ml (1½ tbsp) base oils, with smaller quantities of rosemary (for example, two drops of rosemary to four drops of melissa). For fast relief add four drops to a handkerchief and inhale at regular intervals.

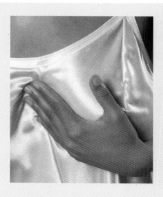

solar plexus stroke
A marvellous way of unlocking tension by calming the main nerves that run through this area. Use your left hand (for calming) to stroke the solar plexus (located just below the breast bone) in anti-clockwise circles. Close your eyes as you do this and try to empty your mind. It can help soothe you even if you're clothed, but the effect is enhanced if you use a relaxing oil such as lavender or geranium. Try it while your bath is running, or when lying in bed before you go to sleep.

headaches

Often one of the first signs of stress and a regular affliction for many people. Cold compresses of lavender or geranium across the forehead provide pleasant relief. Add five drops of one oil to a small bowl of cool or warm water, soak a cloth in the water wring out and lay it across the forehead. To ease a headache caused by tension in the neck, try a sandalwood compress across the neck. Scalp massage is soothing, or try the shiatsu headache relief steps on page 372.

depression

The blues can hit us all from time to time, as financial, emotional or work problems hang over like a dark cloud. In the long term, if problems are not resolved, more serious depression can develop, lowering the immune system and leaving you prone to a

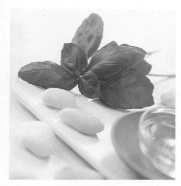

△ Basil is useful for its effects on the nervous system. It can help to dispel fear and jealousy.

jealousy

Most jealous feelings are negative. Jealousy is often linked with anger and/or resentment, and may arise out of an inability to share our friends, family and possessions, or else out of a craving for things that we do not have, which other people (particularly those around us) seem to have. A woman may covet her friend's physical attributes, her successful career, or her conflict-free partnership. Although jealousy is often the most difficult emotion to admit to, it is one of the most deadly, where we stand to hurt not only others but also ourselves. Positive thinking and the use of essential oils which will detoxify or destroy fungi and kill viruses can help to overcome this self-destructive emotion.

Secondary emotions can also be helped by essential oils and are sometimes linked with a primary emotion like fear. Lack of

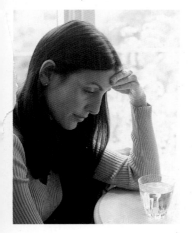

confidence or a sense of under-achievement may involve fear, and mood swings may involve anger and/or irritability.

lack of confidence

Many women suffer from a lack of self-confidence. It can be difficult for women who return to work after being at home bringing up children, or for a woman who is working with people to whom she feels (or is made to feel) inferior. Positive thinking is necessary here, along with neurotonic essential oils which will boost your morale by strengthening the nervous system. These stimulate the mind and will help you to achieve things you never thought were possible. Sweet thyme may help to promote bravery and instil drive and assertiveness due to its many tonic properties. The most effective methods of use are by tissue or vaporizer inhalation, and in the bath.

◁ Water with lemon and peppermint can help to dispel apathy and lift feelings of depression.

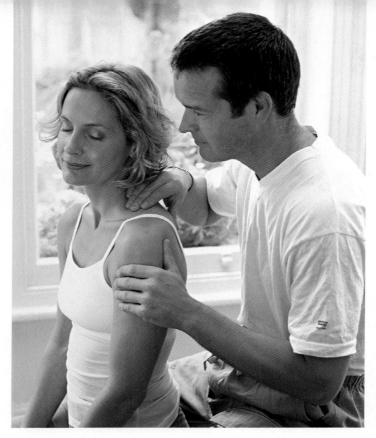

△ A shoulder massage using juniper oil can help when you are feeling emotionally drained.

moodiness

As well as being able to relax or stimulate the nervous system, essential oils can also induce slight mood changes. This makes the use of essential oils suitable for women who are inclined to be temperamental, and for the unpredictable mood swings and irritability suffered during PMS.

loss of sensual awareness

Feelings of indifference, apathy and general loss of libido can be directly related to stress and/or overwork. Taking an essential oil bath or vaporizing some oils an hour before bedtime will help you to unwind, physically and emotionally. You and your partner may like to give each other aromatherapy back or shoulder massages to help each other relax and to prepare for love-making. Use essential oils which are renowned for their aphrodisiac and uplifting effects.

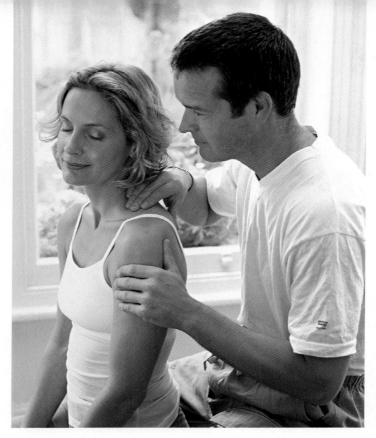

Mood changing aromatherapy

It is all too easy to get dragged down by the ever-increasing, remorseless demands made on you. There never seems to be a moment when you can be quiet and alone, and recharge your batteries. Everything seems stacked against you. But just take a little time out with these oils and you can quickly change your mood, getting rid of the blues and giving yourself a wonderful, refreshing pick-me-up.

uplifting oils

There are unfortunately times in all our lives when we get depressed to some extent, whether due to a specific event or an accumulation of chronic tiredness. As part of a programme of recuperation and restoring your vitality, aromatherapy can certainly be very effective in lifting the mood and giving a boost to your overall energy levels.

For a strong but relatively short-lived effect, try 4 drops bergamot and 2 drops neroli in the bath, ideally first thing in the morning when you are still feeling quite well and relaxed. Do not leave it until too late in the day when the effects of tiredness and stress have taken a strong hold. Aromatherapy stands a far better chance right now of working, and what is more, when it does work it

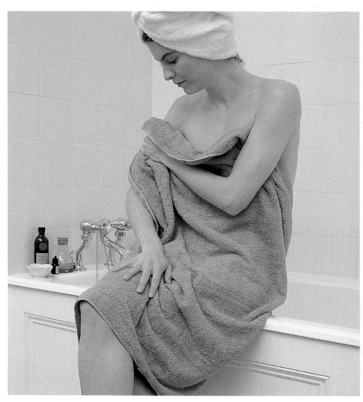

will set you up for the day, giving you renewed confidence. Incidentally, after the bath, gently pat the skin with a soft towel. Do not rub yourself too vigorously.

For a longer-lasting effect, use bergamot or neroli oil in a fragrancer. You will need just one drop of each oil at a time, topping it up throughout the day as necessary.

revitalizing oils

In today's high-pressure world, "high pressure" is exactly what it is all about. We are all expected to pack two lifestyles into one.

△ A bath needn't be just for the evening. A morning bath with warm water and uplifting oils can set you up for the whole day.

Mother and worker, father and possibly chief provider. Nobody gets the right amount of time to themselves to boost their energy levels, or become quietly absorbed in reading or listening to music, for example. The result of trying to juggle too many demands is that nearly all of us reach a state of "brain fag", when mental fatigue and exhaustion grind us to a halt.

Rather than reach for the coffee, or worse still alcohol, which far from being a stimulant is actually well known for depressing the central nervous system, try

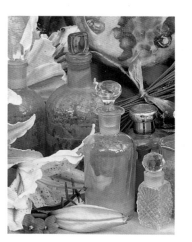

◁ Having a selection of beautifully presented, fragrant bath products can help lift your mood at any time of the day.

using these revitalizing oils. They will give you an instant, revitalizing pick-me-up and make you feel much more alert.

You can use 1–2 drops of rosemary or peppermint oil in a burner. Alternatively, add 3 drops rosemary and 2 drops peppermint to a bowl of steaming water, or use 4 drops of either oil on its own. Give the oils plenty of time to evaporate into the room, and breathe freely. Make sure you then spend some time quietly relaxing, taking in the full benefits of these oils.

invigorating oils

Chronic tension all too often leads to a feeling of inescapable exhaustion, when we just totally run out of steam. At these demoralizing, difficult times we need a sudden boost, and many oils have a tremendous tonic effect, restoring vitality but without over-stimulating in any way. As a group, the citrus oils are excellent for this purpose, ranging from the more soothing mandarin to the highly refreshing lemon oil.

▽ Massage gently all over the body with a light, caring touch. The secret is taking your time, getting the atmosphere right and making sure you choose the right moment.

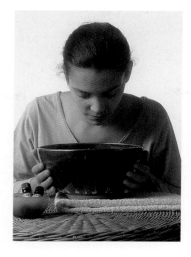

◁ This kind of steam inhalation is a valuable and simple way to receive the benefits of essential oils when either time or circumstance prevents you from having a massage or bath.

Have a warm but not too hot bath, with 4 drops mandarin and 2 drops orange or 4 drops neroli and 2 drops lemon. Alternatively, just add a couple of drops of any of these oils to a bowl full of steaming water. Then sit down calmly, and gently begin inhaling. This will soon help you clear away the tiredness and lift your spirits again.

sensual oils

Tension, anxiety, worry, depression, and loss of confidence and self-belief – these are just some of the many factors that can adversely affect your sexual energy and performance. Sometimes this leads into a no-escape negative spiral of anxiety about sex, leading to less enjoyment, and so on.

The best answer is not to get dragged down, feeling ever more anxious and depressed, until the problem becomes seemingly insurmountable, but to take a little time out of your hectic life. Be together with your partner and have fun; add to your sensual pleasure with an intimate massage session, using one of these excellent blends to release tensions and allow your natural sexual energy to respond freely.

Use whichever of these blends – 5 drops rose and 5 drops sandalwood or 4 drops jasmine and 4 drops ylang ylang – appeals to you both, and include in a massage oil. Use gentle, stroking movements all over the back, buttocks, legs and front.

sleep enhancers

Worries can go round and round inside our heads, usually just as we are trying to get to sleep. Worse, they strike in the middle of the night and get blown out of all proportion. The resulting disturbed and restless night leaves us more prone to stress and anxiety, and a vicious circle can be created. Help break the cycle with a relaxing evening bath. Many oils can be useful – just choosing one that you enjoy for your bath will help you unwind after a long day.

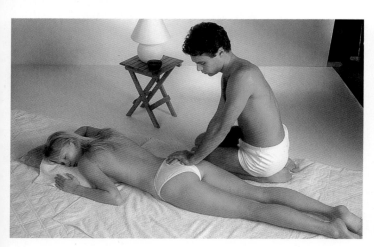

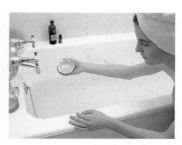

△ Add oils to an evening bath to aid relaxation and sleep. A couple of blends that relax without over-sedating are 4 drops rose and 3 drops sandalwood or 5 drops lavender and 3 drops ylang ylang. Incorporate aromatherapy preparations into your daily bathing routine.

Pre-menstrual syndrome (PMS)

Some researchers estimate that PMS affects up to half of adult women living in modern society. No one knows exactly the cause of PMS, but it is believed that the lowered hormone level in the body after the egg has been released is mainly responsible for the collection of mental and physical symptoms which can become apparent eight to ten days before menstruation. Contributory factors include poor nutrition and stress: women often juggle many responsibilities at the same time, with insufficient time to eat properly and relax.

excessive water retention

Fluid retention is thought to be a crucial factor in PMS, as it affects all the cells in the body. PMS may be accompanied by weight gain and shows itself in the swelling of the abdomen, ankles and breasts, which can become very tender and swollen.

treatment

Diuretic and decongestant essential oils can be used to help reduce swelling.

persistent headaches and sleep disturbances

Both a lack of sleep and regular headaches are draining on the body, and will increase stress levels and the inability to cope.

treatment

Calming, neurotonic and decongestant essential oils can be used to relieve the headaches and/or insomnia by balancing the whole body.

emotional instability

Many women suffer from depression and irritability every month. In some cases, this can be severe and can lead to arguments and difficulties at home and at work.

treatment

Antidepressant and calming essential oils, taken as inhalations and baths, can help.

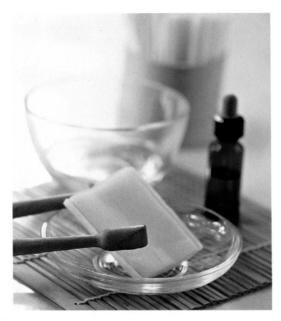

◁ To make a compress, add a few drops of your chosen oil blend to a bowl of water and mix well. Place a piece of cloth on the water's surface and let the oil soak into it. Use as needed.

▽ For sleepless nights, headaches and irritability prepare a mix of Roman chamomile, melissa and lavender. It may be handy to keep some by your bedside.

lifestyle tips for PMS

For the most effective results, a holistic approach to PMS is essential.

• Amend your diet to boost your general health and vitality

• Exercise to stimulate your blood circulation and to relieve congestion: try walking, cycling and swimming.

• Avoid stressful situations wherever possible, and ask for help if home or work responsibilities become too much

• Take your favourite relevant essential oils to work for instant therapy

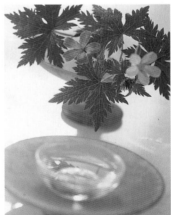

hormonal treatment

Some essential oils have a tendency to normalize hormonal secretions, including those involved in the reproductive system. Cypress is helpful for all ovarian problems. Clary sage and niaouli are oestrogen-like, which makes them useful for the stages in a woman's life when oestrogen production is unstable. To balance your hormones, these oils should be used in applications, baths and inhalations ten to 12 days before the expected start of a period.

Useful essential oils

essential oil	treatment

hormone-like essential oils

essential oil	treatment
Chamomile (German) *Matricaria recutica*	decongestant, hormone-like
Clary sage *Salvia sclarea*	decongestant, oestrogen-like
Cypress *Cupressus sempervirens*	hormone-like (ovarian)
Niaouli *Melaleuca viridiflora*	oestrogen-like (regularizes menses)
Peppermint *Mentha* x *piperita*	hormone-like (ovarian stimulant), neurotonic

painful periods and backache

essential oil	treatment
Basil *Ocimum basilicum* var. *album*	analgesic, antispasmodic, decongestant
Eucalyptus *Eucalyptus smithii* (not *Eucalyptus globulus*)	analgesic, decongestant
Geranium *Pelargonium graveolens*	analgesic, antispasmodic, decongestant
Lavender *Lavandula angustifolia*	analgesic, antispasmodic, calming, sedative, tonic
Marjoram (sweet) *Origanum majorana*	analgesic, antispasmodic, calming, neurotonic
Peppermint *Mentha* x *piperita*	analgesic, decongestant, hormone-like (ovarian stimulant)
Pine *Pinus sylvestris*	analgesic, decongestant
Rosemary *Rosmarinus officinalis*	analgesic, antispasmodic, decongestant

irregular, scanty and/or lack of periods

Mix a blend using the hormone-like essential oils (above).
Other possibilities include:

essential oil	treatment
Chamomile (Roman) *Chamaemelum nobile*	calming, menstrual regulator, nervous menstrual problems
Melissa *Melissa officinalis*	calming, sedative, regularizes secretions
Rose otto *Rosa damascena*	general reproductive system regulator

heavy periods

essential oil	treatment
Cypress *Cupressus sempervirens*	astringent, phlebotonic, hormone-like (ovary problems)
Melissa *Melissa officinalis*	calming, sedative, regularizes secretions

fluid retention

essential oil	treatment
Cypress *Cupressus sempervirens*	diuretic (oedema, rheumatic swelling)
Fennel *Foeniculum vulgare*	diuretic (cellulite, oedema)
Juniper *Juniperus communis*	diuretic (cellulite, oedema)
Sage *Salvia officinalis*	decongestant, lypolytic (cellulite)

low spirits (depression) and fatigue

essential oil	treatment
Basil *Ocimum basilicum* var. *album*	nervous system regulator (anxiety), neurotonic (convalescence, depression)
Chamomile (Roman) *Chamaemelum nobile*	calming (nervous depression, nervous shock)
Clary sage *Salvia sclarea*	neurotonic (nervous fatigue)
Geranium *Pelargonium graveolens*	relaxant (anxiety, debility, nervous fatigue)
Juniper *Juniperus communis*	neurotonic (debility, fatigue)
Marjoram (sweet) *Origanum majorana*	neurotonic (debility, mental instability, anguish, nervous depression)
Pine *Pinus sylvestris*	neurotonic (debility, fatigue)
Rosemary *Rosmarinus officinalis*	neurotonic (general debility and fatigue)

tender, congested breasts

essential oil	treatment
Eucalyptus *Eucalyptus smithii* (not *Eucalyptus globulus*)	analgesic, decongestant
Geranium *Pelargonium graveolens*	analgesic, decongestant

headaches

essential oil	treatment
Chamomile (Roman) *Chamaemelum nobile*	antispasmodic, calming, sedative
Lavender *Lavandula angustifolia*	analgesic, calming, sedative
Marjoram (sweet) *Origanum majorana*	analgesic, antispasmodic, calming
Melissa *Melissa officinalis*	calming, sedative
Peppermint *Mentha* x *piperita*	analgesic, antispasmodic
Rosemary *Rosmarinus officinalis*	analgesic, antispasmodic, decongestant

insomnia

essential oil	treatment
Basil *Ocimum basilicum* var. *album*	nervous system regulator (nervous insomnia)
Chamomile (Roman) *Chamaemelum nobile*	calming, sedative
Lavender *Lavandula angustifolia*	calming, sedative
Lemon *Citrus limon*	calming
Melissa *Melissa officinalis*	calming, sedative

irritability

essential oil	treatment
Chamomile (Roman) *Chamaemelum nobile*	calming, sedative

Common women's health problems

There are several relatively common health problems which can occur at any age and with varying degrees of severity. Stress generally makes all these conditions worse.

irritable bowel syndrome (IBS)

This disorder of the lower bowel usually occurs between 20-40 years of age. The usual symptoms are colicky pains, diarrhoea and/or constipation, and distension of the abdomen, giving rise to noisy rumblings and wind. Emotional factors can play an important part in this disorder, and those who are anxious and over-conscientious are the most likely sufferers. Symptoms can be worse just before a period, especially if PMS is present.

It is useful to experiment with diet. Exclude cow's milk and its products and monitor the result. Foods which contain wheat can also cause problems, as can the caffeine in tea and coffee. Try essential oils which balance the digestive system, used in a variety of ways: by ingestion (*see* Aromatherapy Principles), by application of oils in a carrier base, rubbed on to the abdomen twice daily in a clockwise direction, and by compresses placed over the abdomen.

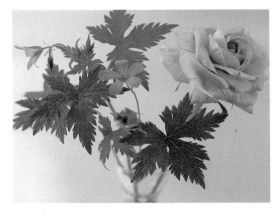

▷ The heady yet gentle aroma of rose is a favourite with almost every woman. Rose helps to lift the spirits and promote feelings of well-being.

▷ An application of fennel, peppermint and/or rosemary can be helpful with IBS. Use in a carrier oil or compress applied to the abdomen area.

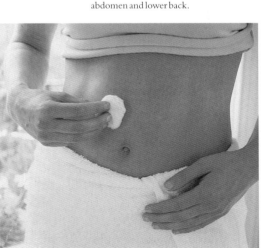

cystitis

This is a common problem that can occur after sex and during pregnancy. Cystitis is an infection and inflammation of the bladder and urethra. It is characterized by a frequent, painful urge to go to the toilet. Treatment is with antibacterial and antiseptic essential oils which have an affinity to the kidneys. Cystitis has been treated successfully using a tea with the relevant essential oils added (*see* Aromatherapy Principles) and by application of the same oils in a carrier base to the abdomen and lower back.

sinusitis

Inflammation of the sinus area around the nose and/or eyes can occur at any time in life after puberty and is often difficult to cure, even with an operation. It causes chronic congestion, catarrh and sometimes headaches. Fortunately, sinusitis can be helped easily and successfully by adding the appropriate essential oils to your regular moisturizer. Allergic reactions or colds can exacerbate the condition, in which case neat essential oils should be inhaled on a tissue or used in the bath. Pressing on the sinus-pressure points on the feet every night while symptoms persist is also helpful.

vaginitis

Inflammation of the vagina, with accompanying irritation, can be caused by leaving a tampon in too long or through use of the contraceptive pill. The most frequent cause is when a yeast-like substance, called *Candida albicans*, a normal inhabitant of the mouth and bowel (and, in women, of the vagina) becomes infected. When symptoms first appear, immediate treatment with essential oils will help. Provided a tampon was not the cause of the inflammation in the first place, try a tampon with 2 drops of tea tree oil inserted into the vagina and left in overnight. Alternatively, taking regular sitz-baths for ten minutes at a time, using a synergistic mix of appropriate essential oils, can also help.

thrush

Infected *Candida albicans* can show as white ulcerous spots inside the mouth (thrush), which can be dealt with using a mouthwash including anti-infectious essential oils. The vagina can also be affected with thrush, giving rise to itching and discomfort. Thrush usually affects women with a low immune system, where it can be due to stress, the overuse of antibiotics or diabetes. Additional symptoms which can present themselves at this time include cystitis, depression and headaches.

With thrush it is helpful if the intake of sugar and refined carbohydrates in the diet is reduced immediately. If the condition worsens, an effective form of aromatherapy treatment involves eating live yogurt containing suitable essential oils: 20 drops of oil to 100ml (6–7 tbsp) of yogurt and, if possible, inserting some of this mixture into the vagina with a tampon applicator.

endometriosis

This condition is when tissue similar to that of the lining of the uterus is found else-where – mostly in the ovaries. The tissue swells and bleeds, causing severe pain before a period and excessive blood loss during it. Conventional treatment may recommend removal of the ovaries (and therefore the

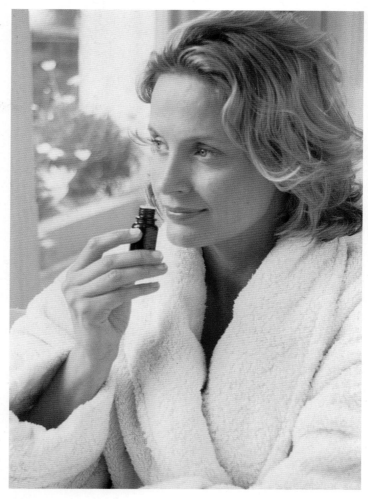

△ **Peppermint is useful for relieving nasal congestion and treating general sinus problems.**

hormone production) so that the uterus is no longer stimulated to produce the extra tissue. The contraceptive pill is often prescribed but this is not always successful.

⁕ Some women prefer to avoid surgery if possible, in which case it is worth trying hormone-like and decongestant essential oils first, as they have been known to help. If surgery is inevitable, then oestrogen-like essential oils will help the body to readjust itself to the loss of the ovaries.

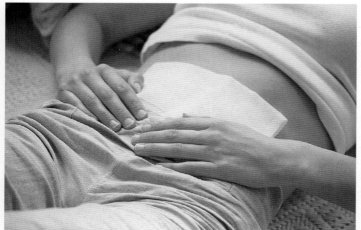

◁ **A compress of clary sage and cypress can be used for problems associated with the ovaries.**

Useful essential oils

essential oil	treatment
stress	
Chamomile (Roman) *Chamaemelum nobile*	calming
Lemon *Citrus limon*	calming, hypotensive
Melissa *Melissa officinalis*	calming, sedative
Ylang ylang *Cananga odorata*	balancing, calming, hypotensive
depression	
Basil *Ocimum basilicum var. album*	neurotonic
Frankincense *Boswellia carteri*	energizing, immunostimulant
Juniper *Juniperus communis*	neurotonic
Neroli *Citrus aurantium var. amara*	tranquilizing (nervous depression, fatigue)
Niaouli *Melaleuca viridiflora*	tonic
Peppermint *Mentha x piperita*	neurotonic
Pine *Pinus sylvestris*	neurotonic
Rosemary *Rosmarinus officinalis*	neurotonic, sexual tonic
stress with depression	
Bergamot *Citrus bergamia*	balancing, calming, sedative, tonic to central nervous system
Clary sage *Salvia sclarea*	balancing, relaxing, neurotonic
Cypress *Cupressus sempervirens*	balancing, calming, neurotonic
Geranium *Pelargonium graveolens*	balancing, relaxing, stimulant (nervous fatigue)
Lavender *Lavandula angustifolia*	balancing, calming, sedative, tonic
Marjoram *Origanum majorana*	balancing, calming, neurotonic
Rose otto *Rosa damascena*	balancing, relaxing, neurotonic, sexual tonic
poor concentration	
Basil *Ocimum basilicum var. album*	neurotonic
Bergamot *Citrus bergamia*	balancing, tonic
Thyme (sweet) *Thymus vulgaris*	cardiotonic, neurotonic, immunostimulant
irritable bowel syndrome	
Fennel *Foeniculum vulgare*	analgesic, antispasmodic, digestive (constipation, diarrhoea, flatulence)
Peppermint *Mentha x piperita*	analgesic, anti-inflammatory, digestive (diarrhoea, flatulence)
Rosemary *Rosmarinus officinalis*	analgesic, antispasmodic, digestive (constipation, flatulence)

essential oil	treatment
thrush (*Candida albicans*) and vaginitis	
Lavender *Lavandula angustifolia*	analgesic, antifungal, anti-inflammatory
Pine *Pinus sylvestris*	analgesic, antifungal, anti-infectious, anti-inflammatory, neurotonic
Tea tree *Melaleuca alternifolia*	analgesic, antifungal, anti-infectious, anti-inflammatory, immunostimulant, neurotonic
Thyme (sweet) *Thymus vulgaris*	antifungal, anti-infectious, anti-inflammatory, immunostimulant, neurotonic
cystitis	
Eucalyptus *Eucalyptus smithii*	anti-infectious, antiseptic
Juniper *Juniperus communis*	anti-inflammatory, antiseptic
Lavender *Lavandula angustifolia*	anti-inflammatory, antiseptic
Thyme (sweet) *Thymus vulgaris*	anti-infectious, anti-inflammatory, antiseptic
sinusitis	
Eucalyptus *Eucalyptus smithii*	anti-inflammatory, antiseptic
Lavender *Lavandula angustifolia*	anti-inflammatory, anti-infectious, antiseptic
Peppermint *Mentha x piperita*	anti-inflammatory, anti-infectious
endometriosis	
Clary sage *Salvia sclarea*	decongestant, oestrogen-like, phlebotonic
Cypress *Cupressus sempervirens*	astringent, hormone-like (ovary problems), phlebotonic
Geranium *Pelargonium graveolens*	analgesic, astringent, cicatrizant, decongestant, phlebotonic, styptic
Rose otto *Rosa damascena*	astringent, cicatrizant, neurotonic, styptic

Sweet scents are the swift vehicles

of still sweeter thoughts.

Walter Savage Landor, 1775–1864.

essential oil	treatment

anger, fear and jealousy

The following essential oils can benefit all of these emotions.
The properties required for each condition are listed first, and the oils
which follow show the properties each possesses relevant to that
particular emotion.

ANGER

Look for oils which are	analgesic, anticatarrhal, anti-inflammatory, antispasmodic, calming, carminative (relieving flatulence), cicatrizant, sedative
Basil *Ocimum basilicum* var. *album*	analgesic, anti-inflammatory, carminative, calming to the nervous system
Bergamot *Citrus bergamia*	antispasmodic, calming, cicatrizant
Geranium *Pelargonium graveolens*	analgesic, anti-inflammatory, antispasmodic, cicatrizant, relaxant
Juniper *Juniperus communis*	analgesic, anticatarrhal, anti-inflammatory
Lavender *Lavandula angustifolia*	analgesic, anti-inflammatory, antispasmodic, calming and sedative, cicatrizant
Lemon *Citrus limon*	anti-inflammatory, antispasmodic, calming, carminative

FEAR

Look for oils which are	antispasmodic, cardiotonic, calming and soothing, digestive, hypotensive, mental stimulant, nausea relief, nerve tonic, respiratory tonic, sedative
Basil *Ocimum basilicum* var. *album*	antispasmodic, cardiotonic, neurotonic
Bergamot *Citrus bergamia*	antispasmodic (indigestion), calming, sedative (agitation), nerve tonic
Geranium *Pelargonium graveolens*	antispasmodic, relaxant
Juniper *Juniperus communis*	digestive tonic, nerve tonic
Lavender *Lavandula angustifolia*	antispasmodic, calming, cardiotonic, hypotensive, sedative
Lemon *Citrus limon*	antispasmodic (diarrhoea normalizing), calming, hypotensive, nausea relief

The flowers anew, returning seasons bring

But beauty faded has no second spring.

From The First Pastoral, *Ambrose Philips, 1675–1749.*

essential oil	treatment

JEALOUSY

Look for oils which are	antibacterial, antifungal, antiviral, cicatrizant, detoxifying, litholytic
Basil *Ocimum basilicum* var. *album*	antibacterial, antiviral, decongestant (uterine)
Bergamot *Citrus bergamia*	antibacterial, antiviral, cicatrizant
Geranium *Pelargonium graveolens*	antibacterial, antifungal, cicatrizant, decongestant (lymph)
Juniper *Juniperus communis*	detoxifying, litholytic
Lavender *Lavandula angustifolia*	antibacterial, antifungal, cicatrizant
Lemon *Citrus limon*	antibacterial, antifungal, antiviral, litholytic

irritability

Chamomile (Roman) *Chamaemelum nobile*	calming
Cypress *Cupressus sempervirens*	calming
Rose otto *Rosa damascena*	calming

lack of confidence

Basil *Ocimum basilicum* var. *album*	neurotonic
Bergamot *Citrus bergamia*	balancing, tonic to central nervous system
Lavender *Lavandula angustifolia*	balancing, tonic
Marjoram *Origanum majorana*	balancing, neurotonic
Rosemary *Rosmarinus officinalis*	neurotonic
Thyme (sweet) *Thymus vulgaris*	cardiotonic, neurotonic, immunostimulant

aromatherapy in pregnancy

Essential oils can bring relief from the many minor troubles which can occur during pregnancy. Discomforts commonly experienced by women include morning sickness, backache, oedema (swollen legs and ankles), constipation, varicose veins, digestive problems (including heartburn), leg cramps and exhaustion. Coping with these discomforts can be especially difficult while the woman is working or if there is a small child or children to look after in the home. Essential oils are also useful during labour, to ease pain and to facilitate delivery.

morning sickness

Nausea, which typically occurs in the morning, is often one of the first signs that a woman is pregnant. Inhalations with a vaporizer can be helpful at bedtime and first thing in the morning. The oils can be left to vaporize overnight in the bedroom. If the sickness persists through the day, prepare a tissue with the relevant oils, and keep it with you at all times.

constipation

This is also another early sign of pregnancy. Prepare essential oils in a suitable carrier base and apply them to the abdomen in a

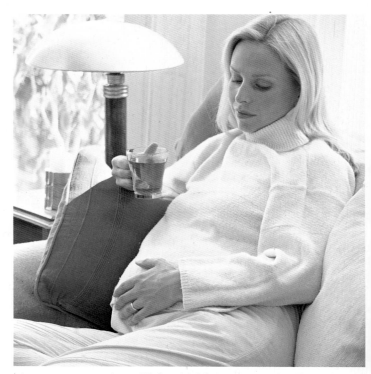

△ As your pregnancy proceeds, you will feel your baby's first movements. Setting aside some time each day to relax and be with your unborn child can help the mother-child bonding process.

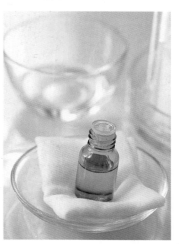

◁ Add a few drops of bitter orange to a bowl of water and make a compress to ease constipation.

clockwise direction. Alternatively, use the oils in the bath and/or on a compress. Eating a healthy diet and drinking plenty of water will help to reduce the risk of constipation.

stretch marks

By the beginning of the second trimester, your clothes will be feeling tighter as your abdomen swells. Halfway through this trimester you will be able to feel the baby's first movements (an exciting moment). Start using essential oils at this time to prevent stretch marks on the skin of the abdomen. Through the correct and diligent application of appropriate essential oils it is possible to maintain a supple and undamaged skin, and you will greatly appreciate your efforts after the baby is born.

Prepare a carrier base (include calendula oil) containing oils with regenerative and skin-toning properties. The mixture should be applied to the abdomen twice daily, morning and night. The area to be covered increases as the pregnancy proceeds, and will include the sides of the body, the groin and on and above the breasts.

backache

As your baby grows, so the likelihood of backache increases. Sitting and standing with correct posture can go a long way to minimize backache, but it will usually occur at some stage and can be helped with essential oils when it does. Prepare a carrier base, then add the appropriate oils and ask a friend or your partner to give you a back massage, ideally at bedtime. Try using the same essential oils (but without the carrier oil) in the bath. Include basil and marjoram in the massage-mix; these can also be used if you suffer from leg cramps later on.

heartburn

The growing baby may also put pressure on your stomach, causing indigestion and heartburn. For heartburn, add 2 drops each of mandarin and peppermint oils to 10ml (2 tsp) carrier base and apply to the painful area. These oils can also be inhaled neat from a tissue or cupped hands, breathing deeply.

varicose veins, swollen legs and ankles

It is as well for all women to watch out for early signs of these conditions throughout pregnancy. Resting with the feet and legs raised is beneficial for all leg conditions. Although the essential oils are different for each condition, the method of use is the same. Prepare a carrier base and add the oils.

Apply the mixture to the whole leg, then bring your hands firmly from the foot up to the knee, before returning to the foot to start again. Massage only in an upward direction, to encourage blood flow to the heart. For varicose veins on the upper leg, massage upwards, going only from knee to groin – not back again – several times.

◁ Your growing baby can cause painful heartburn. Put two drops each of mandarin and peppermint on a tissue and sniff throughout the day.

▽ Backache is a common complaint of pregnancy. Ask your partner for a back massage, using basil and marjoram, before going to bed.

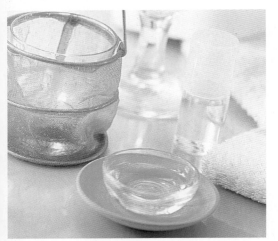

◁ A room vaporizer is a convenient way of inhaling oils. To help with morning sickness, vaporize a combination of lemon, ginger and basil at bedtime and when you wake up.

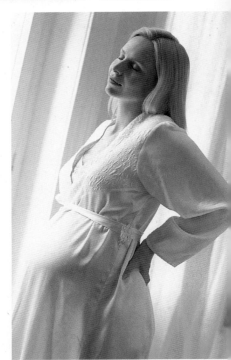

Ante-natal bodycare

During the last trimester of pregnancy, it is a good idea to prepare for labour and to discuss with your midwife or doctor how you would like the birth to proceed. It is helpful to attend prenatal classes, especially if it is the birth of your first child. The classes teach useful exercises to help you relax when the time for labour comes.

preparing for labour

Much of the pain of childbirth, particularly with a first child, is due to the muscles at the neck of the uterus and the perineum being tense and/or inflexible, which means they can tear when stretched. This can be eased by the application of muscle-relaxing essential oils in a vegetable carrier oil. If application is begun daily from several weeks before the expected birth date, the area can be made supple and soft. This will prepare it for the enormous amount of expansion needed for the baby to be born.

Massage a little of the mix twice daily around the perineum area, and try inserting your fingers into the neck of the womb to stretch it, thus helping to prevent tearing.

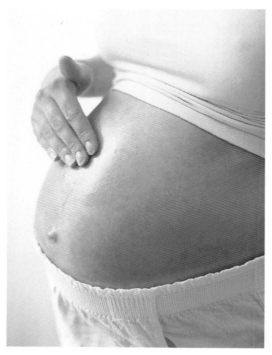

◁ To prevent stretch marks, geranium and frankincense, in a calendula oil carrier, should be massaged on to the abdomen area twice daily.

▽ Massage the lower leg in an upwards direction to relieve aches and oedema.

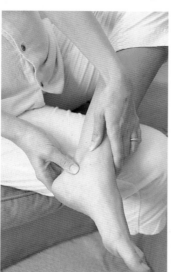

As you get heavier, remember to keep increasing the area to which you are applying your essential oil blend to prevent stretch marks, taking your mix round the sides of your body, on to the upper part of your thighs and above your breasts. It is also important at this time to rest your legs at regular intervals (from every five minutes to half an hour), if you suspect you are likely to develop varicose veins.

As the time for the birth approaches, you may experience conflicting emotions and mood swings. Using uplifting essential oils can give you inner strength to cope with all that is in store for you during this very exciting time in your life.

◁ Make regular checks for oedema on your feet and ankles as your pregnancy progresses. If symptoms occur, a massage plan can help.

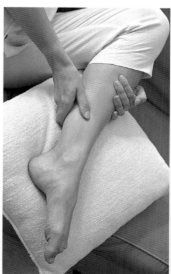

Relief treatments for labour

There are some oils which are particularly useful in labour. In the past, these were limited to lavender and clary sage for their calming and relaxing effects. However, there are a few oils with womb-stimulant and analgesic properties, and these can help with contractions: aniseed, clove bud, nutmeg and sage. These oils are *absolutely not* advocated for the first four months of pregnancy and should not be used until the last week, when labour is about to begin. Used correctly, these oils can help to make the birth easier and quicker, especially for a first-time mother. They are used to relieve pain and induce sleep, and will have a soothing, dulling, lulling effect. Clove bud is particularly analgesic and nutmeg an effective sedative.

treatment

Try a mix of two drops each of any two of the oils with four drops of lavender on a tissue, and inhale between contractions. Some women like to put the tissue into the switched-off gas and air machine, which seems to have the psychological effect of making the oils more efficient.

Alternatively, blend three drops each of aniseed, nutmeg and peppermint with eight drops of lavender into 50ml (2fl oz) carrier oil, and ask your partner to massage your feet and lower legs every half hour. Apply the same mix to your own hands and shoulders, if preferred.

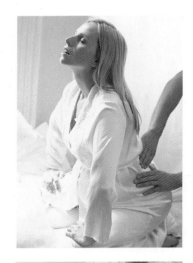

▷ **Lower back pain can be eased by massage. Ask your partner to rub the painful areas.**

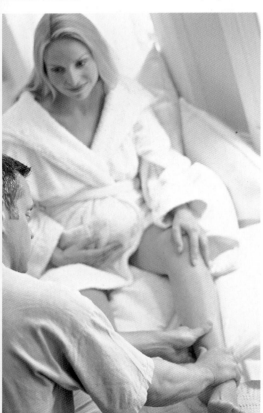

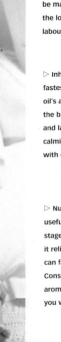

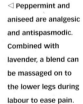

◁ **Peppermint and aniseed are analgesic and antispasmodic. Combined with lavender, a blend can be massaged on to the lower legs during labour to ease pain.**

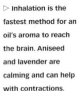

▷ **Inhalation is the fastest method for an oil's aroma to reach the brain. Aniseed and lavender are calming and can help with contractions.**

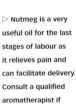

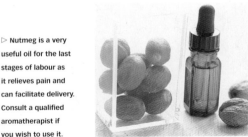

▷ **Nutmeg is a very useful oil for the last stages of labour as it relieves pain and can facilitate delivery. Consult a qualified aromatherapist if you wish to use it.**

Post-natal bodycare

Essential oils can be used to help with the common emotional stresses and physical problems arising as a result of the birth.

Use 6 drops of the appropriate essential oils blended in 20ml (4 tsp) of calendula oil for application. Alternatively, use them on their own for inhalation or in the bath.

birth wounds

During the birth, the perineum may be bruised and/or torn, and can be very painful afterwards. Using the three perineum oils, gently apply them several times a day. If the area is too painful to touch, use a compress (*see* Aromatherapy Principles).

breast feeding problems

Always apply the appropriate essential oils immediately after each feed, so that they are completely absorbed by your body before the baby's next feed is due.

Insufficient milk: fennel oil encourages milk production. Fennel will also help to keep the baby's excreta normal and can help to relieve any wind.

Too much milk: 2 drops of peppermint oil with 4 drops of geranium oil can be used in a massage all over the breasts.

Cracked nipples or mastitis: use 2 drops of each essential oil listed opposite.

emotional difficulties

After the birth, it will take a while before your hormones return to normal. This can be a stressful time as you have a new baby to care for just when you are feeling in need of care yourself. Fatigue, anxiety, despondency and emotional imbalances are common. Essential oils can help before post-natal depression sets in. Blend oils for use by inhalation, in the bath or by application.

treating your baby

Essential oils can help you and your baby cope with the everyday, minor ailments which many babies are subject to, such as

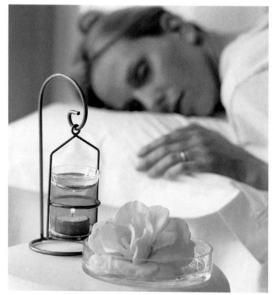

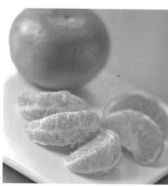

△ The gentle action of mandarin makes it a good choice for treating colic and digestive disorders.

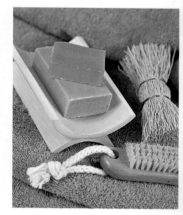

◁ After a long and exhausting labour, and with a new baby to look after, make sure you get enough sleep. Burn lavender through the night to relax and refresh you.

▽ Once your baby is born, pamper yourself and invest in some good quality skincare products.

indigestion, colic, constipation and/or diarrhoea, minor infections and nappy rash. For nappy rash, use 15ml (3 tsp) base lotion with 5ml (1 tsp) calendula oil, mixed with one drop of peppermint and up to three drops of any other selected oils.

Babies can benefit from massage with essential oils. The massage will relax them and can help to strengthen the bond between mother and child. For application to babies, use one drop of essential oil per 5ml (1 tsp) carrier lotion or oil. For sleep problems, try two to three drops of oil in a vaporizer in the baby's room, or try them on a tissue which is pinned to the baby's clothes or placed inside the pillowcase.

Useful essential oils

essential oil	treatment	essential oil	treatment
hormone-like essential oils		**labour**	
Chamomile (German) *Matricaria recutica*	hormone-like	Aniseed *Pimpinella anisum*	analgesic, antispasmodic, calming (gentle narcotic), emmenagogic, oestrogen-like, uterotonic
Clary sage *Salvia sclarea*	oestrogen-like		
Niaouli *Melaleuca viridiflora*	oestrogen-like (regularizes periods)	Lavender *Lavandula angustifolia*	analgesic, antispasmodic, calming (anxiety), sedative
backache		Nutmeg *Myristica fragrans*	analgesic, sedative (narcotic), neurotonic, uterotonic
Basil *Ocimum basilicum* var. *album*	analgesic, antispasmodic	Peppermint *Mentha* x *piperita*	analgesic, antispasmodic, hormone-like (ovarian stimulant), neurotonic, uterotonic (facilitates delivery)
Lavender *Lavandula angustifolia*	analgesic, anti-inflammatory, antispasmodic		
Marjoram (sweet) *Origanum majorana*	analgesic, antispasmodic		
constipation		**perineum**	
Ginger *Zingiber officinale*	analgesic, digestive stimulant	Geranium *Pelargonium graveolens*	analgesic, cicatrizant (wounds)
Mandarin *Citrus reticulata*	antispasmodic, calming, digestive stimulant	Lavender *Lavandula angustifolia*	analgesic, antiseptic (bruises)
Orange (bitter) *Citrus aurantium* var. *amara*	calming, digestive stimulant	Rosemary *Rosmarinus officinalis*	analgesic, anti-inflammatory
Rosemary *Rosmarinus officinalis*	analgesic, digestive stimulant	**breast milk**	
nausea		Fennel *Foeniculum vulgare*	lactogenic (promotes milk), oestrogen-like (insufficient milk)
Basil *Ocimum basilicum* var. *album*	digestive tonic, nervous system regulator	Geranium *Pelargonium graveolens*	decongestant (breast conges- tion – for too much milk)
Ginger *Zingiber officinale*	digestive	Peppermint *Mentha* x *piperita*	antilactogenic (prevents milk forming)
Lemon *Citrus limon*	anticoagulant, antispasmodic, calming, digestive		
stretch marks		**cracked nipples or mastitis**	
Frankincense *Boswellia carteri*	cell regenerative, cicatrizant (scars)	Chamomile (German) *Matricaria recutica*	cicatrizant (infected wounds, ulcers)
Geranium *Pelargonium graveolens*	cell regenerative, cicatrizant (stretch marks)	Geranium *Pelargonium graveolens*	cicatrizant (burns, cuts, ulcers, wounds)
Lavender *Lavandula angustifolia*	cicatrizant (scars)	Lavender *Lavandula angustifolia*	cicatrizant (burns, scars, varicose veins, wounds)
fluid retention		**nappy rash**	
Fennel *Foeniculum vulgare*	diuretic (cellulite, oedema)	Patchouli *Pogostemon patchouli*	anti-inflammatory, cicatrizant (cracked skin, scar tissue)
Juniper *Juniperus communis*	diuretic (cellulite, oedema)	Peppermint *Mentha* x *piperita*	analgesic, anti-inflammatory, soothing (skin irritation, rashes)
Lemon *Citrus limon*	diuretic (obesity, oedema)		
varicose veins		**post-natal depression**	
Clary sage *Salvia sclarea*	phlebotonic (circulatory problems, haemorrhoids, varicose veins)	Basil *Ocimum basilicum* var. *album*	nervous system regulator (anxiety), neurotonic (convalescence, depression)
Cypress *Cupressus sempervirens*	phlebotonic (haemorrhoids, poor venous circulation, varicose veins)	Chamomile (Roman) *Chamaemelum nobile*	calming (nervous depression, nervous shock)
Niaouli *Melaleuca viridiflora*	phlebotonic (haemorrhoids, varicose veins)		

Aromatherapy during menopause

Although a large percentage of women have no problems with the menopause, many do experience some discomfort.

night sweats

These are best tackled through preventative treatment. Try taking an aromatherapy bath with the relevant oils each night before bedtime. Alternatively, try massaging the oils in a suitable carrier base into the body.

hot flushes

Put 20 drops of the same blend of essential oils in 1 litre (1¾ pints) of spring water in a screw-topped bottle. Fit the lid, shake well and transfer some into a purse-size spray and some into a small bottle that you can carry around with you. As soon as you feel a flush coming on, drink two mouthfuls of the water and spray your face and neck. Vitamin E is also said to be effective.

water retention and bloating

To reduce water retention and cellulite, the relevant essential oils should be added to a suitable carrier base and applied daily to the affected areas. The same oils can also be used neat in the bath.

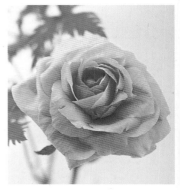

△ Rose otto can help with haemorrhaging. It is also useful for both loss of libido and dry skin.

hair and skin

The condition of the hair and skin can be affected by the hormonal changes of the menopause. Both will become thinner and drier, and it is a good idea to adapt your daily care regime to compensate.

hair

For hair dryness, use a good conditioner. You may like to add appropriate essential oils to give extra shine. For thinning hair, try a daily scalp massage with essential oils (see Aromatherapy Principles).

skin

This not only becomes drier, but is more prone to wrinkles. Try a product containing essential oils or prepare your own mix.

haemorrhaging

Occasional and sudden bleeding can occur when you least expect it. Although essential oils can reduce the amount of blood loss, as far as we know, they do not seem to stop it happening. As a preventative measure, try using styptic and/or astringent essential oils if you are prone to haemorrhaging.

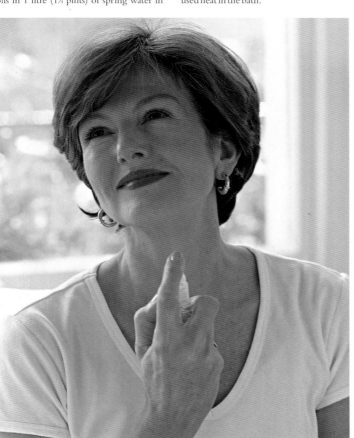

◁ Peppermint and cypress are useful for hot flushes. Make up a mix and use it in an atomizer.

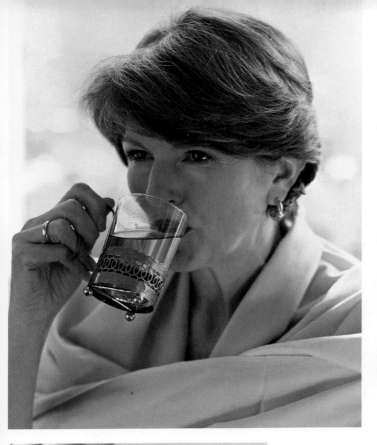

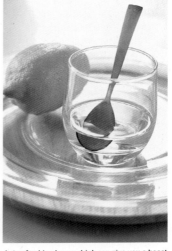

△ A refreshing lemon drink can give you a boost and relieve depression. As always, special care should be taken with oils for internal use.

△ If you are having difficulties sleeping, a soothing cup of sweet marjoram and chamomile tea in the evening can help.

◁ Make your own beauty products by adding combinations of your favourite oils to quality base creams and lotions.

heart and circulation problems

In developed countries, arterial disease is the commonest cause of death for women over 50, killing one in four. This is almost twice as high as the death-rate from cancer.

There are as yet no essential oils known to treat problems with the heart, and it is advisable to check with your doctor and your family history to see if you are at risk. In the meantime, you can help to prevent heart and blood-pressure problems by giving up smoking, avoiding fatty foods and drinks high in caffeine, eating a low-cholesterol diet and taking enough regular exercise. There are also some carrier oils reputed to reduce cholesterol levels.

vaginal dryness

This can cause both emotional and physical discomfort. There are no known essential oils to increase vaginal fluid. Vitamin E is reputed to improve vaginal secretion, and daily application of sunflower oil all round the vaginal opening may also help.

Emotions during menopause

For many women the menopause will coincide with their children leaving home. It can represent a new lease of life as a woman suddenly finds that she has more time for herself. However, as with any major life change, the menopause is often accompanied by mixed feelings, and a woman's new-found freedom may be marred not only by physical symptoms but also by emotional disturbances.

stress-related headaches and sleep disturbances

These disturbances are not necessarily linked to the menopause, and may be stress-related. However, should either of them bother you, inhalation and application of the appropriate essential oils can help.

weight and diet

Appearance is often important to a woman throughout her life. It is not surprising, then, that poor self-esteem and a lack of confidence can be triggered by the physical changes happening in her body at this time.

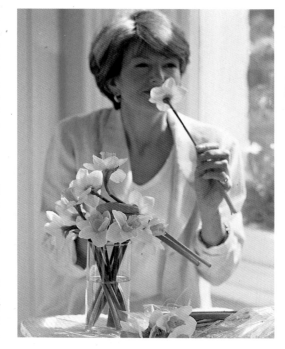

◁ **During the menopause, you may experience strong mood swings. Try to keep things in proportion and take pleasure from the simple things in life.**

△ **When you are feeling tired and irritable, a head massage can help you to relax and unwind.**

Water retention can lead to bloating and weight-gain which, in turn, will exacerbate any feelings of low self-esteem. Tackle this with a positive frame of mind and healthy eating habits – these two things combined will improve self-confidence. Essential oils used for low spirits may help weight loss by stimulating the nervous system.

emotional disturbances of the menopause

- Irritability
- Lack of confidence
- Anxiety and depression
- Poor concentration, forgetfulness and memory problems
- Decrease in self-esteem: through weight gain, lack of interest in sex, changes in physical appearance

tips for healthy eating and drinking

- Drink plenty of water.
- Limit alcohol intake to two units a day.
- Cut down on caffeine drinks.
- Cut down on, or avoid, sugary foods and foods high in fat.
- Eat more fish and less meat (especially red meat); eat plenty of fruit and vegetables, especially those rich in Vitamin C.
- Include foods rich in calcium.

loss of sex drive

For some women, the menopause is marked by a decrease in sex drive (conversely, some women also report an increase in libido). The reduction in vaginal fluid can make intercourse painful, and this can lead to a change in sexual desire.

Several essential oils are reputed to help with sexual problems and to increase desire. These oils relax the mind, relieving it from pressures and tensions and, at the same time, can stimulate the emotions. Use the appropriate oils in a vaporizer for an hour before retiring, in both the living room and the bedroom. Alternatively, sprinkle a few drops of the oils on to your pillow and exchange a gentle back and shoulder aromatherapy massage with your partner.

relationship difficulties

The physical and emotional difficulties of the menopause can put a strain on your relationship with your partner. If your children are leaving home, now may be a good time to re-define your partnership. It can help to blend stress-relieving essential oils with oils which correspond to your emotions, such as anger, fear or jealousy.

▷ **Emotional upsets are stressful and can lead to muscular tension. Rub oils on to your shoulders and neck to help restore your equilibrium.**

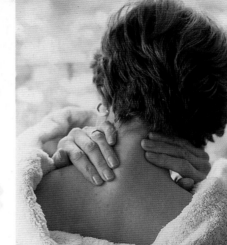

Useful essential oils

essential oil	treatment
hot flushes and sweating	
Clary sage *Salvia sclarea*	antisudorific, oestrogen-like (sweating)
Cypress *Cupressus sempervirens*	antisudorific (excessive perspiration)
Peppermint *Mentha* x *piperita*	cooling
Pine *Pinus sylvestris*	antisudorific (sweating)
reputed sexual stimulants	
Peppermint *Mentha* x *piperita*	neurotonic, reproductive tonic
Rosemary *Rosmarinus officinalis*	neurotonic, sexual tonic
Rose otto *Rosa damascena*	neurotonic, sexual tonic
Thyme (sweet) *Thymus vulgaris*	cardiotonic, immunostimulant, neurotonic, sexual tonic
Ylang ylang *Cananga odorata*	reproductive tonic
low spirits (depression) and fatigue	
Basil *Ocimum basilicum* var. *album*	neurotonic debility, mental strain, depression
Chamomile (Roman) *Chamaemelum nobile*	calming (nervous depression, irritability, nervous shock)
Clary sage *Salvia sclarea*	neurotonic (nervous fatigue)
Cypress *Cupressus sempervirens*	neurotonic (debility)
Frankincense *Boswellia carteri*	antidepressive (nervous depression)
Geranium *Pelargonium graveolens*	neurotonic (debility, nervous fatigue)
Juniper *Juniperus communis*	neurotonic (debility, fatigue)
Marjoram (sweet) *Origanum majorana*	neurotonic (debility, anguish, agitation, nervous depression)
Rosemary *Rosmarinus officinalis*	neurotonic (general debility and fatigue)

essential oil	treatment
fluid retention and cellulite	
Cypress *Cupressus sempervirens*	diuretic (oedema, rheumatic swelling)
Geranium *Pelargonium graveolens*	decongestant (lymphatic congestion)
headaches and sleep problems	
Chamomile (Roman) *Chamaemelum nobile*	antispasmodic, calming (migraines, insomnia, irritability)
Lavender *Lavandula angustifolia*	analgesic, calming (headaches, migraines, insomnia – low dose)
Marjoram (sweet) *Origanum majorana*	analgesic, calming (agitation, migraines, insomnia)
headaches and migraines only	
Peppermint *Mentha* x *piperita*	analgesic (headaches, migraine)
Rosemary *Rosmarinus officinalis*	decongestant (headaches, migraine)
irritability	
Chamomile (Roman) *Chamaemelum nobile*	calming (irritability, nervous depression, nervous shock)
Cypress *Cupressus sempervirens*	calming (irritability), regulates sympathetic nervous system
haemorrhage	
Cypress *Cupressus sempervirens*	astringent, phlebotonic (broken capillaries, varicose veins)
Rose otto *Rosa damascena*	astringent, styptic (wounds)

Aromatherapy in the later years

Physical health problems, minor or major, can become a source of worry and anxiety for an aging person, and can affect their overall mental and emotional health.

headaches and migraines

The reason for these, especially in the elderly, is not always apparent. It is therefore a good idea to use two or more essential oils, to make best use of their synergy. Put the relevant essential oils into your moisturizing cream and use twice daily. This helps both to relieve and prevent the problem, and will benefit the skin at the same time. If headaches persist throughout the day, try inhalation. If the headaches frequently recur, consider that it may be due to a food allergy, such as caffeine. If home treatment is unsuccessful it may be worth visiting a qualified aromatherapist.

shock

The emotional impact of shock can be particularly traumatic for an elderly person. Very often the shock is accompanied by fear, especially in the case of someone who lives on their own. Shock-induced trauma can be helped immediately by inhaling or applying essential oils with a sedative effect.

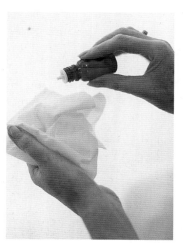

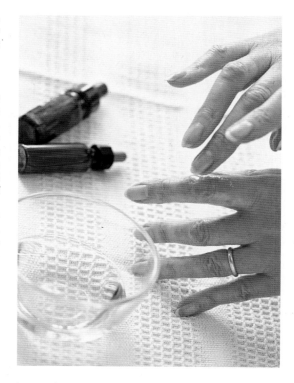

◁ Oils for fear and anger can be a useful support for cancer patients. Use juniper, lemon and geranium in a base lotion and apply the mix to the hands and body.

insomnia

Insomnia is fairly common amongst older people, and can get worse as age advances. Sometimes, there is no clear explanation for it – older people seem to need less sleep. However, the problem may be caused or exacerbated by anxiety and worry. Cramp in the leg muscles or arthritic pain during the night can also disturb the sleep pattern. The traditional essential oil used to help insomnia is lavender, although care should be taken with the dose, as too much will keep you wide awake. Lavender oil, used alone or in a synergy with two or three oils, has been used successfully by some hospitals to treat insomnia.

◁ Lavender and sweet marjoram oils can help with grief and fear. Inhale them from a tissue.

cancer

Aromatherapy cannot cure cancer but it can be used in a supportive role and can greatly improve the quality of life for many cancer patients. Fear of developing cancer can be a big worry for someone who has already lost a relative through the disease, and for cancer patients whose cancer is in remission. Use oils which are good for stress conditions (*see* Stress Soothers), and apply by inhalation, compresses and direct application in a carrier lotion.

dementia

Some people, more often in old age, suffer deterioration of their mental faculties, and are unable to think clearly or to concentrate for any length of time. The memory can become unreliable and confused, and some

▷ **Persistent headaches are debilitating and stressful. Massaging the shoulders with Roman chamomile and lavender will have a sedative and calming effect, while peppermint and rosemary will be energizing and uplifting.**

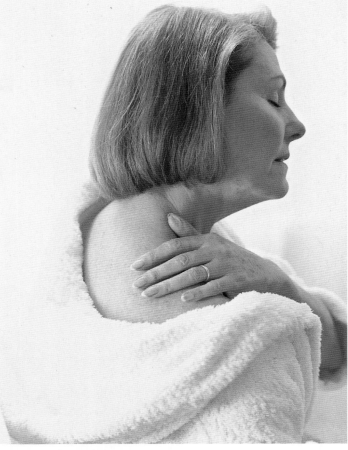

speech difficulties may develop (this is particularly true after a stroke). Alzheimer's disease may develop if the nerve tissue (which cannot regenerate itself) withers and dies in the brain. Try using essential oils which stimulate the mind and improve memory. Some oils are also thought to be able to trigger past experiences, which is helpful for people with Alzheimer's.

Parkinson's disease

The cause of this debilitating, progressive disease is unknown, but a lack of the chemical substance, dopamine, which is needed for co-ordination of the brain muscles, seems to be responsible for its symptoms. Parkinson's disease is character-ized by tremors, muscular rigidity and emaciation, and causes difficulty in speech and movement. Strong drugs are available to replace the dopamine; these help for a while, but they gradually lose efficiency as the body gets used to them. This necessitates a regular increase in dosage levels as the years pass, until, finally, the maximum dose loses its effect, and nothing more can be done to help the patient.

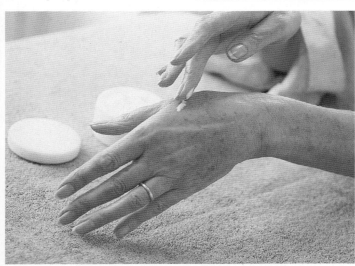

Side effects of the drugs include nausea, insomnia and constipation, all of which can be helped by aromatherapy. One study has also shown that essential oils can alleviate muscular problems, occasionally reducing the degree of slurred speech and tremors. Daily application of a lotion containing essential oils, plus daily aromatherapy baths (where possible) were used in the study. The symptoms which cause the most problems seem to be anxiety, lack of energy, muscular pains and stiffness. Others are constipation, insomnia, cramp, rigidity, tremors and slurred speech. Choose essential oils on the basis of the symptoms causing the trouble.

◁ **For sufferers of Parkinson's disease, a hand and body lotion containing clary sage, sweet marjoram and rosemary can help the condition.**

Useful essential oils

essential oil	treatment

poor circulation

essential oil	treatment
Clary sage *Salvia sclarea*	circulatory problems, haemorrhoids, varicose veins, venous aneurism, cholesterol
Lemon *Citrus limon*	poor circulation, thrombosis, varicose veins
Rosemary *Rosmarinus officinalis*	decongestant, poor circulation, hardening of the arteries

arthritis and rheumatism

Chamomile (Roman) *Chamaemelum nobile*	anti-inflammatory, stress-relieving
Clove bud *Syzygium aromaticum*	analgesic (severe pain), anti-inflammatory, neurotonic (use sparingly – *see* The Essential Oils)
Lavender *Lavandula angustifolia*	analgesic, anti-inflammatory, stress-relieving
Marjoram (sweet) *Origanum majorana*	analgesic, stress-relieving
Niaouli *Melaleuca viridiflora*	analgesic, anti-inflammatory, neurotonic
Rosemary *Rosmarinus officinalis*	analgesic, anti-inflammatory, decongestant, neuromuscular action, neurotonic

bronchial asthma and bronchitis

Marjoram (sweet) *Origanum majorana*	antispasmodic, anti-infectious, expels mucus, respiratory tonic
Niaouli *Melaleuca viridiflora*	anticatarrhal, anti-infectious, anti-inflammatory, expels mucus
Peppermint *Mentha* x *piperita*	anti-inflammatory, breaks down and expels mucus
Pine *Pinus sylvestris*	analgesic, anti-infectious, anti-inflammatory, decongestant, breaks down and expels mucus
Rosemary *Rosmarinus officinalis*	breaks down mucus, anti-inflammatory, decongestant, expels mucus

headaches

Chamomile (Roman) *Chamaemelum nobile*	antispasmodic, calming, sedative
Lavender *Lavandula angustifolia*	analgesic, calming, sedative
Marjoram (sweet) *Origanum majorana*	analgesic, antispasmodic, calming
Melissa *Melissa officinalis*	calming, sedative
Peppermint *Mentha* x *piperita*	analgesic, antispasmodic
Rosemary *Rosmarinus officinalis*	analgesic, antispasmodic, decongestant

essential oil	treatment

influenza

essential oil	treatment
Eucalyptus *Eucalyptus smithii*	anti-infectious, antiviral, prophylactic
Cypress *Cupressus sempervirens*	anti-infectious
Lemon *Citrus limon*	anti-infectious, antiviral
Pine *Pinus sylvestris*	anti-infectious

insomnia

Basil *Ocimum basilicum* var. *album*	nervous system regulator (nervous insomnia)
Chamomile (Roman) *Chamaemelum nobile*	calming
Lavender *Lavandula angustifolia*	calming, sedative
Lemon *Citrus limon*	calming
Marjoram (sweet) *Origanum majorana*	calming
Melissa *Melissa officinalis*	calming, sedative

shock

Bergamot *Citrus bergamia*	balancing, calming, sedative, tonic to central nervous system
Chamomile (Roman) *Chamaemelum nobile*	calming, sedative
Lavender *Lavandula angustifolia*	balancing, calming, sedative, tonic
Melissa *Melissa officinalis*	calming, sedative

incontinence

Cypress *Cupressus sempervirens*	astringent
Lemon *Citrus limon*	astringent

pressure sores

Chamomile (German) *Matricaria recutica*	cicatrizant (infected wounds, ulcers)
Chamomile (Roman) *Chamaemelum nobile*	vulnerary (boils, burns wounds).
Frankincense *Boswellia carteri*	cicatrizant (scars, ulcers, wounds)
Geranium *Pelargonium graveolens*	cicatrizant (burns, cuts, ulcers, wounds)
Lavender *Lavandula angustifolia*	cicatrizant (burns, scars, varicose veins, wounds)

constipation and diverticulitis

Ginger *Zingiber officinale*	analgesic, digestive stimulant, general tonic
Mandarin *Citrus reticulata*	antispasmodic, calming, digestive.
Orange (bitter) *Citrus aurantium* var. *amara*	calming, digestive

essential oil	treatment
Rosemary *Rosmarinus officinalis*	analgesic, anti-inflammatory, digestive (constipation, sluggish or painful digestion)

diarrhoea

essential oil	treatment
Geranium *Pelargonium graveolens*	anti-inflammatory (colitis), antispasmodic (colic, gastroenteritis), astringent
Lemon *Citrus limon*	antispasmodic, astringent, stomachic (gastritis, stomach ulcers).
Marjoram (sweet) *Origanum majorana*	analgesic, anti-infectious, antispasmodic (colic), stomachic (enteritis)
Niaouli *Melaleuca viridiflora*	anti-infectious, anti-inflammatory, antiviral (viral enteritis), digestive (gastritis)
Peppermint *Mentha* x *piperita*	anti-infectious, anti-inflammatory (colitis, enteritis, gastritis), antispasmodic (gastric spasm), digestive

indigestion (dyspepsia)

essential oil	treatment
Basil *Ocimum basilicum* var. *album*	analgesic, carminative (flatulence, sluggish digestion)
Lemon *Citrus limon*	digestive (nausea, painful digestion, flatulence, appetite loss)
Marjoram (sweet) *Origanum majorana*	analgesic, calming, digestive - (flatulence, indigestion)
Orange (bitter) *Citrus aurantium* var. *amara*	calming, digestive
Peppermint *Mentha* x *piperita*	analgesic, carminative (flatulence), digestive (nausea, painful digestion)
Rosemary *Rosmarinus officinalis*	analgesic (painful digestion), carminative (flatulence)

dementia and Alzheimer's disease

essential oil	treatment
Basil *Ocimum basilicum* var. *album*	neurotonic (mental strain)
Clove bud *Syzygium aromaticum*	mental stimulant (memory loss, mental fatigue), neurotonic
Marjoram (sweet) *Origanum majorana*	neurotonic (mental instability)
Peppermint *Mentha* x *piperita*	mental stimulant (concentration), neurotonic
Rosemary *Rosmarinus officinalis*	neurotonic (loss of memory, concentration)

Parkinson's disease

essential oil	treatment
Clary sage *Salvia sclarea*	antispasmodic, calming, regenerative (cellular aging), neurotonic
Lavender *Lavandula angustifolia*	analgesic, antispasmodic, calming, sedative (anxiety, headaches, insomnia), neurotonic
Marjoram (sweet) *Origanum majorana*	analgesic, antispasmodic, digestive tonic, calming (anxiety, insomnia),
Rosemary *Rosmarinus officinalis*	analgesic, antispasmodic, digestive (constipation, sluggish digestion), neurotonic

… 'Tis the hour

That scatters spells on herb and flower

And garlands might be gathered now

That turn'd around the sleeper's brow.

From Light of the Haram, *Thomas Moore, 1779–1852.*

Reiki Principles

Reiki is a very simple system of healing, carried out by placing hands on or over a person with the intent to channel healing energy. Originating in Japan, there are now many thousands of Reiki teachers and practitioners. This chapter will introduce the basic philosophy behind this ancient healing art.

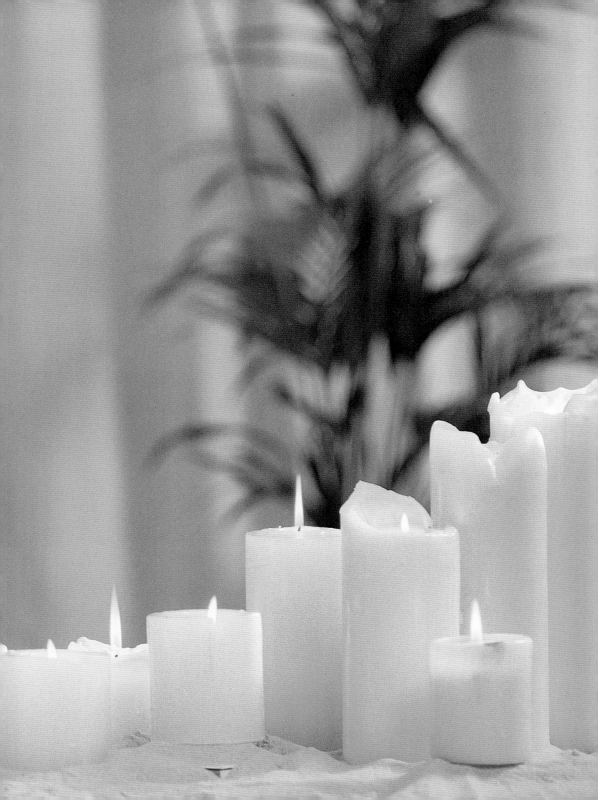

Reiki is love

To experience Reiki is to experience the communication of love from the Universe to all beings. Instinctively tactile, we know from birth the joy that comes from the loving touch of another person. The sensation of touch is present in many of the wonderful healing arts available to us, and we feel the comfort of a person's touch before their healing skills benefit our bodies and uplift our spirits. To receive Reiki, through your own hands or those of another person, is to be held and supported by the life force of the Universe itself. It is to receive cosmic energy which flows through everything on the Earth.

communication and the cosmos

The origin of Reiki is the same loving Universe that gives us breath each second. Reiki invites us to open up to this great love, trusting it and allowing it to flow through us. "Rei" can be translated as universal, or spiritually guided; "ki" is the energy or life force present in everything. Reiki is literally energy (ki) guided by divine wisdom (rei). Having its own intelligence, Reiki has no boundaries, yet it knows where it is most welcome. The energy that passes through a Reiki practitioner's palms is impossible to hold on to because it belongs to everyone and everything, and no-one can harness it – it is intangible. In the modern world Reiki flourishes everywhere, and what is tangible to the many who enjoy it is the physical, emotional and spiritual healing which blesses all it reaches. Reiki brings comfort from pain, creativity when we feel stifled and love when we feel separate.

reiki is for everyone

Whether your life seems lacking or you live it to the full, and whether you are a spiritual seeker, a single-minded materialist, experiencing a period of depression or adapting to change, Reiki embraces and enriches. The energy which permeates the Cosmos is divine wisdom and truth. It transcends time and space, and all religions. It is enjoyed by people of many faiths and of no faith, and promotes positive living and compassion for all.

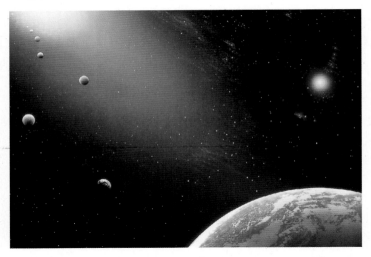

△ Infinite and unconditional; Reiki is the energy of all life – guided by the wisdom of the Universe.

▷ The effect of Reiki is similar to the sun shining on the earth, and we should remember this when we enjoy the intense heat of the sun on our bodies, in the same way as Dr Usui carried a bright lantern in order to remind himself of Reiki's intense healing energy.

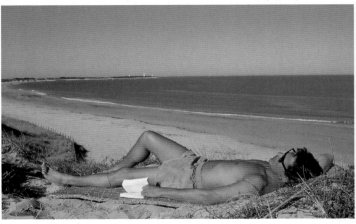

There is a light that shines beyond all things on earth,

beyond us all, beyond the heavens, beyond the

highest, the very highest heavens.

This is the light that shines in our heart.

The Chandogya Upanishad

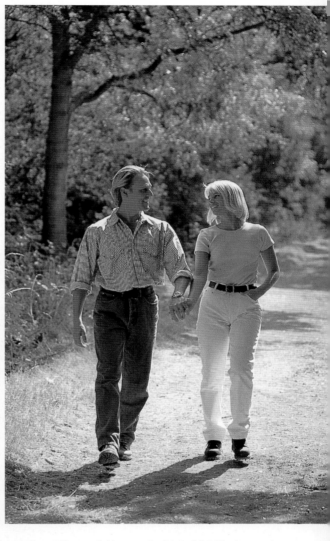

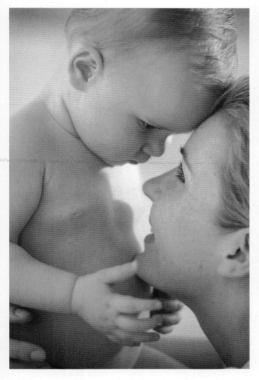

△ **Whether your life seems lacking, or you live it to the full, Reiki embraces and enriches you and the people around you.**

◁ **All ages respond to the healing touch of another, but perhaps the most physically loving bond is that between a mother and her baby.**

universal law

In many different ways, Reiki shows us the happiness we can feel by living in harmony with the laws of the Universe. Love, if you want to be loved; give willingly and you will receive many times. The person channelling Reiki is never drained, as the energy reaches the healer before it reaches the person being healed. We are eternally replenished, which shows us that there is enough of everything to go round. Reiki has been found to be a non-polar energy – it has no opposite. It can only be used to bring good, and if, in a moment of weakness, we attempt to use Reiki to manipulate an outcome which is not for the highest good, it simply does not work. You need no intellectual skills to use Reiki, or to receive it – only an open mind and the intent to heal. Following a Reiki attunement, the ability to channel the power of Reiki is instant and everlasting. Reiki is unconditional love in a world often beset by conflict, and it begins with you.

The story of reiki

Essential energy of the Universe, Reiki is infinite in flow, past and future, and unfettered by concepts of time and space. No-one knows for certain when Reiki was first channelled to heal self and others. Some Reiki practitioners feel that Reiki was known and used for spiritual benefit in the legendary civilizations of Lemuria and Atlantis, while others suggest that Reiki has been the loving energy behind many kinds of healing miracles throughout the ages.

the rediscovery of reiki

The story of how Dr Mikao Usui rediscovered Reiki was originally passed down in oral tradition. The story is still told to classes and each Reiki master/teacher still relates in turn the story they have been taught. It is due to this oral tradition that there are variations in the story of Reiki, but it does not matter if we do not know the exact details of Dr Usui's quest for Reiki or the exact circumstances in which Reiki reappeared to the world. Reiki's story has symbolic value – above all, it tells of a quest from the heart and that is always relevant, today more than ever.

Mikao Usui was born on 15 August 1862, in southern Japan. Although he never received formal training as an allopathic doctor, he was bestowed with this title in his lifetime, in recognition of his commitment to heal wherever he saw suffering. He has been depicted as both a practising Buddhist and a devout Christian; alterations may have been made to suit the politics of the day, or perhaps this illustrates his universal and all-embracing approach to sharing the gift he found with those in need of love everywhere. The story told by my Reiki master says that it was while teaching at a school in Kyoto that Dr Usui was first prompted to seek a method of healing through touch. His young students had been taught the scriptures and had heard with fascination Jesus's words, "You will do as I have done and even greater things." The students asked why ordinary people could not heal through touch and they felt strongly that the legacy left by great healers was the message that everyone could heal if they truly sought the answers. Dr Usui promised to find these answers. He resigned his teaching post, and his quest began.

in search of a formula

In order to find answers, Dr Usui began years of study in monasteries and libraries in the United States, China, India and Tibet. He learned Sanskrit and read the Buddhist

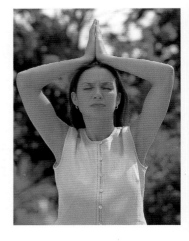

△ **Today you can choose to be attuned to Reiki outdoors in beautiful surroundings.**

teachings in the ancient sutras, or spiritual texts. During this time many wonderful blessings were revealed to Dr Usui, but he wanted to be able to put his new knowledge into practice. All the secrets revealed to him were experienced in an intellectual sense, and Dr Usui knew he must translate what he had learned into action if it was to heal. Yearning to discover a physical formula, he decided he would meditate on his desire to do this, and travelled to sacred Mount Koriyama in northern Japan.

the 21 stones

On reaching Mount Koriyama, Dr Usui gathered 21 stones and made a pile, intending to throw one stone away at the end of each day. The number 21 is quite significant here, and occurs in the ancient writings of many religions. During this

◁ **Before meditating on the mountain, Dr Usui made a calendar of 21 stones to mark the days. After attunements, Reiki takes three days to rise up through each of our seven energy centres or chakras.**

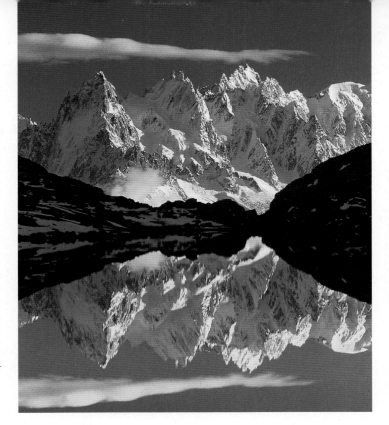

▷ Reiki is the essential energy of the Universe, and it was while he was meditating on the mountain that Dr Usui was blessed with the knowledge of Reiki.

time, he contemplated all he had learned, read and experienced, and meditated on the symbols he had seen in the scriptures. Dr Usui had still not found his answers when the first light of the 21st day began to dawn. As he stood on the mountain looking into the dark sky, he could see a light hurtling straight towards him. He did not move, and the ball of light grew and grew until it finally hit him between the eyes. Dr Usui was convinced he was about to die when he saw millions of tiny bubbles in every colour of the rainbow. The symbols and the very essence of their meanings were contained within the bubbles, and Dr Usui immediately understood them. He said, "I remember." The answers to his prayers had landed on his sixth chakra, the seat of insight and intuition. Reiki had been discovered once more.

four miracles

On his way down the mountain Dr Usui stubbed his toe. Instinctively, he placed his hands over the wound, to relieve his injury. When he removed them, the bleeding had stopped and the toe was healed. It was the first of four miracles. On his way to share his joyous new discovery, Dr Usui saw a place to eat at the roadside. After 21 days without food, the owner advised him to eat little and to avoid overloading his system. Ravenous, Dr Usui ignored his advice and ate until he was full. The man looked on, incredulous at the strength of Dr Usui's digestive system. That was the second miracle of the day. After his breakfast, Dr Usui noticed that the owner's granddaughter was in great pain from a toothache. Dr Usui placed his hands on either side of her face, and the pain disappeared: the third miracle of the day.

When Dr Usui reached the Zen monastery, he went to find the abbot, who was suffering from arthritic pain. Dr Usui placed his hands on the abbot, who felt immediate relief. That was the fourth miracle of the day.

into the world

Dr Usui then decided to take the gift of Reiki to the places where it was needed most. The slums of Kyoto became his clinic for several years, and the healing power of Reiki was very successful at treating many physical disorders. It was with great surprise that Dr Usui saw the same beggars on the streets time and time again, and he wondered why they did not make their way in the world once they were fit and healthy. Perhaps it was because the beggars had not given anything in exchange, and did not appreciate the Reiki; perhaps they did not feel empowered themselves because someone else was healing them; or perhaps they were following their own personal path by begging. Dr Usui realized he could attune others to heal themselves, and began a new life travelling and teaching, and healing with Reiki. He is buried in Kyoto cemetery, where the beautiful inscription on his gravestone is a testament to people's gratitude for his deep commitment to and love for all living things.

the three grand masters

One of Dr Usui's greatest friends was a young man named Chijiro Hayashi, a naval officer. Dr Usui decided to pass on the lineage of Reiki to Hayashi, and he became the Second Grand Master. Hayashi formed the three degrees of Reiki; Dr Usui had previously passed on all of his knowledge of Reiki at once.

Mr Hayashi ran a Reiki clinic in Tokyo, and there the Third Grand Master discovered Reiki. Mrs Hawayo Takata, ill from cancer, was referred to Hayashi's clinic by her surgeon. Mrs Takata received Reiki healing, and after her recovery she persuaded Hayashi to accept her as a pupil. She studied with him for a year, after which she returned to her birthplace of Hawaii, where she was later made Grand Master.

Mrs Takata was the 13th and last Reiki master attuned by Mr Hayashi. Before her death in 1980 she had attuned 22 masters in the USA and Canada. Today, Mrs Takata's granddaughter, Phyllis Lei Furumoto, is Usui Reiki Grand Master.

Reiki ethics

The ethics of living in the spirit of Reiki were formed by Dr Usui after working in the slums of Kyoto, which taught him much about human nature and the world around him. The Reiki principles are thought to have their origins in the philosophy of the Meiji Emperor of Japan. The five principles are really a guide to living with a happy heart, whatever your path in life, and promoting harmony with the world around you, and they can be considered a healing treatment in themselves. Today, there are many variations on the five Reiki principles, so you can find one which

▽ Greet the day with a salute to the sun; adding an element of ritual to your morning routine will create a happy day.

The Spiritual Principles

Just for today do not worry

Just for today do not anger

Honour your parents, teachers and elders

Earn your living honestly

Show gratitude to everything

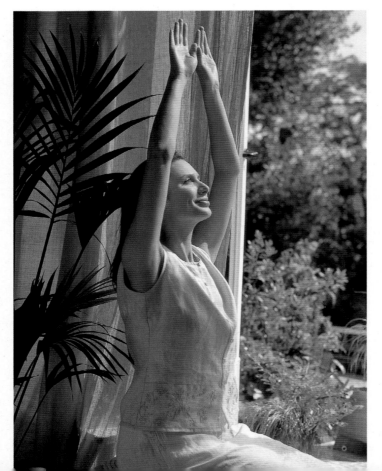

"speaks" to you. The following version was laid down by Hawayo Takata. Dwell on and in them, and allow them to filter through your consciousness.

just for today do not worry

If, each morning, you choose to wake up trusting that whatever the day brings will be a valuable and wonderful experience, you are living this principle. Worry can take up much of our lives – if we are not worrying over past mistakes, we are often fearing the future. We are brought up to compete and to struggle, and this breeds in us an inherent lack of trust in the world around us. We can see the big picture much more clearly when we place our trust in the Divine Plan.

just for today do not anger

Anger can be transformative, and we do not need to hang on to it if we learn that it has such a positive use. What are we angry about? Maybe we feel trapped by a situation or a person. We may fear harmful results for ourselves and others. Recognize how you feel, acknowledge that we are all learning together, and know that all is well. The ability to stand back from our own feelings is empowering. Anger can be a destructive force, but analyzing it can be a catalyst for positive change.

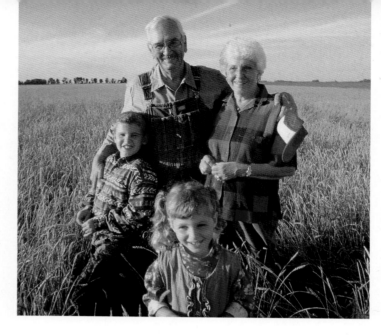

honour your parents, teachers and elders

Everyone can teach us something. Parents, elders and children too, if we listen. If you decide to become a teacher of Reiki you will soon discover how important and enriching it is to bless and thank your students for what they, in turn, teach you. This principle is also helpful in recognizing the value of being non-judgemental in life. Whatever someone's path, it is theirs and as valid as your own. Acknowledge and respect this and create freedom for yourself and others.

earn your living honestly

So many ethical questions abound in the world of work today that living with integrity is important if we are to be at peace with ourselves and our own truth. No matter how small the job, it is our present moment nonetheless, and if we put our hearts into it and do it with love, we will be giving and getting the most from that moment. This principle can also inspire us to have the courage to find work in a field we truly love, fulfilling our purpose.

show gratitude to everything

It is a thrilling revelation to discover how an attitude of gratitude enhances life – and how swiftly. The moment we wake up feeling "thank you" instead of "please", the universe begins to echo our positive new thought patterns – and send some more of it our way. The last of the five Reiki principles, this goes a long way towards living all of them, and creating our own reality. Bless your life and it will be even more joyful.

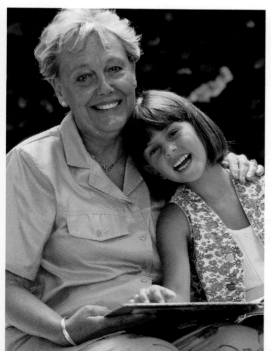

◁ Our teachers are sometimes younger than us, when we honour the wisdom of life in all its stages and all its forms.

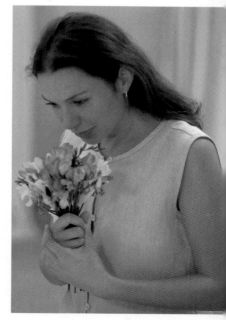

▷ Enjoying the beauty of life is at the heart of Reiki – take time to appreciate nature's gifts and use your senses to the full.

Reiki schools – the many in the one

reiki principles

There may be as many as 30 different variations of Reiki being practised in the world today. Many branches of Reiki are practised and enjoyed today, all descending from, or linked to, the Usui System of Natural Healing. The human mind is great at separating, and there is some argument today as to what is traditional and what is accepted in the Reiki world. Included here are brief descriptions and explanations of the origins of some of the many Reiki schools thriving today. Follow your heart and you will find what you are looking for.

rainbow reiki

Rainbow Reiki was developed as a healing system by Walter Lubeck and, as the name suggests, Rainbow practitioners use many tools with which to empower and complement the Usui system. Crystals are often used for healing purposes and can be powerfully complemented with a Reiki energy charge. Rainbow Reiki aims to put us in touch with our Inner Child, and is a fruitful and enjoyable way to rediscover untapped creativity, happiness and a clear perception of where we are in our lives. Its practices include the unique Powerball Technique as well as aspects of shamanism.

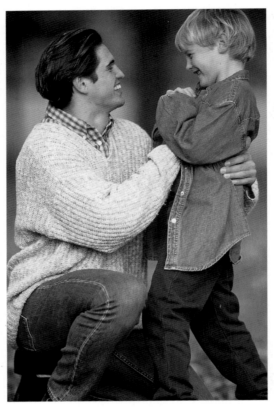

◁ Rainbow Reiki is a powerful healer. It can be used to reconnect us with our inner child, who still knows our dreams and aspirations even when the logical mind feels out of touch.

There is nothing on earth so curious for beauty

or so absorbent of it as a soul.

Wassily Kandinsky

karuna reiki

Karuna Reiki is often described as the Reiki of Compassionate Action. It was developed by William Lee Rand, and is considered among Karuna practitioners to be the next step on from Usui Reiki, with Karuna attunements available only to Reiki practitioners who have already attained master/teacher level. Karuna is a Sanskrit word meaning "a compassionate action intended to relieve suffering from all sentient beings". A total of 12 Karuna Reiki symbols are taught at two levels of proficiency, each symbol possessing a precise energy and used for healing at deep, cellular levels.

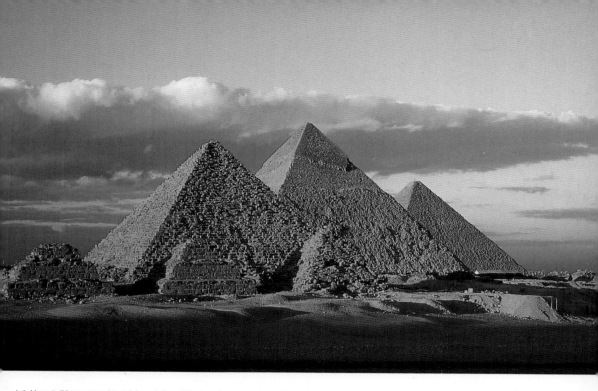

△ Sekhem Reiki, as opposed to Seichem, is thought to have been reconstructed from the reincarnated memories of the life of an Egyptian high priest.

seichem reiki

Seichem Reiki is said to have its roots in the same sutras in which Usui was given the traditional Reiki symbols. Seichem practitioners claim that not all the information of Reiki is passed on in the Usui system. Apparently, an Usui master and a Seichem master met and exchanged their information and ideas. Seichem was found to have two additional symbols, used to profound healing effect. Dr Usui is said to have attuned many people during his lifetime, and Seichem was one of many schools which later grew from his teachings. Seichem works in harmony with the elements of earth, air, fire and water, as well as ether, which connects to the higher realms of existence.

tibetan reiki

Tibetan Reiki is sometimes taught in conjunction with Usui Reiki, mostly on request and to facilitate empowerment. Some of the symbols used are very similar to the symbols used in Usui Reiki, with almost identical pronunciation. They are

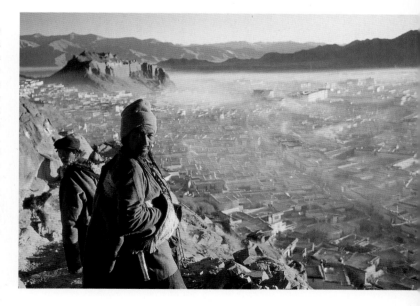

also possibly of shamanic origin, like many symbols from the ancient world still used today. Tibetan Reiki is often said to be the closest to Usui Reiki.

△ Hands-on healing in association with powerful symbols has been part of the spiritual knowledge of Tibet for thousands of years.

Having a healing

What might prompt your first experience of receiving Reiki? Perhaps you are in physical pain or discomfort. Perhaps you are feeling under pressure and are looking for a soothing relaxation method. You might want to complement other therapeutic skills which you have already tried. Maybe you are just curious to know more about this all-round healing phenomenon, or maybe you feel this is the right channel for your own healing powers. All of these reasons could spur you to seek out a Reiki practitioner, and details are easily found in the windows of holistic health shops, the pages of New Age magazines or by word of mouth. Send up a wish to the heavens – everyone has a different story of how they found Reiki, and often it seems that Reiki finds you once you are interested.

finding a tailor-made service

What are you looking for in a Reiki practitioner? Some of us are happy to make an appointment over the phone and to turn up on the day, others may have special considerations to take into account. Although Reiki is strictly a clothes-on, hands-on affair, you may want to choose a Reiki practitioner with whom you feel comfortable and gender may be a part of this issue. If you are not mobile, you may be looking for a practitioner who is; many carry portable couches and will visit your home, in which case will there be noisy children running about when you need peace and quiet? Alternatively, they may practise from theirs. Available times must be arranged, of course, and you may want to know the duration of the Reiki session,

usually about an hour. Make enquiries about charges – rates vary widely, and many practitioners offer concessions or are willing to make an exchange for special skills or services.

the reiki experience

Your Reiki practitioner will probably want to know a little bit about your general health and your lifestyle before he or she begins. They will ask you to take off your shoes for comfort, and perhaps any metal jewellery in case it interrupts the Reiki flow or prevents your free movement. Even if you have a specific injury, you will receive a full-body treatment working from head to toe with the traditional hand positions. However, if your body won't allow free access, don't worry – the Reiki will get

◁ **On the first meeting a Reiki practitioner may give you a questionnaire to fill in, or you might have a chat about your general health and well-being.**

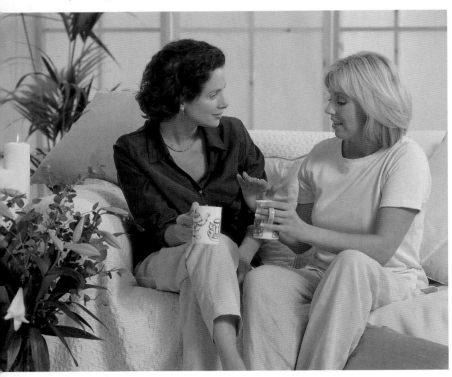

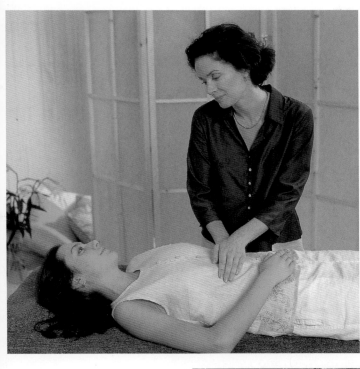

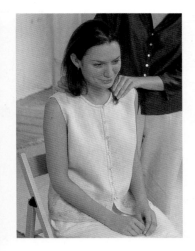

△ Whatever your reason for seeking Reiki, you will receive a full body treatment, usually beginning at the head and shoulders.

◁ Feel free to talk to the Reiki practitioner during a session, as things often come to light when you relax and allow your own healing to happen in this way.

there anyway. The practitioner will usually remain quiet during the session; this is because it is your time, to relax and to let the gentle power of Reiki flow into your being. However, as you relax you may want to ask questions, or express yourself, or laugh or cry or giggle – there is no right or wrong reaction to Reiki. It simply facilitates holistic healing and promotes well-being.

surprising results

Maybe during your Reiki session you felt tingly, or saw beautiful colours or felt wonderfully relaxed, but find that your back is still painful or your knee still stiff. Remember, part of the holistic nature of Reiki is that it heals the whole. And remember, the beauty of Reiki is that it knows already where to go – in fact, the only thing that can possibly direct it is your higher self, in co-operation with the Reiki energy. Many people are surprised when they go home and fall asleep for 3 hours. Sometimes a rest is just what the body needs to process and digest experience, or allow natural energy levels to recuperate. Conversely, many people say that after

Reiki they return home and clear out all the junk in their house, or spend the afternoon working in the garden. Reiki certainly nurtures imagination and creativity too.

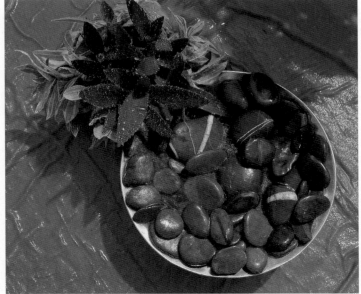

△ Purples and blues and dreamy images are commonly seen by the person receiving Reiki, as the whole being opens like a flower in response to the loving nature of this energy.

Reiki attunements

You may decide you would like to be able to give yourself Reiki or help others with it, or both. Attunements are a prerequisite to practising Reiki, and an element of the teachings that set Reiki apart from other healing systems. Reiki will not work if you have not been attuned by an initiated master, even if you already have other wonderful healing skills, and these will be complemented once you have been attuned. An attunement to the Usui System of Natural Healing is very often a landmark in a person's life, so profound and wide-ranging are the results. In choosing to be attuned, you are embarking on a journey towards healing your own being – physically, mentally, emotionally and spiritually. In short, a Reiki attunement often helps people realize their potential in whatever way they choose to do so.

an ancient bond

The relationship between master and student is part of many ancient practices but unique to Reiki in the Western world, where information is so readily accessible. Dr Usui received his Reiki attunement "direct" and it has been passed on one-to-one ever since. Attunements are a meaningful experience for both master/teacher and student; no two are the same, and students can teach the teachers a lot about the nature of Reiki. They are a blessing for both – it is a wonderful thing to be able to share with someone else, and to know that another person is empowered to share Reiki with themselves and others. A student will always remember his or her attunement to Reiki with great affection, for both the experience and the teacher's compassion and communication at this time.

preparing for attunements

There are beneficial things a student can do to prepare for attunements, psychologically and physically, at first, second or master/teacher level. For a few days before your attunement drink as much water as you can, to cleanse your system, and eat fresh, organic and unprocessed foods as much as possible. If you use recreational drugs, including cigarettes and alcohol, reduce your intake as much as you can. If you give yourself time to relax and contemplate your stepping into Reiki, you may want to experiment by putting your hands on yourself and feeling the sensations, so that you have something to compare with after the attunement. Take the opportunity to be in touch with any existing healing powers you may have which will be enhanced by a Reiki attunement.

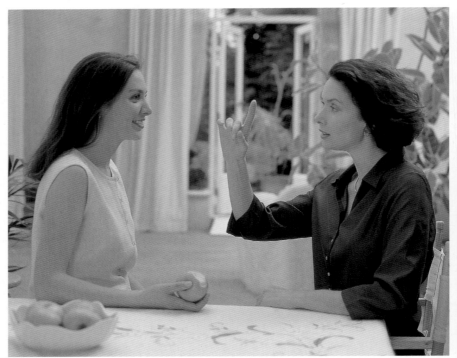

▷ A Reiki teacher sits with her student and draws one of the symbols in the air as she explains its dynamic nature.

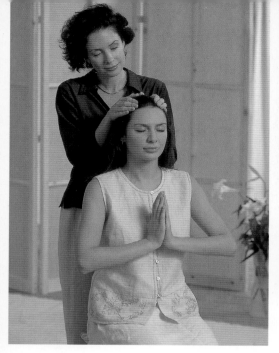

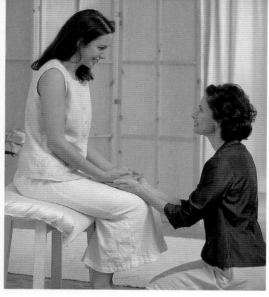

◁ **Reiki attunements can take place lying down, standing, or sitting on a chair with eyes closed.**

△ **Receiving a Reiki attunement is like receiving an ancient blessing on your life.**

the physical attunement process

During all attunements, the Usui Reiki symbols are used to open the chakras and allow the person to become a Reiki channel. In the First Degree there are four attunements, but in the second and third degrees there is only one, so they are more brief. The student sits on a chair, eyes closed, with their hands in the prayer position, and the Reiki master/teacher moves round the chair throughout the attunement process. During your attunement relax and savour the moment. You may feel many wonderful sensations, from the exhilarating and emotional to the more subtle. Afterwards, you will be given time to absorb your experience and to return to the moment.

after an attunement

In the 2–4 weeks following an attunement, your system will be adjusting to your new gift of Reiki and integrating the energies into your being. You may experience a healing process, and this is nothing to fear.

▷ **Many people feel a conscious connection to all life forming in their hearts following their attunement.**

Many people have all the symptoms of a cold, except the discomfort, as the body cleanses and balances its new energy system. Sometimes the effect is emotional and you may remember things you had forgotten, or feel tearful or light-headed and giggly, or completely go off cigarettes and alcohol.

Now is the time to treat yourself with Reiki. If you don't use it for years, it will still be there on demand – "Hands-on, Reiki-on, hands-off, Reiki-off", as Mrs Takata used to say. But the more you use Reiki, the more you will feel its healing benefits as your whole being begins a new lifestyle.

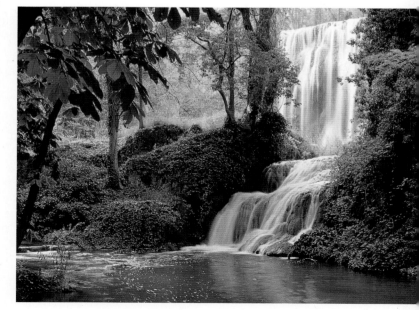

The endocrine system and chakras

The hand positions taught in the Usui System of Natural Healing aim to treat the recipient as a whole. If this is not possible for some reason, the Reiki energy will reach the parts most in need. Attunements are created by placing the Reiki symbols in the chakras to open the body as a channel, so chakras are important in that respect. They are also vital in the understanding of healing the whole.

Chakra is a Sanskrit word meaning "wheel", and it is not unusual to feel a spinning motion in the area of a chakra, through your own hands or someone else's. Chakras are multidimensional, layered energy centres in our bodies, and, since the earliest Eastern representations, often depicted as lotus flowers. Most people cannot see chakras, although this talent can be developed. They are arranged in a central line along the body, going from bottom to top when numbered. They can be treated from the back or the front and are often felt as balls of energy. The functions of the chakras are many, and we are learning more about them all the time as we have further insights into the dynamics and significance of vibrational healing in all its forms. Chakras perform their many duties in perfect synchronicity with our endocrine systems. This amazing system controls the functions of the body at a cellular level through seven major glands in the body, each of which is associated with a particular chakra. The glands of the endocrine system are responsible for the correct amount of chemical nutrients, or hormones, fed to each of our organs, and if one of them has an imbalance it can be felt. In the case of an illness caused by such an imbalance, for example hyperthyroidism, holistic healing methods recognize that physical symptoms are just the visible result of imbalance in energy manifested at a more subtle level at an earlier time. The area of the weakest energy flow would be the area in which an illness manifests, an unbalanced chakra being the weakest link in the chain.

THE CHAKRAS AND THEIR POSITIONS
The following table lists the chakras and corresponding endocrine glands, and where they can be found on the body.

chakras	glands	site
coccygeal/root	gonads/ovaries	base of spine
sacral	leydig	5–7.5cm (2–3in) below navel
solar plexus	adrenals	between ribcage and navel
heart	thymus	centre of chest beside the heart
throat	thyroid	middle of the throat
third eye	pituitary	centred just above eyebrows
head/crown	pineal	crown of the head

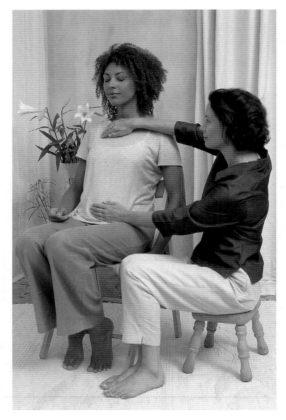

◁ A chakra balance is a comprehensive way to treat the body when there is not much time available. This kind of balancing is good for alleviating stress, and problems with health sometimes come to light.

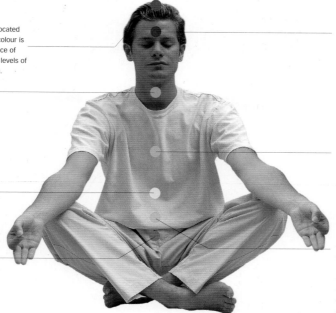

The seventh chakra, the crown, is located just above the top of the head. Its colour is violet and it maintains overall balance of the chakra system, stimulating fine levels of perception, intuition and inspiration.

The fifth chakra, associated with blue, is located at the throat, and its concerns are communication, personal expression and the flow of information.

The third chakra, associated with yellow, is at the solar plexus, just below the ribcage. It identifies and assists in the sense of identity, self-confidence and personal power.

The first chakra, or base chakra is located at the base of the spine. Linked with red, it is concerned with physical survival, energy distribution and practicality.

The sixth chakra, often called the third eye, is at the centre of the brow. Its colour is indigo and it is concerned with understanding, perception, knowledge and mental organization.

The fourth chakra is located at the centre of the chest and is associated with the heart. Its colour is green and it deals with relationships, personal development, direction and sharing.

The second chakra, linked with orange, is based in the lower abdomen, just below the navel. Its functions are creativity, feelings, sexual drive and pleasure, as well as exploration.

the art of synergy

The energies absorbed by our etheric bodies vibrate at a higher energetic level than those in our physical bodies. One of the main functions of the chakras is to decrease the rate of these energies as they filter downward, to an appropriate rate that our organs can deal with and use. In turn, the endocrine system sends out signals and relays energy to the chakras. Once in the form of chemical hormones, they can then be absorbed and processed by our endocrine system and used in various amounts to nourish our organs and tissues.

a web of life

Chakras operate on many levels; they are a feature of the entire Web of Life on a microcosmic scale in every one of us. While they are communicating with our endocrine system, they are also nourishing every part of our bodies with subtle, life-force energy, or "ki" as it is also known. Chakras are connected to each other and to our physical cellular structure by threads of subtle energy, called "nadis". At the same time, our chakras are fine receptors of psychic energy, picked up by our astral and mental bodies, which vibrate at an even higher rate than our etheric bodies. In this

way, chakras are considered to have an important part to play in our spiritual evolution, as all energies picked up by our spiritual, mental, astral and etheric bodies are transmitted through the crown chakra situated on the top of the head and down to the lower chakras, which then distribute the energies to our organs. The energy

frequencies at which our organs vibrate varies, as do the frequencies of our chakras. It has been found that organs with a similar vibration are grouped together with the chakra of a similar frequency. Each chakra therefore has several organs to which it gives vibrational nutrition, one cycle in a system of symbiotic flow.

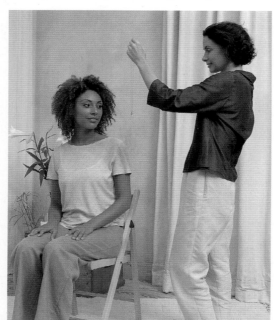

◁ **Sometimes Reiki practitioners use a pendulum to dowse the energy field of a person they are going to treat.**

The use of symbols

The use of symbols is familiar to people of all cultures. Our first examples are often wizards and witches in fairy tales, and later we learn that these tales have evolved from symbols in our own subconscious. If our dreams puzzle us, we can often decipher them and realize that our subconscious minds are using symbols in the form of archetypes, which are the inspiration for the fairy-tale allegories we loved as infants. The psychologist Carl Jung rediscovered these archetypes after learning that the same symbols were significant to cultures the world over. They seem to be in the subconscious of the planet as a whole, and appear to have evolved with us. In our everyday lives, the exchange of rings is a symbol of eternal love, a circle with no end. And when we hold our hands in the prayer position, we are symbolically sending up our wishes and thanks to the heavens.

It is the intention behind a symbol which creates its energy, and endows it with so much significance. In a second degree Reiki class, students feel the thrill and power of the symbols even before they are brought up to the level of the conscious mind by the attunement process. Walk into the power symbol or the mental/emotional healing symbol after drawing it in the air and you can feel the energy right down to the tips of your toes. The human race has reached the age when sacred knowledge is no longer the same as secret knowledge. Experiencing the symbols personally is an exciting and direct confirmation of their subtle power, today as much as ever.

A symbol can express a thousand words in a geometric or pictorial form. Many of us have seen a Reiki symbol or an astrological glyph and felt as though we have seen it before, or even doodled it ourselves, at some time in our lives. We may have thought we had done this absent mindedly, but can we be certain, once we have begun to research a little deeper into our psyches? The sign of the cross is recognized by everyone, but it also represents the flat, horizontal line and plane of the Earth, penetrated to its core by divine power descending from above. As above, so below, we learn in the Lord's Prayer, and this rich message is conveyed by just two lines.

Reiki master William Rand cites the ancient male and female Antahkarana symbols as the link between our physical brains and our spiritual selves. Rand's insights led him to believe that the Antahkarana is a carrier of vital, Kundalini life-force energy from the Earth. It is also said to carry ki (or "chi" or "prana") from the eighth chakra in our subtle bodies back down to the Earth again, making a full connection. This Kundalini energy is said to rise up our spines as we evolve in awareness. The Antahkarana symbol, whose origins are unknown, takes the form of a geometric shape, or "yantra", long used in meditation in Tibet and India. The male version is compact and focused, a symbol of channelled, directed energy. The female representation is expansive, showing a balanced and dispersed energy. Both are reminiscent of the ancient Hindu swastika and can be seen as cubes within a circle; if you look at them long enough, you can grasp the multidimensional qualities and sense of perpetual forward motion. The essential energy of the Kundalini is again represented in Tibetan Reiki, in which the symbol of Raku, the Fire Serpent, is used to balance chakras from the head downwards to the root or base chakra. This symbol also comes to us from China and other parts of Asia, and is used by practitioners in healing and prior to attunements.

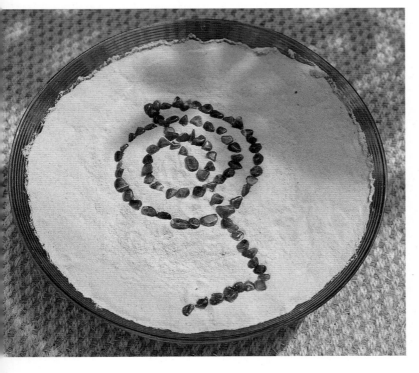

◁ The power symbol, cho ku rei, can be read clockwise or counter clockwise, and its potency means it can be used in every aspect of life.

The Usui distant healing symbol proves time and again that there is more to space and time than our current concepts of physics allow. This symbol is used for absentee healing, bringing past, present and future into oneness. It has been translated as "The spirit in me honours the spirit in you". Today attunements to Reiki are offered on the Internet. It is not necessary for a Reiki master/teacher to be present if we can use the distant healing symbol to such incredible effect.

The Usui Reiki power symbol has been found to work in healing with the spiral turning in clockwise and counter clockwise directions. It empowers everything for the highest good, even other symbols.

Symbols cannot always be fully appreciated by looking at them on the page. Draw them in the air, visualizing them and imagining them in their multidimensional forms. Often you will find you imagine them in the colours of healing (gold or purple) as you are creating them. When you do this, you are playing your part in the creative manifestation of universal healing.

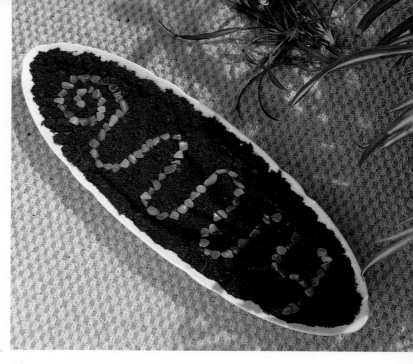

△ **If you are meditating or focusing on your energy and raising your awareness, why not make a physical manifestation of this shape? Raku is the symbol of life force or Kundalini energy.**

REIKI SYMBOLS

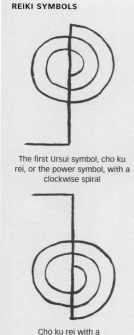

The first Ursui symbol, cho ku rei, or the power symbol, with a clockwise spiral

Cho ku rei with a counter clockwise spiral.

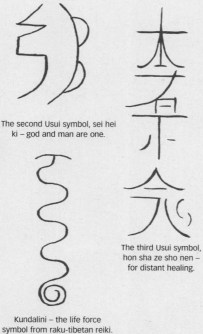

The second Usui symbol, sei hei ki – god and man are one.

Kundalini – the life force symbol from raku-tibetan reiki.

The third Usui symbol, hon sha ze sho nen – for distant healing.

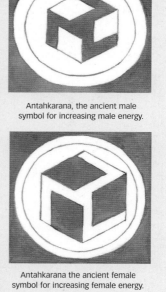

Antahkarana, the ancient male symbol for increasing male energy.

Antahkarana the ancient female symbol for increasing female energy.

Intuition and bodyscanning

As you become more familiar with the practice of channelling Reiki for yourself and others, you will feel your intuition becoming clearer and the moments when you are aware of it will become more frequent. Getting acquainted with your intuition is one of the most exciting things you experience after an attunement to Reiki. It grows just like any other part of your expanding self and its relationship to All That Is. Reiki gently frees old patterns of thinking, sometimes without you even noticing, and without the need for the brain to become involved. In so doing, the power of Reiki creates new space for continuing growth and awareness.

using your intuition

When you are channelling Reiki for a recipient, you may feel that a specific place on the body wants attention. Sometimes an area of the body can feel noticeably hotter or cooler than others. Your hands or fingers could start to tingle, or you might feel that you don't want to move your hands at all even if you have been holding them in a certain position for the usual five minutes or so. These are all signs that a particular part of that person needs the energy more than other parts. While we know that Reiki reaches everywhere, it is perfectly all right to wait until these feelings decrease before you move on and continue the full treatment.

Avoid scaring the recipient if you feel the presence of an imbalance or blockage. Rather than asking if she is suffering any pain or discomfort, enquire if she would like you to focus anywhere in particular. If she volunteers information about an illness or a specific problem, recommend that she visits a doctor.

You may already be in touch with your inner voice or higher self or spirit guides, and perhaps you would like to ask for help from all light beings, or Reiki angels, to bless your session together. It is vital to ask the spirits for their help or blessing – if you remain silent or wait for them to come to you, you could be waiting for a long time. The spirits never impose on us, but wait patiently to be consulted. If it seems that nothing is happening, and you don't feel any

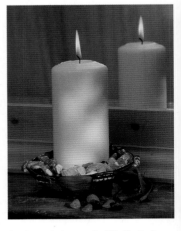

△ Beings emit the warmth of life, like the flame of a candle, and this can be felt when scanning.

warmth to tell you that Reiki is flowing, be assured that they are with you. A true request to the Universe always gains a response, so have faith.

Although the Reiki energy needs no help, I have asked the Reiki angels for love

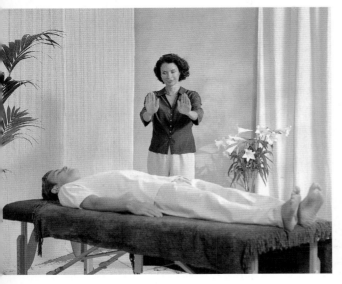

Reiki angels

Angels and spirit guides do not impose themselves

on us. Introduce yourself and ask for their

help and blessings.

◁ Beaming from a fews steps away means that the whole body can be treated at once, rather than a specific point.

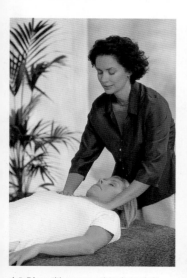

△ Reiki practitioners sometimes leave their hands for longer over parts of the body where they perceive hotspots, as these can denote tension. Cold spots can signify blockage.

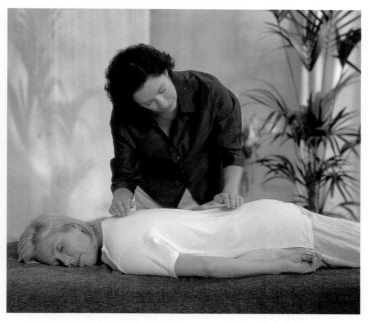

and clarity during attunements, and my more perceptive students have said afterwards that they had sensed that there was someone with me during the whole process, even though I myself had no idea they were there.

bodyscanning

Once the recipient is on the couch some Reiki practitioners like to scan a body as a way of introduction before a session. Some like to do it afterwards, and some do it before and after, to record any changes. If you explain your actions to the recipient, she will be more aware of changes too. The recipient may not have heard of this practice, so put her at ease.

To scan a body, begin at the head or the feet. Holding one hand a couple of inches above the clothes, pass slowly over the length of the entire body, making a mental note of your observations. This is good to practise in a group at healing circles, where you can discuss your Reiki discoveries. You can get the same clues from your own body, as you pass your hand over yourself. Practising on yourself will help you to explore, and to gain invaluable trust in your own being. Giving yourself Reiki is an exciting way to learn.

△ A Reiki master will keep her mind open for messages and will listen to her spirit guides and request their help during a treatment.

▽ An energy sweep is a balancing and refreshing way to end a Reiki session.

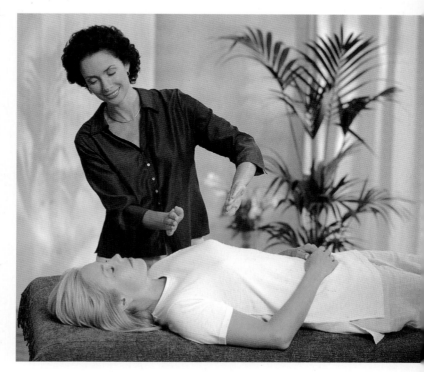

Choosing a master

If you have enjoyed receiving Reiki, and would like to channel the energy for the benefit of yourself and others, you may one day decide to learn how to perform attunements yourself. For now though, you need to find the right Reiki master for you, someone who will gladly share their experience with an open heart in a way which appeals to you practically.

Today there are so many Reiki schools to choose from, and so much information within easy reach, that you can find us everywhere. However, as with many things, word of mouth is often the best way of ensuring you make the right connection. Although it is not always true that what a friend likes will appeal to you, many Reiki masters find that an attunement to Reiki is followed by enquiries from the recipient's friends and relations. Recommendations reach like-minded people, who are attracted to an energy akin to their own. "I had been wondering about learning Reiki for some time, and when I heard about you, I just knew this was the time for me. I had to ring you. Will you attune me?" is a common

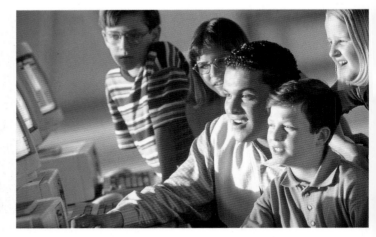

response from people excited about practising Reiki themselves. It is often the case that someone mentions a new experience that you have been thinking of trying yourself. Reiki seems to find people, at the right time, in the right place, with the stunning synchronicity we are now learning is the nature of the Universe. Why else

△ Small teaching groups in any discipline or skill offer a close teacher and pupil relationship. You might prefer this setup for your Reiki class.

would people say with such certainty that they knew something was meant to be? It is good advice to say to someone seeking a master, "Ask the Universe, or God, or however you see the creative principle of life, for some guidance in finding your Reiki master. You will know when it is right for you."

something for everyone

If you thumb through the pages of health and healing publications, you will come across adverts offering Reiki attunements on a particular date, where a Reiki master attunes classes of up to 20 or more people over the course of a weekend. For first degree classes, two of the four attunements are given on each day, with the rest of the time spent discussing the theory of Reiki and exploring the multitude of ways in which you can use it. In the case of second

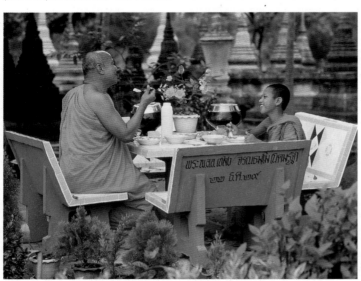

◁ The bond between master and student is traditional and ancient, and can still be found one-to-one today, if you choose.

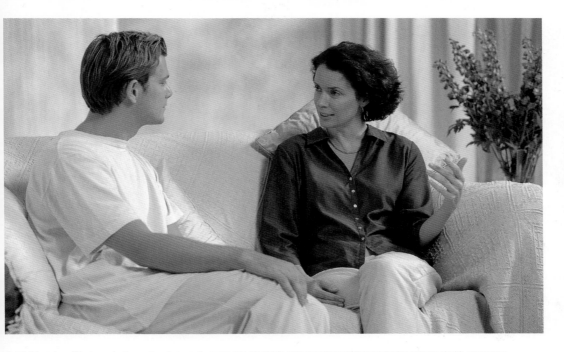

△ A Reiki master will be happy to discuss the attunement process and other Reiki matters with you before you decide to proceed with a treatment.

and third degree classes, there is just one attunement; the extra time is spent either on the uses for Reiki symbols, or on expanding experience and learning how to perform attunements to the best of your ability and for the benefit of your own future students. Some Reiki masters offer the first and second attunements together in one day or over the course of a weekend, so it is well worth discussing this possibility.

Being part of a large class can be very stimulating. You will get to know other people who share your interests and with whom you can continue to network, or maybe even set up your own Reiki sharing group afterwards. Attunements are a powerful healing process in themselves, and often an emotional one, where hidden feelings may surface, so a large class can be exciting and supportive for all involved.

If you think you would prefer not to share your innermost feelings with people you do not know, a smaller class of two or three people may be more appropriate for you. Sometimes friends choose to share the experience of an attunement, and you could

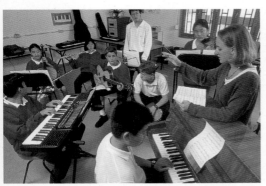

◁ Just as a music class of several pupils offers more scope for harmony and resonance, so a large Reiki class can be exciting and stimulating for some. Others may prefer the intimacy of a smaller class.

get a small group together if you all feel the same way. A Reiki master may be willing to visit your home, or you may be welcome at his/hers. This creates a special occasion in an informal and comfortable setting where you can eat, drink and chat your way through the experience.

meet your reiki master

Many Reiki masters hold open days to encourage people to share questions, discuss issues surrounding Reiki and experience some Reiki healing. Reiki manuals written by the teacher will often be for sale or on loan, and this is a valuable way of finding out more about your compatibility with your prospective Reiki master. Reiki masters will be happy to make an appointment to talk about their attunement methods, or you can talk over the telephone. You can discuss things like financial charges or exchanges for a Reiki attunement, as well as where it will take place. If you feel the master is not for you, wish him or her luck and say so. Whether you want an attunement on the eve of a full moon or under a waterfall, there will be someone, somewhere, who can do it for you.

Reiki Routines

Reiki works on many levels and can be administered by laying hands on a person or by simply channelling energy in their direction. In this chapter, the key hand positions are described for self-help treatment, and for treating others. How Reiki works with other healing therapies, such as reflexology and meditation, is also discussed.

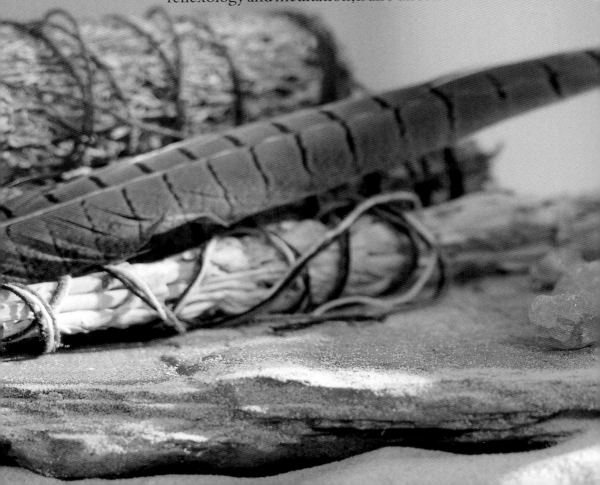

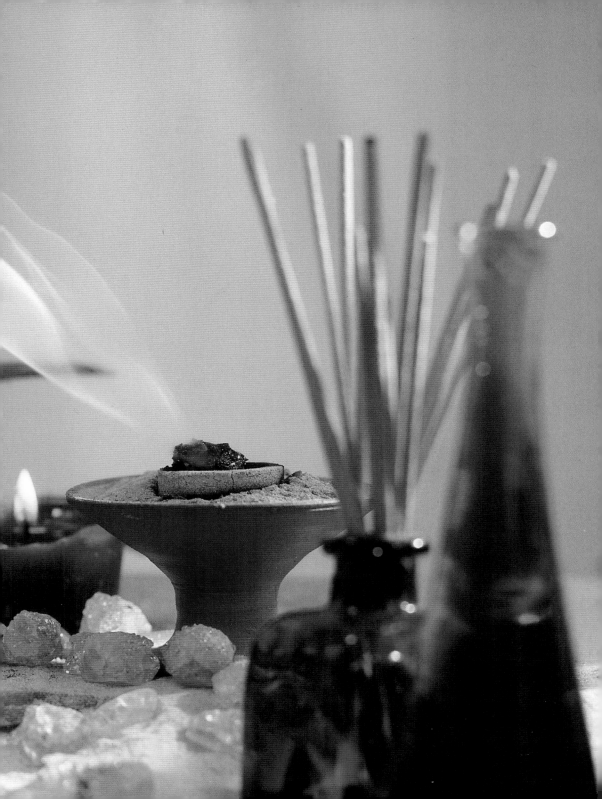

The first degree

After the attunements to First Degree Reiki, you will be empowered to channel it for anything with which you have direct contact. Anything you place your hands on will receive Reiki simply by the intention to heal, and as you use it more and more this may happen automatically as it becomes integral to your being.

There are four attunements carried out in the First Degree, and it is often after the first of these that people feel a hitherto unknown sensation in the hands and a tingling in the feet. Sometimes the Reiki attunement prompts people to shed tears, or giggle or yawn, sometimes they feel slightly "spaced out", and sometimes it makes no discernible difference. The latter is often the case if the student has already been introduced to energy/vibrational healing at an earlier date. However you respond – and remember there is no right and wrong in Reiki – it is always a joyous experience and frequently a deeply moving and spiritual one. It is said that Reiki is a remembering, rather than an acquiring of anything new. This feeling of being completely at one with

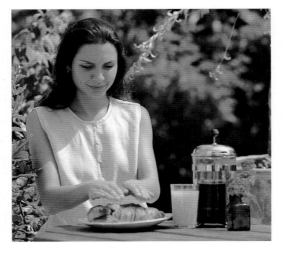

◁ You can bless all things with Reiki hands, including your food and drink.

or at home during an attunement is sometimes accompanied by seeing colours, or images of people or beautiful landscapes.

after attunement

Depending on your Reiki master and the size and duration of the class, some of the many different ways of applying Reiki will be discussed and explored after the attunements. Your concepts of hands-on healing will be expanded as you learn you can give healing not only to yourself, and other people, but also to pets, plants, food, drink and inanimate objects such as batteries, letters and computers. Anything energetic will benefit from Reiki.

Students taking the First Degree will have the opportunity to try out the traditional Reiki hand positions on themselves and each other during the class. They will also be given examples of short- and long-term treatments, and perhaps examples of appropriate positions for particular conditions. It is the most

incredible landmark to be given the gift of healing, and it can be overwhelming at first. If you go home after an attunement only to sink into a spell of gloom or fly off the handle, don't worry – it's all part of the process. Place your hands on your stomach or head, or anywhere that feels comfortable,

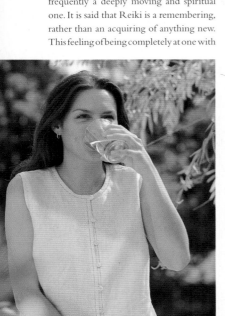

◁ Drink as much water as possible before and after attunements, to help the body assimilate this new energy.

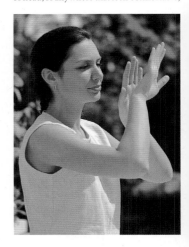

△ They look the same, but they feel different: sometimes people feel heat or tingling in their hands after an attunement.

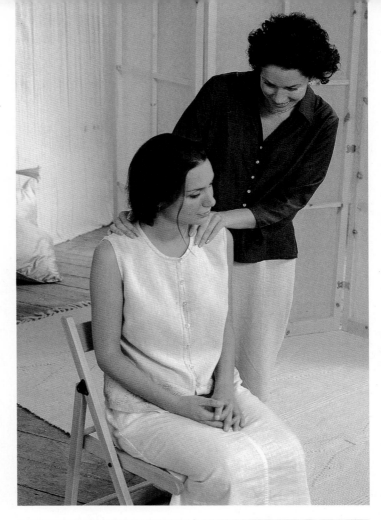

▷ During the First Degree, your Reiki teacher
will show you how to position your hands when
channelling for another person or for yourself.

and think "Reiki Go!". At this very special
time, Reiki will accelerate the healing
process in an exciting yet gentle way,
helping you to take responsibility for
yourself by giving and accepting the gift
of healing.

the next step

Although Dr Usui is reputed to have passed
on all his Reiki knowledge in one go, it is
unusual to find a Reiki master who feels
comfortable about passing on Reiki in this
way. Although there is nothing intellectual
to "learn" about Reiki, after an attunement
to any of the three degrees a 21-day
cleansing process takes place in the body as
energy filters and adjusts in the Reiki
initiate. This process is reminiscent of how
Dr Usui spent 21 days on Mount Koriyama,
seeking the Reiki formula that would allow
him to activate the energy. This period
occurs as the Reiki is absorbed into each of
the seven main chakras in the physical and
etheric bodies (three days for each chakra).

These days, many Reiki masters advise
prospective students to wait at least three
months between accepting the First and
Second Degrees, and often longer before
deciding to become a Reiki master themselves. This is intended to allow the student
time to process the experience of attunement, physically, emotionally and mentally.
Some people also feel they would like to
acquaint themselves with the physical experience of activating Reiki before becoming
involved with the symbols and distant
healing. Other people have continued very
happily after receiving attunements to the
First and Second Degrees, feeling it has given
them more to work with. You can listen to
the experiences of Reiki practitioners, but
in the end you must allow yourself the
freedom to follow your own heart.

▷ After the First Degree you can enjoy your
Reiki wherever you are, and can even give it
to yourself as you relax with a hot drink.

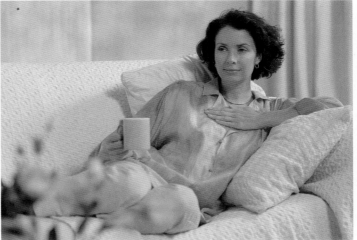

The second degree

The Second Degree enables the practitioner to increase the power of hands-on Reiki, as well as sending healing across time and distance using the Reiki symbols given to Dr Usui on Mount Koriyama. Attunement to this level brings the symbols placed in the subconscious mind in the First Degree up to the conscious level, so that they can be used with awareness in as many aspects of your life as you wish.

the attunement

There is just one attunement in Second Degree Reiki, the student having already taken the major step of accepting the Reiki energy in his or her physical body during the First Degree. This opens the chakras even more to receive and channel the Reiki healing energy. This degree works on the level of the mind and emotions, which brings new opportunities to heal and to transcend mental and emotional problems. This, in turn, creates space in one's mind for expansion and growing spiritual awareness.

keys to creating energy

Following an attunement to Second Degree Reiki, students are shown pictures of three of the four symbols used in healing. (The fourth is taught at master/teacher level.) Traditionally, Usui teachers instructed their pupils to destroy any representations of the symbols before they went home, but now sacred no longer means secret, and the symbols are available for all to see on the Internet and in books, some of them in this book. The teacher's main objective when explaining the nature of the Reiki symbols is to convey the multitude of ways in which they can be applied. As the fundamental key to the activation of Reiki, they are all-embracing and can be used for every circumstance in our lives.

the first symbol

The first symbol to be learned is the power symbol, cho ku rei. When invoked by someone who is attuned to Reiki, this creates the energy "God Is Here". As this suggests, this amazing phenomenon can be used to lovingly empower and bless yourself, other living beings, anything you take into your body, situations and occasions, inanimate objects and just about anything else you can think of, to startling effect. This symbol is often visualized on the backs of the hands while giving a treatment to yourself or others. It can also be drawn in

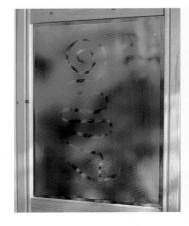

△ Draw a symbol in the steam of a mirror to give yourself added energy or a healing space.

the soil of an ailing plant, and in food with your fork. It is effective for clearing a house where trauma has occurred, or to welcome a new home. Paint it over your walls to give a joyful aspect to interior design, or in the bath for an invigorating start to the day, or in the classroom for a lively lesson – this symbol brings positive energy and life to every possible situation.

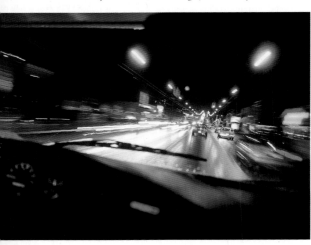

◁ Some people use Reiki symbols to help clear their way of obstacles – even busy traffic on the road can be affected.

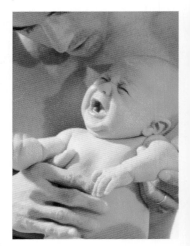

▷ Using the Reiki symbols can help create a calmer environment. Try them on a crying baby.

the second symbol

This symbol, sei he(i) ki, promotes mental and emotional healing wherever it is called to help. One of the first successes I enjoyed with this symbol was visualizing its creation between the eyes of a boisterous dog during the lunchtime of my attunement to Second Degree Reiki, immediately after my Reiki master had cited this use as a good example. The dog was bounding towards us and just as I finished saying the name of the symbol for the third and last time, it stopped in its tracks and padded on peacefully. This healing symbol can also be drawn in the air near a crying baby, as its energy is soothing and clearing. Draw it over or under your bed at night, or on a piece of paper to place under your pillow, and in places where there is conflict of any kind.

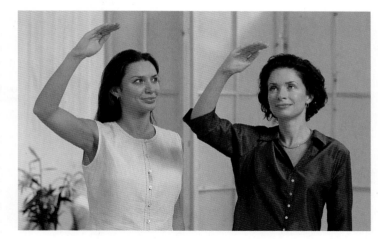

△ During the Second Degree you will learn how to draw the symbols, and explore exciting ways of using them to enchance daily life.

the third symbol

This symbol, hon sha ze sho nen, is the only one needed to send Reiki healing over distance or time, and it transcends both, acting in the past, future and present simultaneously. The name of this beautiful symbol can be interpreted as "May the Buddha in me reach out to the Buddha in you to promote harmony and peace." In this way, we really reach the essence of the object of our healing intent. Many people insist that people must ask for healing, and that you should not send it of your own accord. Use your own judgement in this matter. Perhaps someone is too ill to reach you, and you know the healing would be accepted with gratitude. Proceed with the best intentions and send your thanks to the Universe.

sending reiki

This can be done in as many ways as you can imagine. Here are a few tried and tested aids to channelling distant Reiki:

- Hold a picture of the person to whom you wish to send Reiki, or place it close by, and focus on the image while sending Reiki.

- Write the person's name on a piece of paper, as well as the date and time when you wish to send Reiki, and the place where they will be when the healing is intended to take place. You can speak these instructions too, inwardly or out loud. Draw the distant healing symbol, and the other symbols if you wish, over these written intentions.

- Give yourself a self-treat, and as you do so send it to another by saying inwardly or aloud, "As I heal myself, I am also sending Reiki to [the person's name]." You could continue, "My left side represents [person's] back, and my right side the front of their body", or any part of them on which you wish to focus.

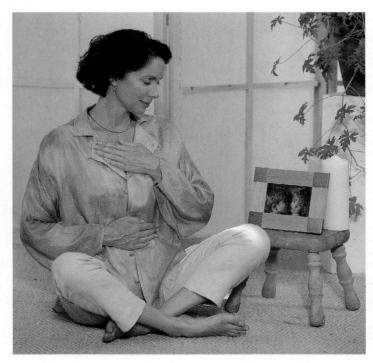

△ Sending distance healing while giving yourself Reiki is a very effective way of practising.

The third degree

Many people practise Reiki happily for years without ever feeling the desire to become a teacher themselves. Others decide to take the Third Degree for healing purposes only, to enhance their activation of Reiki with the master symbol. As with the decision to accept any of the three Reiki Degrees, there are many schools and attitudes to choose from when you are considering becoming a teacher and passing on attunements yourself.

the right moment

Judgement is sometimes passed by Reiki masters about whether a student is sufficiently aware to embark on the Third Degree, but, whatever anyone may tell you, this decision should ultimately be made by the student – even if that decision is to be guided by the master as to when the right time is reached. If you have spent some time sharing Reiki with others, whether for friends, professionally, or both, you may well feel it is the right time for you. That is the

time to contact your Reiki master, or to look for another master to attune you to the Third Degree. Although First and Second Degrees are sometimes given during the same course, it is advisable to wait a while until becoming a Reiki master yourself, simply so that you know what you are passing on to others – it is difficult to teach otherwise.

commitment to evolution

Making the decision to become a Reiki master does not mean you should let yourself be pressurized by suddenly being thought of as a "guru", and open for advice 24 hours a day – asked for or otherwise. What we are really doing when we ask for Third Degree attunement is making a commitment to the spiritual evolution of ourselves and others on the

All shall be well,

all shall be well,

and all manner of things shall be well.

St Julian of Norwich

planet, for we are all learning together. Taking the Third Degree is a commitment to our intention to live within the Reiki ideals. The Reiki principles were written to empower us towards our own happiness, and they are included in every other spiritual teaching and religious school of thought in one form or another.

different approaches

More and more people are taking Third Degree since the explosion of Reiki in the Western world during the 1980s. There are so many kinds of Reiki to choose from that if you follow your intuition you will find one that is right for you.

Traditionally there is a period of training as a Reiki master, which usually lasts about a year. An Usui Reiki master may ask a candidate to accompany him or her on First and Second Degree courses, for which you may be asked to pay in the region of $10,000 (£6,000), the figure recently confirmed by the Reiki Association as a fair financial

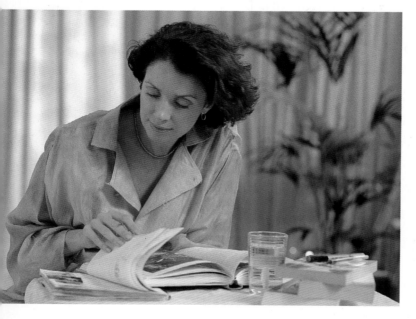

◁ **There is nothing academic about Reiki, but there is much to learn from the experiences of other philosophies and practitioners.**

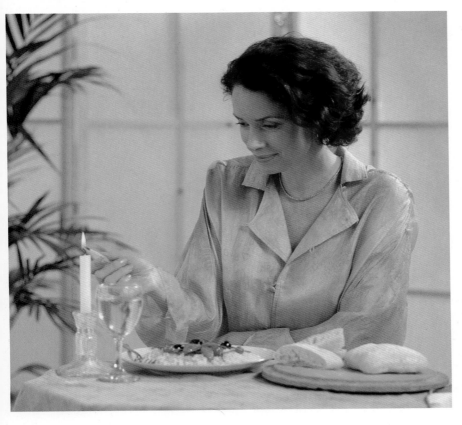

◁ As with all attunements, you will benefit from giving your system cleansing space at this time. Make special moments by adding an element of care or ritual to everyday activities.

exchange for master-level attunement. During your apprenticeship, you may be asked to send essays on Reiki to your Reiki master, who will mark them for you.

There are also other Reiki masters who are in love with Reiki themselves and recognize the wish to be able to pass it on, especially at a time in the world when the more healers there are the better. Their courses may last a weekend only and you can shop around for a suitable fee or exchange.

Everyone who decides to take the step towards Reiki mastership does so having found joy in living within the Reiki principles. They are honouring an inward promise to continue evolving along that path because they have found it constantly returns love and happiness to their lives. The desire to become a Reiki master signifies trust in the Universe, and the underlying wish to shed the constrictions of the ego gently and with as little conflict and as much love and acceptance of oneself and others as possible.

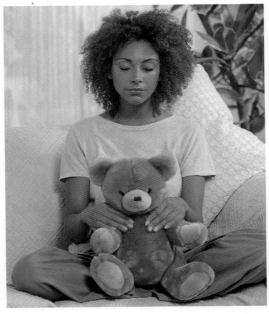

▷ Keep practising your attunements and hand positions, even when you have reached master level, on willing friends or family members, or even a co-operative bear.

Hand positions

The hand positions used in Reiki have been passed down through the lineage of masters and practitioners in the traditional Usui System of Natural Healing, and have many physical and metaphysical benefits, which will be explored on the following pages.

During a treatment, the hand positions are usually followed in sequence from head to toe, though occasionally people begin at the feet and finish at the head. Following these positions gives the attuned practitioner a comprehensive method of treating the whole person in a comprehensive way. The positions are designed to care for the whole being – physically, mentally, and also spiritually, as you will remember that the etheric body has seven chakras of its own which correspond to the seven main energy centres of the physical body.

I have met people who were informally attuned to Reiki, for instance at a summer music festival. They were simply passed the attunements to channel Reiki, but were given no history of Reiki or any other theory. It appears that the Reiki hand positions are so straightforward that these new practitioners were able to discover them entirely through their own experience and intuition, without the aid of books. They subsequently were surprised to find in books the identical hand positions to those they had been using. They had found that the positions simply seemed the most natural way to give a Reiki treatment to the whole body.

get over it

It is worth including a note on the sensitive subject of hand positions and breasts. No guidelines exist and most practitioners treat breasts as more or less invisible during a Reiki session, probably feeling that recipients would prefer it that way. However, with breast cancer rates soaring in the western world, I feel it is worth asking female Reiki recipients if they would like some Reiki on their breasts too, not just above and below them. Our breasts are in the

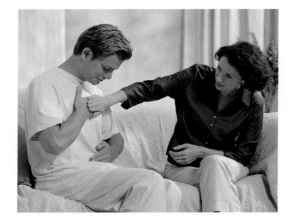

◁ The hand positions in Reiki are easily taught, and seem to be part of the intuitive, natural process of healing when they are explained by a master or teacher.

area of the heart chakra, and are nourished by this centre, but they are also intended for nurturing, and we are not nurturing them psychologically by constantly ignoring them during healing opportunities.

If you are a Reiki practitioner yourself, you will know how wonderfully warming this direct contact with the breasts is during a self-treatment, and the willing recipient will benefit greatly from the very fact that she is caring for this part of her body. Most women will probably not mind another woman placing hands horizontally across her breasts, as we are acquainted with more intimate health check-ups. If you are too bashful to ask, or your recipient refuses, you could simply hold your hands a few centimetres above the bust and treat her at an auric level, which is still beneficial.

We need to stop separating parts of our bodies into sexual and non-sexual – the symbolic gesture of Reiki attention here will be of great benefit both to our bodies and our psyches.

how to hold your hands

Your attunements to Reiki allow you to channel healing through the palm chakras, and in order for the energy flow to be focused, practitioners keep their fingers and

thumbs together, and their hands flat or very slightly cupped. This may not be possible in certain circumstances, for example, at the scene of an accident, or during a couch treatment when you may feel that your thumbs are in the way around the throat area. In cases like these, don't worry about the physical detail, the Reiki will still be flowing outward.

how long?

Reiki guidelines recommend three to five minutes spent in each hand position. Sometimes, you can feel intense heat or cold when you place your hands on a particular spot. Sometimes, your hands can tingle or feel heavy as the recipient draws in the energy, and sometimes you may feel nothing, in which case be assured that the Reiki is still working perfectly.

If any particular feeling in your hands has not dissipated after five or six minutes, you can leave your hands in position until it does – although often if you leave then return to a "hotspot" after carrying out the remaining hand positions, you will find it no longer thirsts for the Reiki so strongly. This is because an imbalance may have been created elsewhere, and has now been healed at the source, or vice-versa.

Hand positions for reiki using a couch

Begin by tuning in to Reiki and breathing calmly in the present moment, with your hands on the recipient's shoulders as he lies face up on a treatment couch or massage table. This moment or two gives the recipient time to settle in and become accustomed to your touch and the treatment room. Once you have hand contact with the recipient, try to maintain contact until the treatment is over. The recipient will be more relaxed if he is aware of your body position throughout the session.

▷**1** Place the palms of your hands over the recipient's eyes, with your wrists just above the forehead, thumbs meeting at the bridge of the nose and fingers on either side of the nose on the cheeks. Gently lower your hands until you are touching his face. Centring around the sixth chakra, this position energizes the eyes, and aids clear vision, including the intuition. You will also be treating the emotional stress release points just above the arch of the eyebrows.

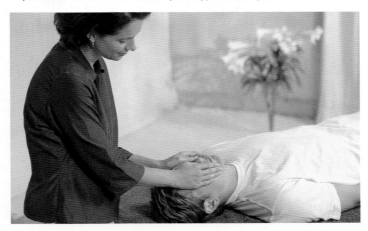

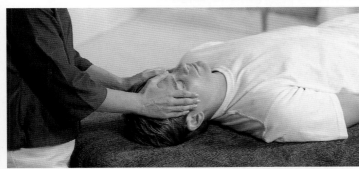

◁ **2** Gently part your hands and slide up and sideways until your palms are on the temples, and your fingers just on the ears and the jaw area. This position helps to dispel tension in the face.

▷**3** Slowly slide your right hand from the recipient's ear on to his cheek, and with your left hand, gently roll his head on to your right hand, so that this hand is now flat. Slide your left hand underneath his head just above the neck so that you are cradling it. Your right hand can now roll the right side of his face toward the left and slide underneath the right side of his head. Achieving this position change fluently can take practice, but once you are there you will notice how relaxed the recipient is when he allows the weight of his head to rest on your hands. It is quite comfortable to perform, and amazingly soothing, balancing the energy in both sides of the brain and releasing mental tension. You can visualize drawing the mental/emotional healing symbol on the backs of your palms while you are changing position, or just beforehand, and this will further enhance the benefits.

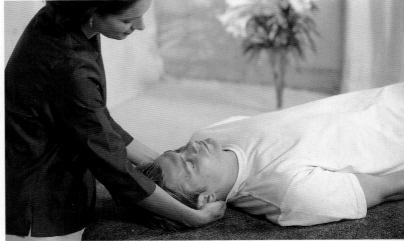

▷

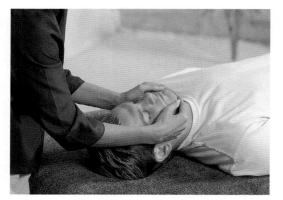

◁ **4** With your left hand, gently roll the recipient's head to the right, so that your right hand supports it, and move your left hand down to the bottom of the chin and throat as you slowly slide your right hand out from underneath and guide the head so that it is again centred on the couch. Rest your elbows on the treatment couch so that you are steady, and do not place pressure on the recipient. Place your hands with the heels of your palms on the side of the neck and your palms and fingers lightly on the throat, overlapping. Alternatively, you can lightly place the thumbs on the bottom of the jaw and interlace your fingers over the throat if the recipient is not very relaxed. Either way, be aware that the throat is a very sensitive place, where the fifth chakra known as the "centre of the will" resides. The throat stores emotional memory and communication, so it is important to respect this. Be aware that in this position the recipient may get a lump in his throat, or tears may well up as healing occurs, releasing trauma and emotion.

▷ **5** Still resting your elbows on the couch, or standing if this is more comfortable, slide your hands below the throat, lightly outward on to the chest and towards the arms. Stop when the palms are on the armpits. This is not a traditional hand position, but I have included it because so many people love it and visibly relax, absorbing the Reiki into the lymph region. This is a great help in ridding the body of toxins. The position also treats the lungs and clears the chest, great for smokers and asthmatics.

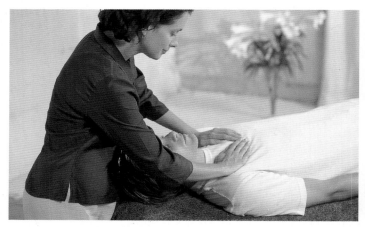

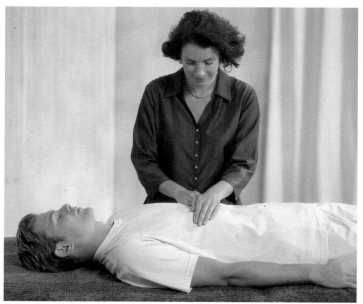

◁ **6** Now stand if you weren't already, and move to one side of the chest. Place your two hands in a straight line across the sternum. This is now the fourth chakra or heart area and Reiki here helps to encourage the recipient to love – both oneself and others. You can also hold BOTH hands on either side of the body, always staying near the centre, for three to four minutes anywhere in this area.

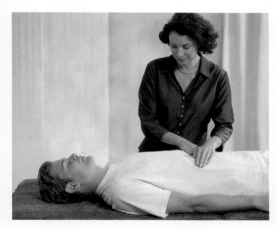

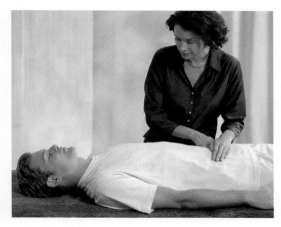

△ **7** Hold your hands, again one behind the other, over the chest area, continuing to give Reiki to the heart and lungs as you move downwards.

△ **8** Next, move the hands down, resting across the solar plexus area where emotions are stored. Continue downwards, resting the heels of your hands either side of the pelvis, with your fingers pointing upwards towards the navel. This benefits the pelvic area, and all organs near the second chakra. Finally, move one hand slowly up to the centre of the chest, ending the treatment for the front of the upper body.

▷**9** You can then treat the legs, moving downwards in as many stages as your time allows. These positions relax muscles all the way down the lower body, and create a balancing effect.

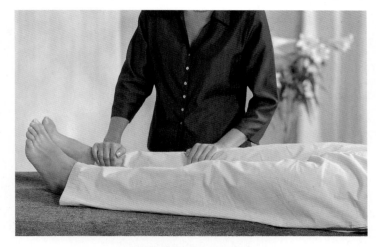

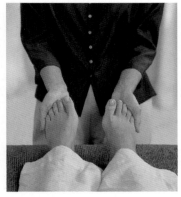

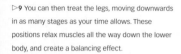

◁**10a** Treat the tops of the feet to bring awareness to the whole body, and to ground the recipient as he may feel slightly heady.

◁**10b** The soles of the feet being so sensitive, this position can help to bring round a sleepy recipient at the end of a treatment.

Hand positions with recipient face down on a couch

Reiki sessions can be successfully carried out just treating the front of the body, but you may like to treat the back directly, especially if the recipient is having problems in this area. Ask your recipient to gently turn over on the couch for the second half of a body treatment using the following positions.

▷ **1** When your recipient has turned over, place your hands on either shoulder, moulding your hands to their shape. As well as introducing the beginning of the back treatment, this position soothes and melts away deep-seated tensions stored in the neck and shoulder areas.

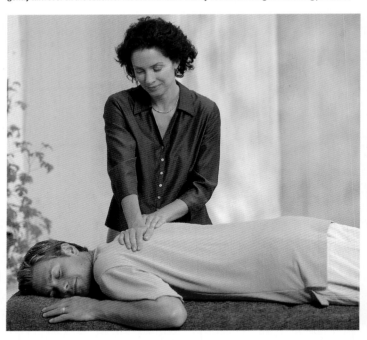

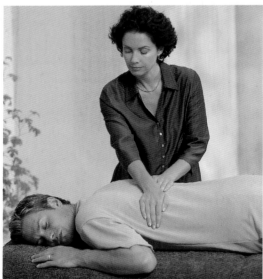

△ **2** This is not a traditional hand position, but again, it's much loved and, appropriately, works on the heart chakra. You can also follow this by making a T-cross, with one hand placed vertically underneath so that the heel of the hand is nearer the solar plexus.

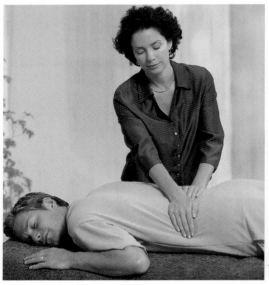

△ **3** Gently move your hands outward, so that they are positioned on either side of the abdomen and solar plexus, moving down towards the kidneys, until your hands are either side of the ribcage. This position is a fabulous boost to kidneys and adrenal glands.

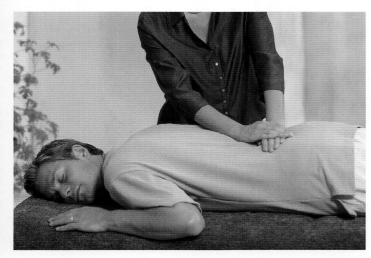

◁ **4** Slide your hands down and together, so that they are in a small T-cross at the base of the spine. Complete the upper body positions by moving one hand to the top of the spine, with the other at the base. This will act like a spirit level, balancing the energy along the spine and gently rejuvenating the recipient.

▷ **5** As when giving Reiki to the front of the body, you can move down the legs and further relax muscles and joints. You can ask if there is anywhere the recipient would like you to focus.

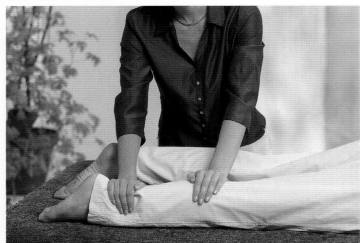

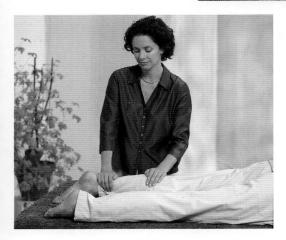

◁ **6** When you have worked on one leg, use the same positions on the other.

winding down

End this part of the treatment by moving down to the feet, crouching on a level with them, if that feels comfortable. Rest your hands lightly on the recipient's soles, and then visualize the creation of the mental/emotional healing symbol. Then, keeping your hands where they are, imagine the outline of the power symbol on the backs of your hands. Now would be a good time to use the distant healing symbol before the other two, and send the recipient more Reiki for a further hour following this hands-on treatment.

Hand positions for others using a chair

Sessions in a chair are often preferred by people who are new to Reiki, they are also great for spontaneous Reiki treats, and also for anyone who finds it a struggle to get on and off a couch. Recipients should be seated straight, but relaxed, and the Reiki practitioner should find an ideal height with shoes on or off, or back strain can occur. Check that you can move around the chair freely for all the hand positions you intend to use. Again, these positions are intended as a guide, so go with your intuition.

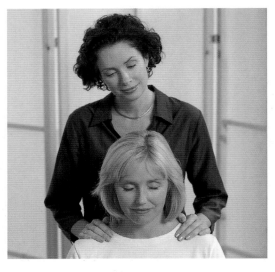

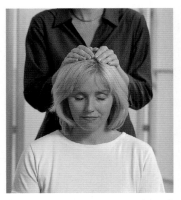

◁ **1** First of all, lay your hands on the shoulders of your recipient as you stand behind her and tune in as before, taking a few deep and gentle breaths and resting your hands lightly on her body. Now is a great time to draw the distant healing symbol in the air over the recipient's head, in order to send healing while you are also enjoying a hands-on session.

△ **2** Put your hands very lightly on or over the top of the recipient's head, as this position can be very stimulating. Only hold this position for two or three minutes, as this is the area of the crown chakra and is very delicate.

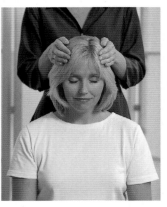

◁ **3** Move your hands to either side of the recipient's head as you stand behind her. This position is very supportive, even though the recipient is sitting, and you can strengthen the treatment by drawing in your mind the mental/emotional healing symbol on the backs of your hands, followed by the power symbol on top of this. This position balances energy in the brain and is good for stress.

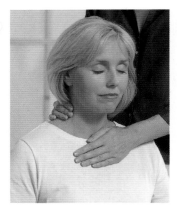

◁ **4** Now move one hand and gently lay it on the throat area with the other hand at the base of the neck. You can continue to move down the torso like this, hands on the front and back, covering the chest and solar plexus.

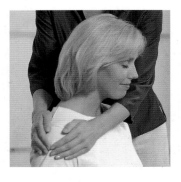

◁ **5** Now reach across the recipient to finish the treatment with the shoulders. Complete the treatment with one hand at the top of the spine and one at the base for the balancing "spirit level" position. You might need to crouch for this one.

ADDITIONAL WINDING DOWN

Use this hand position on the recipient's feet, especially if they are feeling slightly light-headed. Crouch in front of her, or sit on a chair facing her and take one or both of her feet in your hands, channelling Reiki on to either the tops or the soles of the feet. This will help to ground the person and completes a full-body treatment.

Self-treatment hand positions

Giving yourself a treatment in a chair is a great way to spend a free quarter of an hour. You could do a couple of the positions while sitting at your desk at work or in a quiet moment at home. If you have longer, use the time – it's never wasted if you're using Reiki. You might find that you only mean to give yourself ten minutes but then just don't want to stop. Let the Reiki take you where it wants to go and don't rush away.

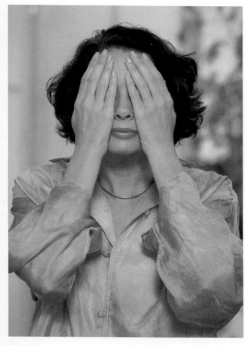

◁ **1** Place both your hands over your eyes and feel refreshed. This hand position helps to restore clear vision in strained eyes, and is effective for headaches and sinus trouble too.

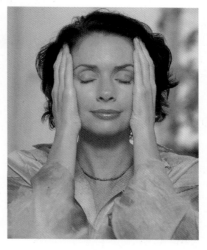

△ **2** Place your hands on your temples to help to clear an overactive or tired mind. You can also treat your ears and jaw muscles like this. If your arms get tired, rest your elbows on your knees.

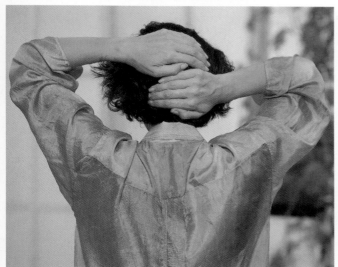

△ **3** Move your hands round to the back of the head and the neck area, dispelling tension and refreshing the brain. You might need to be in a more supportive armchair for this position, as your arms can tire.

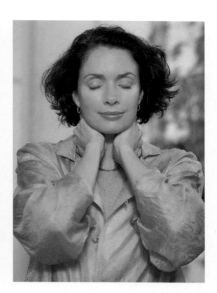

△ **4** Now put your hands either side of the neck, benefiting the area of the thyroid glands, associated with communication and self-expression. This position treats the throat chakra.

▷

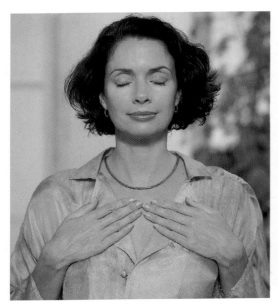

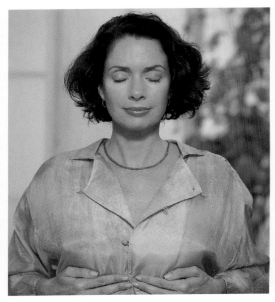

△ **5** Place your hands above the breasts on either side of your chest. This position is very good for lymph drainage and clearing toxins from the body, so it sometimes gets very warm.

△ **6** Place your hands on your chest, fingers meeting in the centre at the heart chakra. This helps to transform emotion in the solar plexus to the heart area of unconditional love.

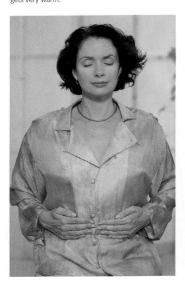

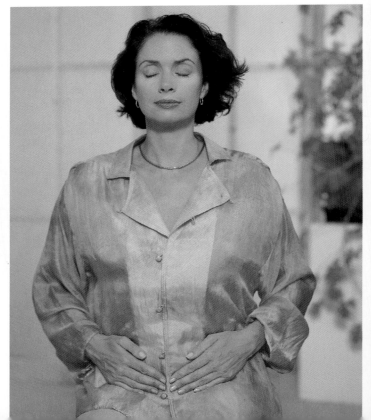

△ **7** Moving downwards, put your hands on your ribcage, giving Reiki to the solar plexus centre and all governed organs nearby.

▷ **8** Place your hands about an inch below your navel, the location of the sacral or second chakra. This position is good for stabilizing and releasing sexual tension, and also treats the spleen.

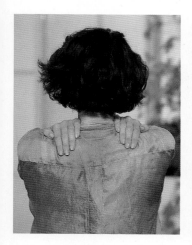

△ **9** Place a hand on each of your shoulders. This benefits the neck, shoulders and back. If this position feels awkward try crossing your arms in front before putting your hands in position.

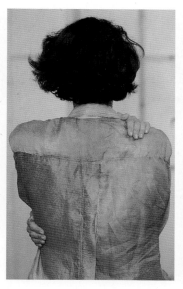

△ **10** Cross your arms and place one hand on your shoulder, and the other at the side of your ribcage, spreading the flow of Reiki downwards.

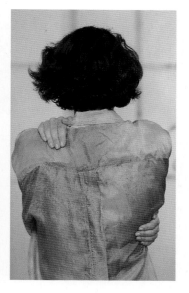

△ **11** Now repeat these hand positions on the other side of your body.

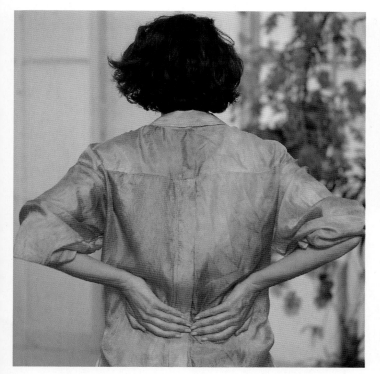

△ **12** Move your hands round to your lower back and place them over the kidneys, treating all organs cared for by the third, sacral chakra, including the adrenal glands.

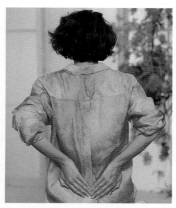

△ **13** Finally, move your hands lower to the base of the spine. Whether treating from the back or the front of the body, this position is beneficial for issues surrounding survival, the will to live and fight-or-flight instincts.

WINDING DOWN

To balance yourself and bring yourself back to the present moment, place your hands on the tops of your feet for a few minutes. You can also finish a self-treatment by placing one hand on the forehead and one near the first chakra at the base of the spine.

Treating self

There is one important rule about using Reiki on yourself – do it as much as you can. It will enhance your being in a myriad of ways, and we all know that the happier and the more whole we are feeling, the more good things we want to give to others.

Sometimes it may seem difficult to fit yourself in when friends and family are queuing for relief from physical and mental bumps and bruises. You may have even been motivated to channel Reiki so that you can use it to help someone close to you. However, this is a case of "Physician, heal thyself." The Reiki will leave you feeling as if you have had a refreshing shower each time you channel it through your being, but it is also important to nurture yourself with a long, deep soak. You will find that the symbolic gesture of giving Reiki to yourself is indeed a significant part of your own healing process. However, we are not always as comfortable about receiving things as we are about giving them. We may not feel that we need healing, and many of us hold the belief deep down that we are not worth it and don't deserve it. Reiki gently shows us that we are loved unconditionally by the Universe. It works just as well on a

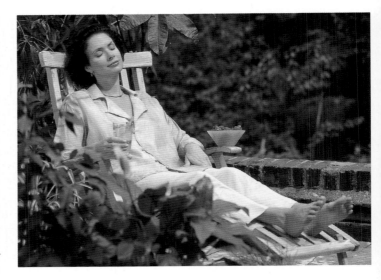

△ Spend some time each day enjoying life's gifts – sitting in the sunshine for a few moments will raise your spirits and link you to the Universe.

hangover as it does on a cold, making no judgements: our own concepts of what is self-inflicted and what is not are completely irrelevant to the Universe. One of the first joys of the gift of Reiki is the enlightening feeling of being "at one" that unfolds and envelops us, and is there anything more welcome in today's world than that?

Everyone is different, but when you give Reiki to others you will have more understanding of their responses if you have experienced it yourself. During our attunements, we learn that Reiki heals even when it is called on for the first time after five or ten years. You don't have to "practise" because you already have it, and there is nothing for your brain to "learn". The more you give Reiki to yourself, however, the more you can feel its effects, which is very exciting, and good for your confidence

when using it with others. So it really is totally unselfish to begin with yourself, in fact it is vital. In this way, putting yourself first brings benefits not only to you, but to others too.

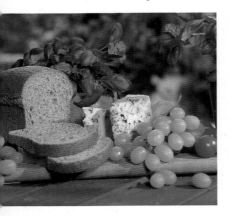

△ You may find yourself eating healthier foods after Reiki attunements, as part of a greater commitment to life.

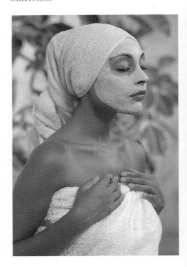

▷ Give yourself a quick Reiki treat at any time, even during a regular beauty routine. You can also do it in the bath or in the shower.

There is no substitute for setting aside a full hour for a Reiki self-treat. Set your alarm clock if you have appointments, and switch off the telephone. As we shall explore later, Reiki works beautifully with other therapies, so you can incorporate it into a foot massage or beauty treatment. If you are having a busy day, give yourself Reiki as you go along – some of the hand positions are inconspicuous enough to enjoy as you stand queuing in the supermarket. Just put your palms anywhere on yourself and think, "Reiki Go!" If you are watching television, you can put your hands on yourself and give some Reiki. Even if you have a drink in one hand and put the other hand on yourself, you will benefit your whole being by treating your body and what you are about to take into it at the same time.

Some people choose to give themselves Reiki at the beginning of the day. This is the perfect time to thank the day for all the wonderful experiences it will bring, and will help you to live and grow in the Reiki principles. Just before going to sleep at night is also a great time for a self-treat – if you fall asleep, the Reiki will filter through. If you feel sleepy and want to avoid nodding off,

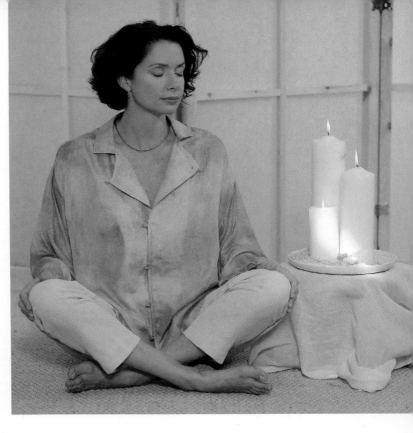

sit in a chair instead. You can also visualize the mental/emotional symbol above your bed if you are feeling stressed, and wish to wake up refreshed and renewed. Any time you have your hands on yourself and are channelling Reiki, you can also be focusing the healing energy on dilemmas and questions you may have; make this your intention and wish for the best possible outcome. There are as many combinations as you can think of in which to enjoy the benefits of Reiki, so allow your imagination to create your own healing reality.

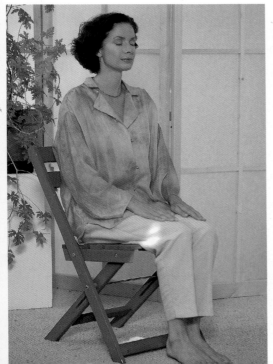

△ Be aware of the sensations you experience from different hand positions, while giving yourself a Reiki self-treat.

◁ Making a self-treatment a part of your everyday life has a multitude of benefits for your mind, body and spirit.

Sitting quietly,

doing nothing, spring comes,

grass grows.

Osho

Treating others

Two conditions must occur before healing can take place. There must be a shift in the consciousness of the recipient – he/she must want to heal and must assist in that process by having an open mind. There must also be an appropriate exchange (of money, of energy or of a gift).

Before your Reiki recipient arrives, there are a few things you can do to create a space conducive to this healing. First and foremost, you will be the one spending the most time in the chosen healing area, so make it a space in which you are happy and relaxed. Before the arrival of your visitor, take a few moments to ground yourself in the present moment, just as you do at the beginning of a self-healing session. Tuning your being into the Reiki energy before the arrival of another person will benefit both of you. You will be calmer and more assured at the outset of the session, and you will be able to focus naturally and with clarity.

"Smudging" or cleansing the air with a sage smudge stick is a fragrant way to prepare a healing room and welcome a spiritual and peaceful ambience. If you have taken your Second Degree, you can do this while also activating the Reiki energy in the room by drawing the emotional/mental healing and

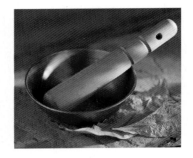

△ Sounding a singing bowl is a lovely way to cleanse spaces before and after a treatment. You can also burn incense or candles.

power symbols in each corner. Another lovely way of doing this is to draw the distant healing, emotional/mental and power symbols in the centre of the room, then visualize gathering up the symbols in your arms and scattering or sprinkling them outwards in all directions. If you draw the distant healing symbol in the air over the couch or chair, you can send your Reiki recipients healing before they arrive and throughout the session itself.

Wash your hands before and after each Reiki session – dirty fingernails are offensive, and your hands will also hold the

scents of the day. Brush your teeth too. Place a box of tissues near the recipient in case they need one; you can also offer to place one over their eyes to absorb moisture and to assist with their focus during the session. There should always be fresh water to drink, and a light blanket in case your recipient feels cold.

Different people like different smells, so remember this if you use incense or essential oils. You could wait and ask your recipient which aromas they like from a selection of oils. Check that you are both agreed on the length of time for the Reiki session, and include a few minutes in which the recipient can return to the present with a hot drink. Sort out payment or exchange for the treatment before the session begins. Ask if they prefer daylight, or the curtains half-drawn or closed with a lamp lighting the room. Ask them to remove glasses, perhaps lenses, shoes and any jewellery. If you think you will want to take your shoes off, do so before you begin.

You could start at either end of the body, but Reiki hand positions usually begin at the head and work downwards, ending with the toes. Position a clock with a face large enough to see easily without having to twist

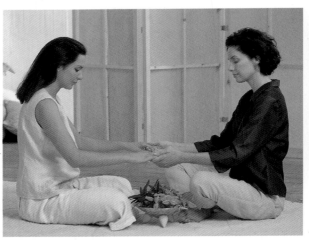

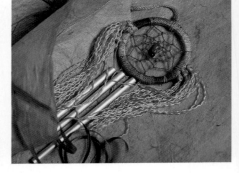

◁ There must be an exchange of energy before a healing, so that both are participating in the experience.

△ Many people give something of significance, such as a dream catcher, rather than money.

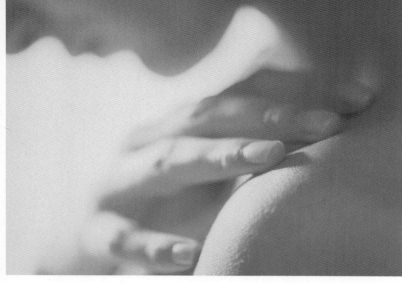

◁ No pressure or manipulation is necessary in Reiki, nor is it necessary to remove clothing, but the touch of Reiki is as loving and natural as the warmth of human touch.

▽ Some people feel it is helpful to cleanse the aura by smudging as part of the ritual and ceremony of a significant healing process. Use whatever you and your recipient feel at ease with to focus your thoughts and energies.

or interrupt the treatment if you are unsure of the time spent on each position. A lightweight chair is useful if you are treating the torso, for example, and can do so effectively sitting beside the couch. Most people are quiet during a Reiki treatment, but sometimes people need to chat, or find themselves shedding a few tears or even giggling. Be responsive to comments, but try and say as little as possible. You can help the healing best just by listening, so resist any temptation to offer advice or anecdotes, as these may be distracting. Make the healing session a time when you pass on only essential and positive information. You are acting as a facilitator and Reiki is doing the healing, so the more supportive you are, the more healing the experience will be. If you wish to know, ask the recipient if there is anywhere they would like you to focus, but avoid negative words such as pain. By the time you are two-thirds of the way through a Reiki session, some people will have dozed off, so whisper when you have finished the treatment. Be gentle, and give them time to drift back into the present.

Afterwards, ask if there are any questions they would like to ask or if there is anything that they would like to share.

When your visitor has left, turn the pillows over, open the curtains and the window for a minute or two, and take time to sit and be still once more. Thank the Universe for the gift of this Reiki session and dedicate it to love.

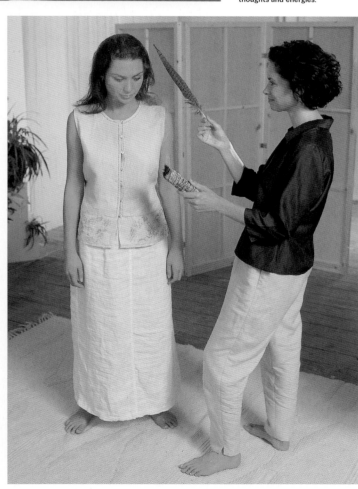

Group healing

Joining a Reiki healing group gives people the chance to enter the unique space that is created when a group of people with the intention to heal gather together. The loving energy emitted by a group of healers is so strong that it is tangible both to the people channelling Reiki and the recipient. Sometimes people say they can see the healing energy of Reiki vibrating around the many pairs of hands while participating in a group healing session.

numbers and positioning

A shorter time is usually necessary for treatments when they are carried out by a group, perhaps half an hour or so. The time allotted to each person will depend on how many there are, but you can always split into two groups using two couches. A group healing session is appropriate for anything from two to ten people, basically as many as can place their hands on a body. This will not usually permit keeping to the taught hand positions, but is wonderful for the recipient. If

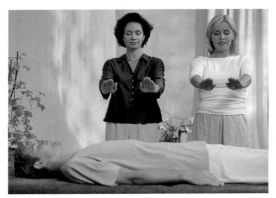

◁ Two practitioners beaming a Reiki treatment at the same time will increase the effect, and a good way to use the combined power is to beam the whole body from a few steps away.

there are only two of you, you can carry out a very satisfactory Reiki treatment in a number of ways, such as working from the head down one side of the body and around to the other side (following each other), or beginning at the head and the feet and working your way up, meeting at the heart and stomach areas. This will harmonize the chakras of the recipient in a balanced and even way.

opportunities to experiment

If there are too many people for one recipient, use the distant healing symbol together in another small group. You could send this healing from a different room or from the hands-on session, as both will activate the Reiki energy and further intensify the healing for the recipient and the rest of the group.

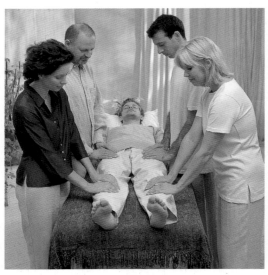

△ There is no ideal number for a Reiki group – many hands are making light work at this healing session.

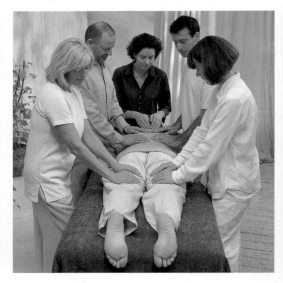

△ A healing group can meet as often as once a week to reap the rewards of powerful Reiki channelling.

Another technique that works well in a group environment is "beaming". Stand a few feet away from the treatment couch and hold your hands out straight, with your palms facing the recipient (and the team in this case). Draw the distant healing symbol, the emotional/mental healing symbol and lastly the power symbol in your mind, and see them floating above the couch. Surround your visualization in a golden light and send Reiki to this healing; feel the energy radiating from your hands, and know it is filling the entire space with love and Reiki. This wonderful and enhancing healing technique treats the aura of the recipient, harmonizing imbalances before they even reach the physical body. "Beaming" is also an ideal way to work with someone seeking relief from a chronic or stubborn complaint, while they are enjoying a hands-on treatment. If there are enough people, the group could work in shifts for two or three hours.

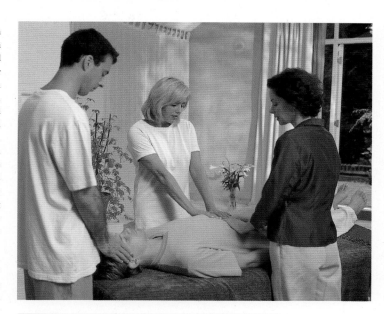

△ Hands can be positioned anywhere on the body or at the request of the recipient.

finding and creating a healing group

There are Reiki healing circles in most areas, and you may be invited to join one already run by your Reiki master. If you can't find a Reiki healing group, go along to your local spiritualist church, which will certainly have a healing circle of its own and may be able to refer you; in any case, healing with other people of different "schools" will be a unifying and expanding experience. You could also place an advert in an appropriate shop window, or on the noticeboard of the local health clinic or complementary healing centre. Ask your friends or place an advertisement in the local newspaper, using a post office box if you prefer. You may find other people contact you wishing to do the same, and you may choose to set up the first Reiki healing group in your town. Whether you find a group or found your own, you will then have the facility to enjoy giving and receiving healing at least once a month, maybe once a week – it's up to you.

setting the scene

Third Usui Reiki Grand Master Mr Hayashi is known to have encouraged and participated in group healings at his Tokyo

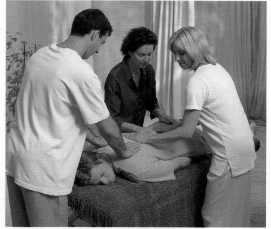

◁ Sometimes the group will work together intuitively, other times there will be guidance from one of the healers.

clinic, and other forms of healing involving group ritual can be found in cultures throughout history. There is a great deal of scope for experimentation and for enhancing your experience of Reiki sharing, complementing it with other systems as the "global village" breaks down more and more barriers between belief systems.

A group healing meeting may begin with a Reiki circle ritual, a prayer to spirit helpers, a space-clearing ceremony, or a chant or song to invoke love and unity for the duration of the healing meeting. Some Reiki groups use tranquil healing music

with a marker every 5 minutes, so that the group knows when to change position. Others find this a distraction and prefer to select someone who will keep time for the rest. Everyone is different, and communication is the key to a harmonious group experience. Sometimes there will be people in your group who are also spiritual healers or shiatsu practitioners, or people who practise different kinds of Reiki. This makes it even more interesting when you sit down and explore your feelings afterwards. Reiki groups are a sure way to discover new ideas and techniques.

The power of groups

There is growing awareness of the power of group healing as we extend beyond individual action in the Age of Aquarius. In this new era the emphasis must surely be on the importance of humanity working as a whole, and this is demonstrated all over the world by thousands of people who share the wish to help alleviate suffering simply by using the power of love.

Some of these groups travel to war-torn areas to aid the emotional, physical and spiritual healing of the victims of conflict. Healing parties of various schools and denominations have been received by world leaders, with whom decisions of universal importance rest. As anyone who has used the Reiki distant healing symbol will know, distant healing, whether sent to an individual or to the planet itself, is just as effective.

The power of prayer has been proved to work beyond doubt. People who have had near-death experiences report feeling and seeing the positive energy created by a prayer said for them. Hospital studies have shown that patients being prayed for enjoy quicker recovery rates than others, even when they are unaware of the prayers.

The common intention shared by so many to raise the vibration of the world literally "lightens" the atmosphere. Motivated by unconditional love, we know we are operating from our hearts. This heartfelt wish has spurred people all over the planet to stop what they are doing at a pre-arranged time on a significant date, and to focus on sending healing to humanity and the Earth itself.

New physics continues to convince us that we are not individuals alone, but

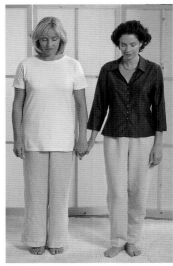

△ **Two practitioners focusing before the beginning of a Reiki healing session, and sending their best wishes for this meeting.**

bundles of energy which overlap and meld with each other. Although there is no danger of contracting another person's ailment during a Reiki healing, people often see the auras of practitioner and recipient flowing into each other during a healing session.

Groups are also playing an increasing role in creating a peaceful planet in preventive ways. There are now academic research teams monitoring the efficacy of distant healing on decision-making processes in matters including nuclear issues. These and other projects are proof that we can enjoy enormous success when we work together, particularly as part of a healing group. Just sharing the intention and vision to heal means that the consciousness of the planet is transformed, because we are creating our own mass consciousness. As time goes on and we learn more, these kinds of exercises may well extend to group healings throughout communities. Teachers and

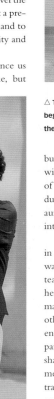

△ **A healing circle provides an intimate way of bonding and charging up the Reiki energy before and after a meeting.**

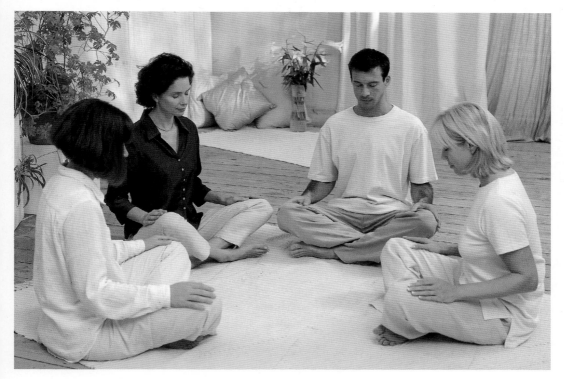

△ **Many people meet at significant times to send distant Reiki and other forms of healing and prayer for the wellbeing of the world.**

children could be encouraged to take part in distant healing sessions at school, and we could see the day when they are accepted practice in hospitals. They would be especially beneficial in government and in the prison system – what a healing phenomenon that would be.

Healing is a conscious effort which is expanding, and it benefits us all to take part, for we are all part of a greater whole and we are creating our own future. If we think about when we have been most miserable, we can see that it is very often the state of feeling separate which causes us loneliness and sadness in life.

A healing circle is both a symbolic and practical way to experience the flow of healing. You could do this with your Reiki sharing group before a session with someone who has a chronic or stubborn complaint. The infinite flow of a circle is bonding and will charge up the Reiki,

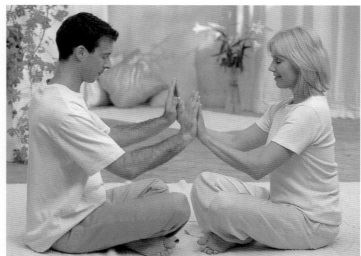

activating it ready for a treatment. Afterwards it will give you all some extra healing time for yourselves, following which you could share your findings and feelings. Start up your own group with a circle of close friends and watch it grow.

△ **A cycle of Reiki flowing between two or more people is thrilling and gently powerful. This sharing can be done for many reasons and at many different times, for support, healing, energizing, visualization and meditation.**

Reiki and nature

There are some very effective ways to complement these beautiful and beautifying therapies with Reiki. The most obvious of these is to Reiki your essences and oils simply by holding them in your hands – a great way of giving yourself two treatments in one. Aromatherapy massages are a heavenly experience on their own, but if you are using lavender oil to counteract stress, for instance, the effects can be enhanced by drawing the healing symbol in the air above the recipient, as you might during a regular Reiki treatment. In the same way, one can complement the healing of emotional issues by using Reiki with flower essences. Each essence has a life lesson encapsulated within. Observing the life lessons associated with each remedy can be a marvellous and speedy way to articulate a confusing emotional issue.

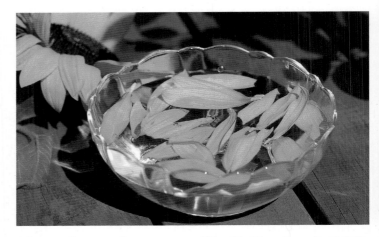

△ If you are making your own flower essences, hold the bowl in your hands for a few minutes so that Reiki will be an added benefit.

▽ Every living thing can be complemented with healing energy guided by the Universe.

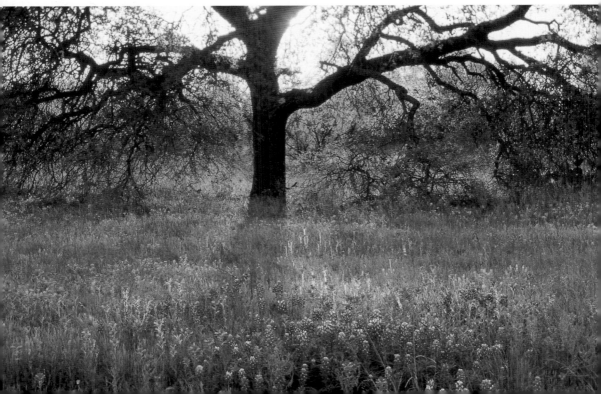

Using reiki with flowers

When you are giving someone a massage with aromatherapy oils, it is natural to treat your recipient to some Reiki as you touch them. In this way, you will be charging the oils with Reiki and lengthening the healing effects of the oils themselves. You can also send Reiki to a treatment, or to your oils before a session. Draw symbols on or in them if you like.

Rescue Remedy, a powerful Bach flower essence, and other flower remedies work beautifully with Reiki, as they are strong and subtle healers. When you are using flower remedies, you can hold the bottles in Reiki hands or send Reiki as you take the essence.

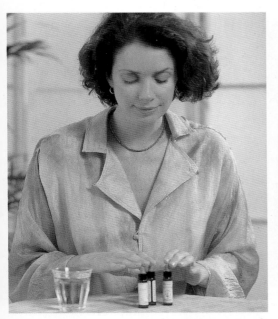

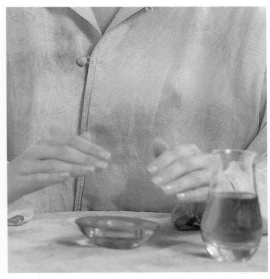

△ Giving Reiki to a bowl of essential oil before giving a massage is a powerful combination of two therapies.

△ The simplest way of complementing your flower essences is to hold your hands above them in a Reiki blessing.

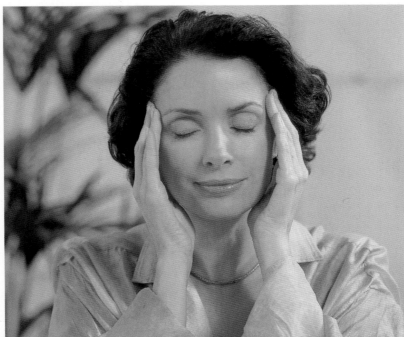

▷ Gently rub the Reikied oil into your temples as part of a complementary self-treatment.

Reiki with colour

There is great scope within Reiki for complementary healing with colour. This can be effectively carried out during hands-on or distant-sending Reiki sessions. Visualizing or sending colours is beneficial for the recipient of Reiki, not least because he or she can actively participate, and can continue to do so at home. Those who ask to receive Reiki are creating their own healing, but whereas we are dependent on a practitioner for Reiki, the healing benefits of colour and positive imagination are bestowed on us from an early age.

People who can see the aura, or energetic field, around living things know that we are truly colourful characters. Our many aspects create energy which vibrates at a certain rate, creating colour in and around our bodies. During the 19th century the Russian electrical engineer Semyon Kirlian discovered how to photograph the energy field, and there are now many Kirlian photographers who can give you a print of your chromatic make-up as it is today. Many people can read auras, seeing the colours surrounding and interpenetrating us as representing our state of health on all levels. This can be very helpful in locating and understanding the cause of disharmony and disease.

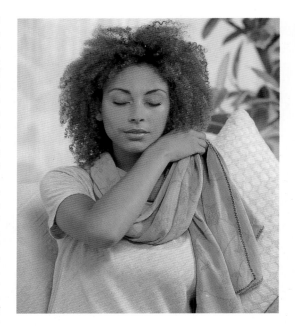

◁ Learning about colour can increase our insight into healing self and others. Blue is the colour of healing in Reiki.

colourful creation

Colour is such a beautifully simple thing to use in healing, making the most of light in all its myriad forms by absorbing it into our beings. This can be done in a number of ways – how many times have you gazed at a colour, breathing and drinking it in as though you could look at it for hours? We are all responsive to colour, instinctively preferring one to another on different days and surrounding ourselves with colours we can live with harmoniously.

The beneficial effects of colours in the treatment of certain conditions is well documented and the chart below illustrates the colours which correspond to each chakra in the body. Always consult a qualified colour therapist with a specific

problem. Next time you have a sore throat, wrap something blue around your neck; the blue light will help to balance and restore your throat chakra and the surrounding parts. You can give it some Reiki as well before you put it on. The colour spectrum is called the "rainbow bridge", linking our planet to higher worlds.

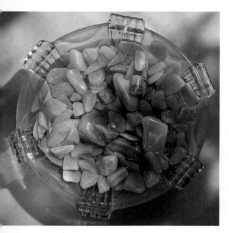

◁ Soak some blue stones in a bowl of water, then drink the water. For added effect give the stones and the bowl some Reiki first.

REIKI AND COLOUR	
chakra	colour
root	red
sacral	orange
solar plexus	yellow
heart	green/pink
throat	blue
pineal	indigo
crown	violet/purple

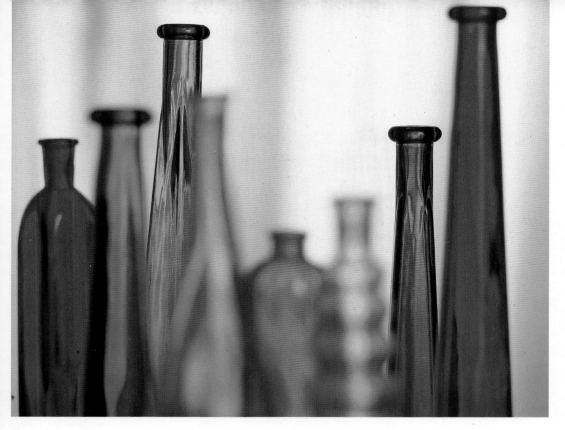

△ Bring more colour into your life, your home and your wardrobe, and benefit from its vibrancy and energy-enhancing qualities.

reiki and colour harmony

- If you are feeling blue, send pink. Enjoy a Reiki self-treat, visualizing pale pink if you are feeling sad, or green if you are irritated or angry. Remember that you can send Reiki to anything, even a visualization. Sometimes, the colour you need is difficult to visualize, so look at a patch of it, consciously soaking it up.
- Literally drink in the healing powers of a colour by leaving spring water in a glass container of your chosen colour. The effects of this "hydrochromatic therapy" is increased if you stand the container in the sunshine for a few hours, or place Reiki hands on the bottle or tumbler. Always sip slowly and gently, and use with caution.
- Paint light bulbs different colours and use them in your own Reiki treatments and for others. Paint each one the colour of a chakra, and keep them available for a lamp in your healing space. Taking 10–15 minutes for each chakra, the colour and the Reiki will balance and restore harmony in the whole person.
- Stand a few feet away from the recipient, holding your palms out straight, and visualize him or her surrounded by gold while you send Reiki. You can also visualize a gold shroud at the beginning and end of a hands-on Reiki session.
- Do this for fun with a friend. "Beam" a colour in the same way as above with your arms out straight, then try and guess which colour is being visualized. You can both finish with white or gold to heal and protect. You can also give this to yourself before a recipient arrives: surround yourself in gold or imagine a pink bubble around yourself to create a positive and loving space between you.

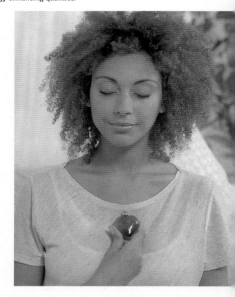

△ Red, worn or seen, can lift depression and motivate.

Reiki with reflexology

Reiki is so inclusive in nature that it complements all other healing arts, especially tactile ones where the benefit of the energy channelled through the hands is at once relaxing and invigorating. Reflexology, the practice of treating the whole body by touching the feet and sometimes the palms, is an especially valuable example of a therapy which complements Reiki successfully.

Reflexology was known to ancient civilizations in India and other regions, and is now acknowledged all over the world as a respected, effective and enjoyable form of healing. These days, many qualified reflexologists use Reiki in conjunction with their own methods, and if you practise Reiki you can give yourself a Reiki reflexology full-body treat by holding your hands on or over the pressure points of the foot.

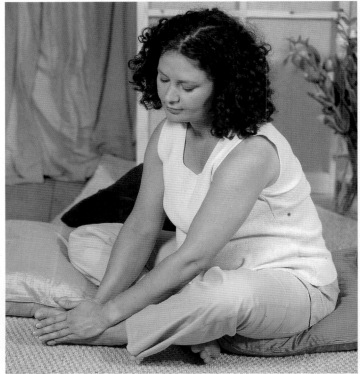

△ Giving your feet gentle Reiki will give the whole body a tonic and is an especially gentle position for pregnancy.

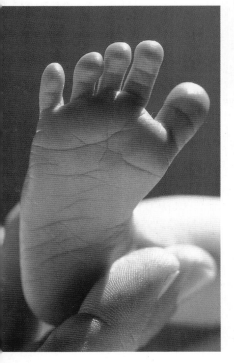

◁ The feet and the hands are maps of our entire systems, from the very first days of our existence to the end of our days.

Every part of the foot is represented by an organ in the physical body. For example, by holding the inside edges of one or both feet, you are in fact applying Reiki to the spine. (This is especially useful for a self-treatment in a comfortable position.) By placing your hands on the outside edge of one or both feet, you are applying Reiki to every joint on the edge of your body, travelling downwards from shoulder, elbow and hip to the knee and ankle on either side. Pressure points for the various organs are fairly close together on the foot, so you may have trouble differentiating which area of the body you

are treating with Reiki. However, this can only be a benefit, as Reiki energy knows exactly where to go, and you cannot overdo it. Some reflexologists use their thumbs to channel Reiki, as this is how they generally hold or massage a pressure point when giving a treatment.

In some instances of serious injury or illness, the body part in need of relief cannot be reached; this applies to complaints such as brittle bone disease. By holding the feet in Reiki mode, you can overcome this difficulty and still be in contact with the location on the body. Another illness

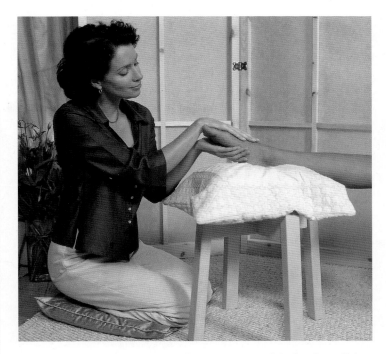

△ Hold the feet of the recipient in cupped hands for an all-over treatment in just five minutes. This is an effective position for someone who needs a gentle Reiki session.

difficult to reach is diabetes but using reflexology and Reiki on the feet is a very gentle therapy for the body, and as helpful as any hands-on full-body Reiki session.

Giving Reiki to your feet is also of benefit to the feet themselves. We often disregard blisters, calluses and other painful complaints because we don't have the time to put our feet up for long and repair the damage. Enjoying Reiki in this way will benefit your body, make your toes tingle and put a spring in your step.

▷ Return your recipient to earth with a grounding experience to connect and refresh.

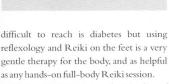

The wave lives the life of the wave

and at the same time, the life of the water.

Thich Nhat Hanh

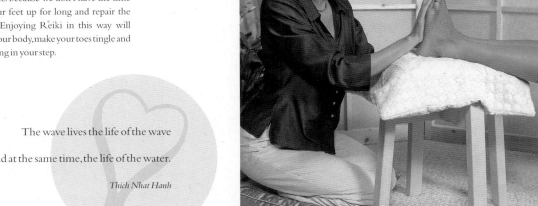

Reiki and crystal healing

Crystals and stones have benign powers of their own. Their transformational and healing qualities have been well-known to people of the many ancient cultures, and we are now rediscovering them, just as Reiki and other healing gifts have returned to us. These powerhouses of the planet heal with no help from us, yet they can be programmed with positive wishes and healing intent. Each gem or stone has a distinct healing function and energy vibration, which is both profound and subtle, and benefits all living things. The vibrational essence of a gem or precious stone has the power to heal at the very source of an illness before the symptoms manifest in the physical body.

magic in multiplicity

Just as crystals are multi-faceted, their powers to heal are also varied and versatile. Colour and structure are both significant elements in their potency to help everything from backache to psychic development. When we hold a crystal or stone on or over a part of the body or in our hand while sending Reiki, it focuses and amplifies our healing wishes. Held on our own bodies, they likewise heal and strengthen, balancing energy within us and promoting positivity, not unlike the way Reiki symbols work.

the origins and history of using crystals

Discoveries of crystal skulls at sites around the world and the technology that gemstones have given the human race today have increased our understanding of crystals and their ability to send, transform and absorb information. In ancient Sumeria, Arab scholars were adept in the arts of astronomy, astrology and alchemy, combining this expertise with their use of gifts from the earth for healing. The qualities contained in the essence of a gemstone were often taken into the body in the form of a gem elixir, drinking water which had had a crystal or stone soaking in it for a day or more.

In Indian and Western astrology, birthstones can be sources of power in a particular aspect of a horoscope, and traditional astrologers place great importance on the appropriate energy of a crystal for an individual. Some people believe it is unlucky to buy your own crystal, and this is probably to ensure it is given in love. These days, we are getting better at giving ourselves love and many people use their intuition, simply holding a crystal and choosing the one which feels best in their hands. If you have never taken much notice of crystals, spend some time holding them and see how you feel. Live with them for a few days and you will appreciate how unique each one is. It is good to share your responses to different stones with others.

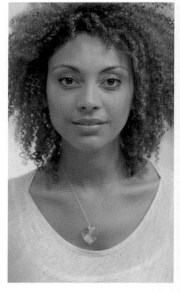

△ Ancient Indian astrologers believed wearing a chosen stone can complement a person's character.

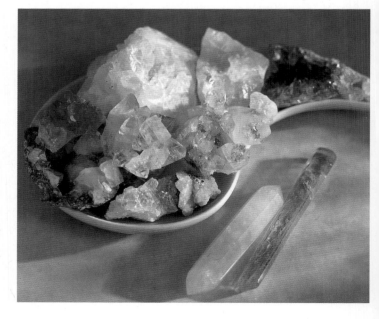

▽ Infusing crystals with Reiki will enrich their own qualities and energize a room or crystal grid.

experimenting with crystals

Notice the marvellous effects of crystals in many aspects of day-to-day life. Experiment with crystals to feel their own power, then charge them with Reiki and observe any changes. You can become intimate with both your crystals and Reiki in this way.

- Cleanse your crystals every now and then by holding them under running water or burying them in sea salt for a few hours.
- Place a clean crystal in your water filter so that you can absorb its healing power when you drink the water. You can charge it with Reiki too, or even send Reiki to your crystal(s).
- Give some Reiki to a crystal and place it in your bath.
- Place crystals on a windowsill late at night so that the first, life-giving rays of the morning sun will cleanse them and nurture their strength.
- When the moon is waning, and especially when it is new, it will bathe and cleanse a crystal placed on a windowsill; when it is waxing or full, it will increase its power. Rose quartz is often used for emotional healing and the moon is associated with our psyches and emotions, so this stone may be particularly responsive to lunar cycles. You can note the astrological sign the moon is passing through, and use a crystal with relevant properties.
- Give a crystal some Reiki and place it in a plant pot or hang it above flowers. Place it in your food cupboard to promote long and healthy life.
- Place a small amethyst on your sixth, "third eye", chakra while you are lying down during a self-treatment. Amethysts are highly regarded by crystal healers as they have special properties which encourage insight and spiritual transformation.
- Hold a quartz crystal which has been charged with Reiki above the recipient's head for a while to focus healing energy and increase insight.

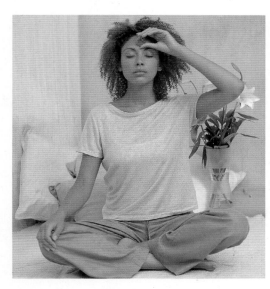

◁ **Holding a quartz crystal on your forehead during meditation or self-treatments can enhance perception and intuition.**

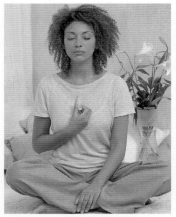

△ Hold a crystal near your heart when making an affirmation.

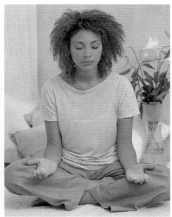

△ Place crystals in your palms to feel a powerful circuit of energy while sending Reiki.

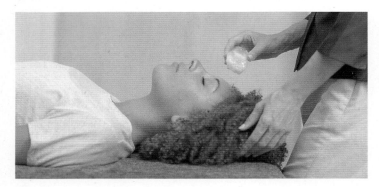

△ You can hold a crystal filled with Reiki above the forehead of your recipient to enhance insight.

Reiki and affirmations

Reiki is a catalyst for growth and positivity in all areas of life, a message from a loving Universe, bringing with it a realization that we are responsible for ourselves and our own healing. It shares with us the revelation that we create our own reality. Our thoughts are forms of energy, just like everything else; people who can see auras say that anger, for example, manifests itself as a red, spiky movement around the body. Technology now enables us to photograph and measure the energy fields our bodies emanate – the visible results of our emotions.

Our personal beliefs, and the thoughts and emotions they breed, are the most important contributing factor to our state of health. We have all experienced the benefits of positive thinking in our lives, and how it helps us to be happier. Research shows that recovery from illness, and immunity from disease, is strongest among people who love themselves, others and life, and who use techniques like visualization. Positivity and the expression of love are as powerful as diet in the treatment of disease.

Practising Reiki for oneself can be described as a healing affirmation on its own, as we are demonstrating that we are worth spending time on. Making time for others comes more easily to many of us, as we are raised to look after other people first,

▷ **Speaking your affirmations to yourself is an interesting way to discover more about yourself. Use a mirror for maximum effect.**

and we can see an hour a day spent on ourselves as indulgent if we are busy. Reiki allows us to feel and recognize ourselves as part of something greater, each of us an expression of the Divine. An affirmation is a positive statement, and a positive statement

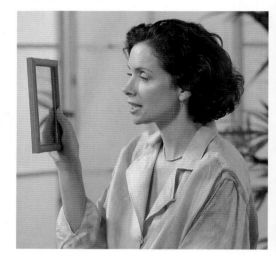

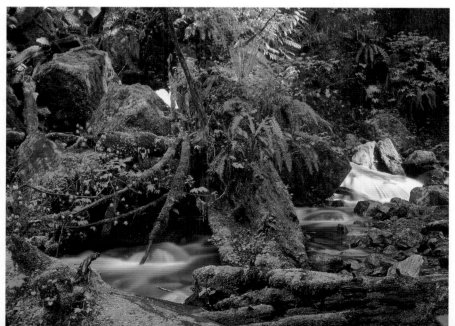

◁ **Affirmations connect us to our universe by showing us we can create our own reality in the very ways we want to.**

made to oneself is swiftly followed by an echo from the Universe, which dislikes an empty space. When we begin each morning feeling thankful and happy with life, we are expecting our lives to be good and full, and the Universe responds, likewise. If we wake up fearful of what the day will bring and feeling desperate, the Universe will respond similarly, making us feel weighed down. What was once dismissed as "all in the mind" is now valued for the same reason.

There is no better time to try out this "attitude of gratitude" than when you are feeling dreadful. This is not because we are seeking sainthood, but because it is really effective at turning a "bad" situation into one of value. Don't hang on to it, take a leap of faith, with as much of an open mind as you can muster, and say, "My life is good and all is well, and things are getting even better and we are growing from here." An important thing to remember about affirmations is to Keep Them Positive. Words like "don't", "can't" and "won't" can be less effective and confusing. Make your affirmation in the present tense. Decide on a positive sentence that is comfortable to you and "feel" it as much as you can while you say it, seeing a positive situation or your smiling self.

Saying an affirmation aloud and with feeling will endow it with more energy, and so will looking into your own eyes in a mirror. Tapping (not rubbing) the thymus gland in the centre of your chest while speaking an affirmation will also empower you. Words spoken with intent are all the convincing your body and the Universe need to hear, and gratitude and trust in life will attract more to be grateful for.

using affirmations

Affirmations on creating health and wealth can be found in texts of all religions and are making a comeback in all areas of life. Here are some suggestions on how and when to use them.

- Reiki can be sent to any affirmation because it is a creative and positive use of our emotions, for example: Reiki sessions: "I dedicate this healing to the highest good." Habits: "I release the need to smoke or use drugs." Emotions: "I am motivated by love. I communicate with love and clarity."
- Write your affirmation on a piece of paper and give it some hands-on Reiki.
- When you begin a self-treat, send some Reiki to your affirmation of the moment.
- Give your Reiki recipient a few moments to think of an appropriate goal they would like to achieve. It could be to conquer a particular fear, in which case an appropriate affirmation would be "I am positive and creative/ I am calm and comfortable."
- Sometimes we are mystified by the cause of an illness or emotional upset. We are suddenly helpless because our brains are vexed. Remember that intent is everything, and by standing back from the situation in our minds it is easier to say something helpful, such as: "I thank my body and the Universe for showing me there is conflict to resolve. I understand and release the belief system which causes this condition."

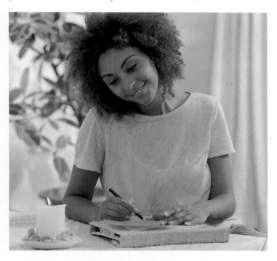

◁ Writing affirmations down and giving Reiki to the written wish is also effective.

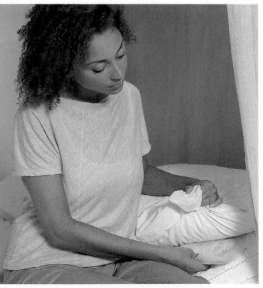

◁ For even greater effect, strengthen your written wishes with a symbol and place the paper under your pillow before you go to bed.

Reiki and meditation

Meditation is used by people of every culture and religion, and is a powerful tool which enhances our health in every way. All you need to begin benefiting from meditation is 15 free minutes each day. If you begin your day in this way you soon find your mind is clearer and calmer, and your body more relaxed and easy. Far from spacing you out, meditation promotes "less haste, more speed" as efficiency increases with mental awareness. Meditating on your own breath or on a positive visualization causes the heart rate to fall, and the immune system to rise by 50 per cent.

Buddhists detach from all but the constant breath in meditation and realize unity with the Universe through chanting mantras, as spiritual affirmations. By doing this they transcend an attachment to suffering in life. The Sufis, mystic Muslims, are famous for their whirling meditations, where one hand is held above the head in a meditation of motion in which they connect with One, Allah. They realize the connection between human and divine, and "die before they die", realizing the impermanence of earthly life through an experience of the infinite. Hindus contemplate the wheel of life, ever-changing, and Christian gnostics unite in the mystery of creation through meditation. Meditating on something or nothing brings increased health and awareness.

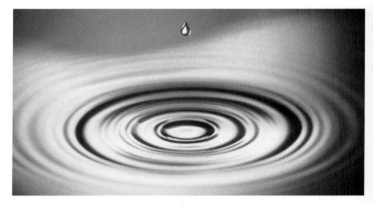

△ We are all part of a bigger whole, like ripples in a pond.

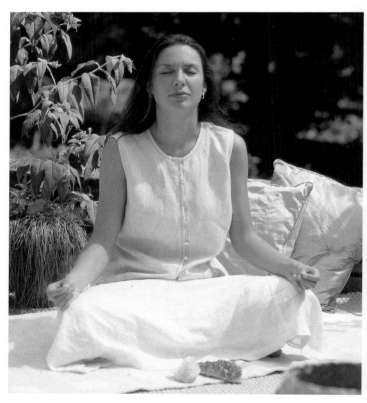

△ Being aware of your breathing rhythms releases finite time and space.

REIKI AND MEDITATION

chakra	musical note	mantra
root	C	lam
sacral	D	vam
solar plexus	E	ram
heart	F	yam
throat	G	ham
pineal	A	ksham
crown	B	om

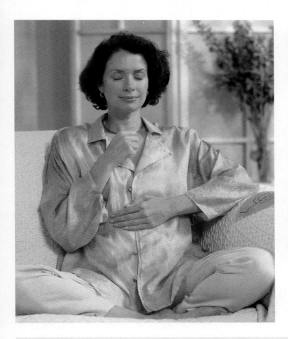

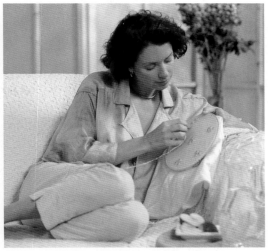

◁ Tapping the thymus gland is a
way of absorbing new chosen
belief systems.

△ Meditation influences all aspects
of your life and is effective in
increasing levels of creativity
and imagination.

ALL IN THE BREATH

You can send Reiki to the following meditations before practising them, and also to intentions
if you are seeking an answer or resolution to something. All of these meditations can be enjoyed
for just ten minutes, or for longer.

• Try this fascinating exercise and discover how much your breath affects your everyday senses.
Stand before a plant and look at it for a few seconds, then close your eyes. Take a deep breath,
filling your body with oxygen and feeling it reach up to your shoulders as you breathe in.
Breathe some more, so that your breaths become natural and relaxed, and be conscious of
breathing from the centre of your being. During an inward breath, open your eyes and look at
the plant, observing what you see. Repeat the exercise, this time opening your eyes as you
breathe out. What differences do you notice, however subtle? Do this before reading on.
A friend told me that he had done this in front of a fir tree in the Spanish mountains – the tree
looked sharper and aggressive with an intake of breath and gentler while exhaling. This
exercise has its origins in Taoism, the practice of breathing and living with the Tao, the Way or
natural flow of life.

• Sit comfortably, cross-legged on the floor or simply in a chair, and place your hands on your
heart chakra or in your lap. Breathe comfortably, eyes closed, and focus on any one of the four
Reiki symbols, seeing it before you in any colour. You could meditate on the mental/emotional
healing symbol for solace and inner peace. Focus now and then on a drawn symbol if you can't
remember the exact form. Visualize the symbol before you, feeling its energy and
contemplating its name and meaning. Meditation on Reiki symbols will encourage creative
insight as well as increased awareness and physical relaxation. You can also do this with all
four symbols, beginning with the master symbol and ending with the power symbol.

• Connect with the core of yourself, seeing it as a golden-white light in your centre. Slowly,
expand the light inside you until it extends to the tips of your fingers and toes. Be aware of
your light overflowing into the room, the building, your town, your world and your universe,
before bringing it home to your being again.

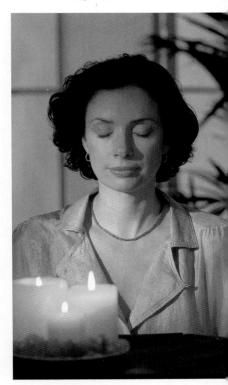

△ Meditating on clarity and love before a Reiki session allows
you to be in the present moment and enjoy it.

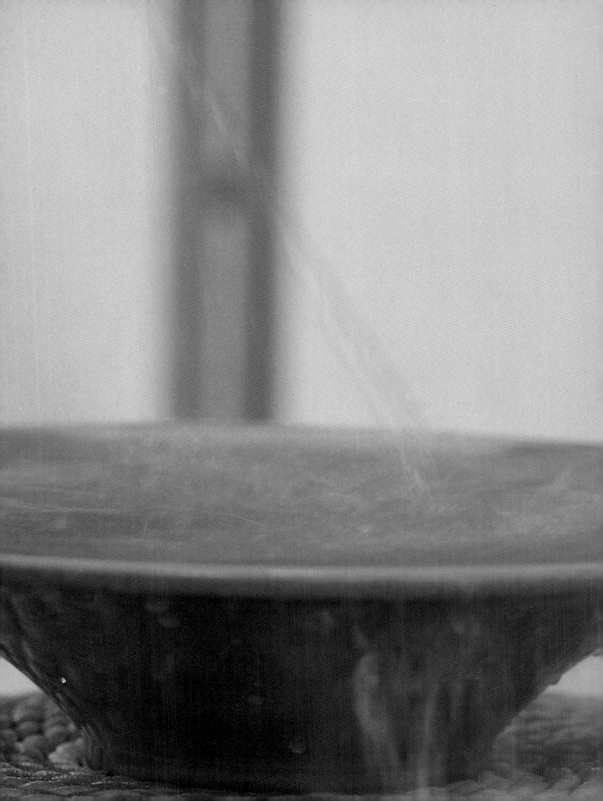

Therapeutic Reiki Treatments

Reiki heals on all levels, physically, mentally and spiritually, and supports the body's natural ability to heal itself. It is very useful for dealing with common disorders such as headaches, colds and backaches, and can be safely used on children, pregnant women and animals.

Reiki with care

Reiki is compatible with just about everything – complementary therapies, different religions, any kind of diet, no matter how unhealthy, medicines from the doctor or chemist, inanimate objects – to sum up, life itself. Reiki can never do harm, and you can never have too much. Reiki practitioners know that even for a healthy body Reiki is beneficial, its wisdom as ever guided by the Universe. I have never known a recipient to have anything other than beneficial effects. However, there are a few situations where contra-indications may be present, and where care must be taken to ensure Reiki is beneficial. For example, Reiki and alchohol definitely don't mix.

The most important things to ensure are that your intention is to use Reiki for the highest good, and that the recipient wants to receive Reiki. If you or someone you know

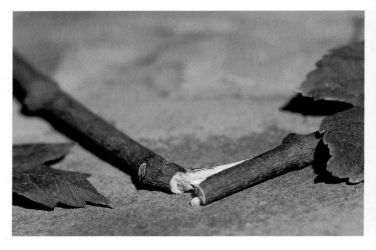

△ Care must be taken with broken bones – you should not treat them until they have been correctly set by the medical establishment.

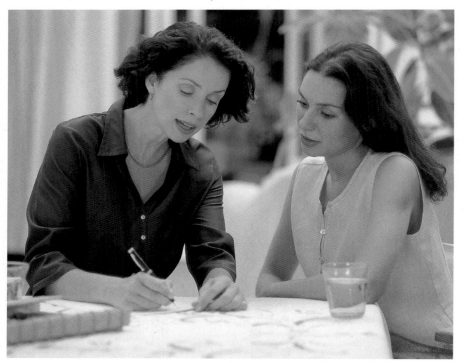

◁ A practitioner will make sure she knows the details of a person's state of health, particularly, the use of any drugs.

is about to have an operation, ensure you send Reiki before or after the time of surgery. Reiki can cause changes in consciousness which may be incompatible with a general anaesthetic. The important thing to remember is not to send Reiki when someone is about to be anaesthetized, is in theatre or is not yet conscious after an operation. When recovering from an operation, though, Reiki will lift the spirits, accelerate healing and do whatever needs to be done, and most hospital personnel are happy to see family and friends helping a patient in this way.

People with diabetes should keep a close eye on their insulin level if they wish to receive Reiki, in case the Reiki causes the insulin in their bodies to fluctuate.

There are different kinds of pace-maker devices to aid the heart, and more care is needed with some than with others. Pace-makers that kick in when the heart rate falls below a certain level are normally compatible with hands-on Reiki and distant healing, and great benefits have been known in these cases. Reiki practitioners need to exercise more caution if the recipient wears the kind of pacemaker that operates all the time, as Reiki could affect the heartbeat mechanism.

Broken bones can heal so quickly under the influence of Reiki that it is essential they are set correctly before a healing session takes place. An ill-set bone may have to be broken and re-set if the Reiki healing takes place too soon.

Not many of us like to touch flesh wounds, but nevertheless, if you are giving Reiki to someone with a gash or burn, make sure you place your hands over it to minimize the risk of infection. Recipients also appreciate this hand position if they are in pain. I have noticed that when I burn myself and channel Reiki, the sensation of being burned returns before the pain calms and then ceases, like a physical mirror-image of the original burn.

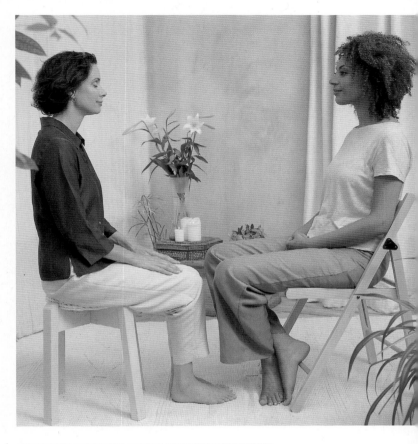

△ If a body is sensitive, or even painful to touch, or the recipient suffers from a condition such as diabetes, Reiki can be beamed or sent.

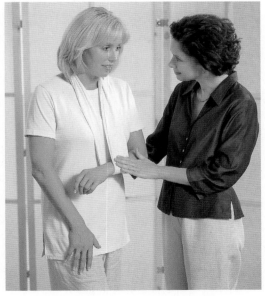

◁ Heat from Reiki can sometimes be felt through bandages, several layers of clothing, and even plaster casts.

Patterns of healing

By wanting to heal, we take the first steps towards transformation and wholeness. With the faith that we can assist our own healing, we create a revolution in our minds, changing our pattern of consciousness from one of being a victim to one of growing empowerment. We are all transformers, and living with Reiki creates change.

If you are receiving Reiki through someone else, or if you are about to be attuned or have recently been attuned, you may find that you experience a healing process. This can be a disconcerting sensation, and there are ways in which you can support your being during healing, to ease this time and speed it up.

First Degree Reiki, empowering a person to channel hands-on healing, is often regarded as a time for physical healing, when a supportive nutritional diet is especially important. Second Degree Reiki, with its use of the symbols and distant healing, is said to be a time for mental and emotional healing. With the decision to take Third/ Master Degree Reiki, you make a commitment to your own spiritual growth. Everyone is different, and you may find something easy while others may not.

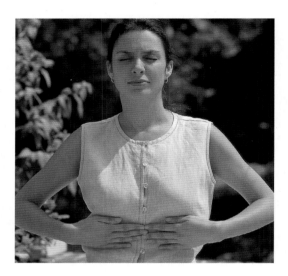

◁ Giving yourself Reiki often will help integrate the Reiki with your being.

Whatever happens, and however strange or fearful a situation might seem, love and be honest with yourself. Thank any symptoms, quietly or out loud, for showing you that something is happening at a more subtle level, and say that you are willing to learn its origin and to release the pattern of thought which is the cause.

patterns and the process

Sometimes after a Reiki healing session there is a resurgence of an old physical pain or emotional hurt. This is why Reiki practitioners generally like you to receive four healing sessions on consecutive days, no matter what the complaint. This gives the practitioner and the recipient time to deal with anything that may re-surface once the healing process has begun, and allows time to dispel the pain or hurt.

For instance, a man who had suffered with migraines for 20 years turned up for our second session complaining of pain in his kidneys. He said he had always intended to drink more water, and now his kidneys were shouting an answer to him. Since he stopped dehydrating, he has not had a full migraine and his headaches are now also rare. Sometimes Reiki can provide the fresh perspective necessary.

A few weeks before my attunement to First Degree Reiki, I hurt my back lifting. A week later I was working in a store with the doors open on a cold day. That night, what had at first felt like a chill in my teeth had spread to my entire face, and I have

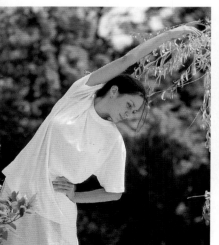

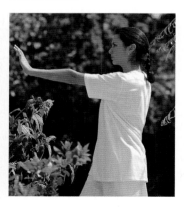

◁△ Gentle exercise helps to cleanse the system too, while increasing awareness of your whole being. If your time is limited, just try some gentle stretching movements each morning.

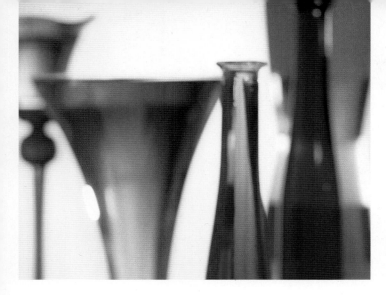

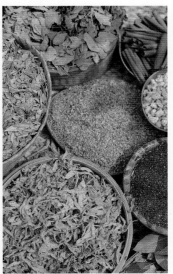
◁ Colour reflects and enhances our mood and
Reiki is often associated with colour
visualization, especially with blue and purple.

463

therapeutic reiki treatments

never felt pain like it. I could not think of a cause, except for the back injury, which was minor in comparison. A few days later, after no relief from prescribed painkillers, I was so exhausted that I began to try various complementary therapies for the first time. The benefits were amazing, even though the pain did not disappear. Reflexology helped ease my back and my body reacted strongly to the lymph system hand position, as it cleared out toxins. However, my entire jaw was still stinging, one day I was in agony when I saw a sign offering Reiki in a shop window. No better time to put Reiki to the

test before my attunement I thought. The practitioner advised me that it was quite usual to have what was known as a "healing crisis" before becoming a channel for Reiki, and the treatment took the edge off the pain. By the time my First Degree date came, the pain had disappeared. It was a milestone for me to recognize that my pain had more to do with mental patterns, and it dawned on me what it meant to take responsibility for myself. With that, my own healing began. Being able to transform pain into an empowering experience showed me what adventure in my life could be about. It also prompted me to ask myself if I really wanted this kind of trial in order to transform.

To cite another example, a woman was diagnosed with lymph gland cancer and her company paid for her to have Reiki to complement the chemotherapy she was receiving. She and her partner had to travel a long way to hospital and back, and their home was repossessed while this was going on. What surprised her was the calm with which she was reacting to everything: "Usually, I would be stressed and worrying, and at the moment, I'm just not. I don't

◁ Reduce your caffeine intake, drink plenty of water and blend your own herb teas as you open up to a new way of living.

▷ Eating organic and raw food as much as possible is refreshing and cleansing.

know for sure if it's the Reiki, but I feel very peaceful and I have also begun to have meaningful dreams," she said. This woman recovered from cancer, has returned to her job and now practises Reiki.

nourishment

Taking responsibility for your own healing is helped by choosing to take good things into your body, and there can be nothing easier than drinking more water. Reiki practitioners often ask recipients to drink more water before and after healing sessions. After an attunement people may not feel like eating processed (or even cooked) foods and they may go off caffeine, alcohol and cigarettes. At this time, we are assimilating and integrating the Reiki energy as it travels though our chakras to the whole of our bodies. Our true selves co-operate with this energy and we consciously choose water and herbal teas, salads and fruits, organic food, less sugar and salt, and so on. We may change again, but at these sensitive times our minds clearly recognize the benefits of Reiki "self-treats".

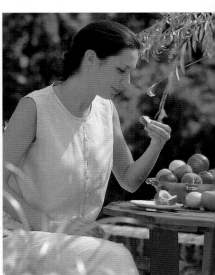

Reiki first aid for accidents

Sometimes we come across the scene of an accident, whether we are in a car or walking in the street. We glance at the ambulances and blankets on the road, hoping the people involved are not badly injured and will be all right. When you practise Reiki, there are things you can do to help in such a situation, whether medical support is there or not. You could help while waiting for the ambulance to arrive or even while you are stuck in traffic waiting to continue your journey. Any Reiki is better than none, and will ensure that people are in a better state when medical help arrives. If you are stuck watching and feeling helpless, this next story gives us all a reason to sit up and take heart.

the positivity of a prayer

A woman who had been in a car accident found herself looking down on the chaos, having left her body as many people do in such cases. She could see grey smog hanging over the cars in the ensuing traffic, but she also noticed that a few cars back, a white

> Man is made by his belief.
>
> As he believes, so he is.
>
> *Bhagavad Gita*

light was rising in the air. Curious, she went to have a closer look. On reaching the roof of the car, she discovered she could slide through it at will and found herself in the passenger seat, next to the driver who was saying a prayer for everyone involved in the accident. The light she had seen was coming from the driver's hands as she held them in the prayer position. Amazed, the woman returned to her own body, but not before she

had made a mental note of the car number plate. After her recovery, she managed to trace the owner of the car and took her a bunch of flowers, thanking her for her efforts and telling her what effect they had had.

This is another wonderful first-hand account of experiencing the power of a prayer from the heart. If you come across an accident and feel helpless, you don't have to be – you can send up healing light energy instead of the negative grey clouds created by feelings of fear and anxiety.

reiki help

If you have taken Second Degree Reiki, you will know that you are also sending a prayer when you send healing over distance or time. By offering your healing intention up to the Universe for the best possible outcome, you are doing exactly that. If you drive past an accident, you can visualize the mental/emotional healing symbol in the air in the surrounding atmosphere. If you are in your car waiting to pass, make the distant

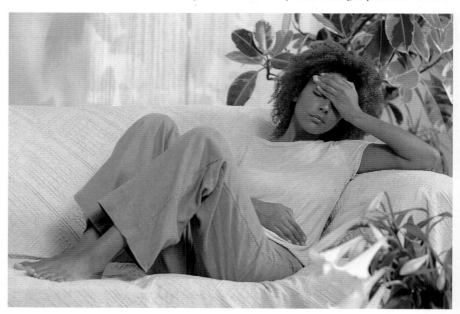

▷ A self-treatment with Reiki can help to alleviate the symptoms of a cold or stomach bug and aid its progress through your system.

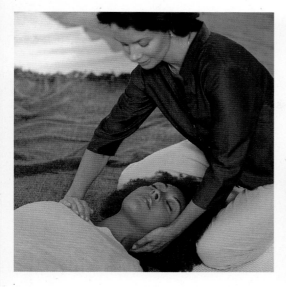

△ Placing your hands in the shoulder and neck area is beneficial for relieving whiplash injuries sustained in a traffic collision.

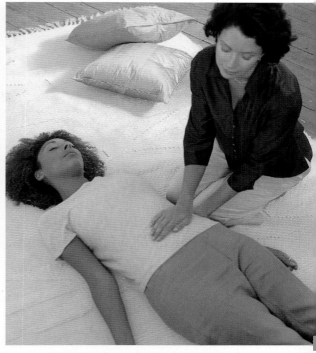

▷ Any Reiki, no matter where you place your hands, is very good for relieving the symptoms and stress of shock after an accident. This can be done at the actual scene of an accident or some time afterwards.

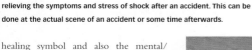

healing symbol and also the mental/emotional and power symbols. Focus on the situation in a neutral way, letting the Reiki flow where most needed.

If you are nearby and can give a Reiki touch to someone feeling pain or fear, so much the better. Your physical contact through Reiki will comfort and heal, no matter where you place your hands. If you carry Rescue Remedy, give the bottle Reiki for a few minutes before giving it to the people involved in the accident. Then place your hands on the person's shoulders if you can, allowing Reiki to facilitate their own healing and to reduce trauma and shock. This position also feels very supportive. Kneel at the person's head, cupping it gently in both your hands. This will comfort, help concussion and stabilize the brain energy. You can also place one hand over the forehead, rather than on it, to cover the emotional stress release points just above the eyebrows.

▷ Keeping the recipient warm in a blanket and the comfort of Reiki will help after a shock or trauma of any kind.

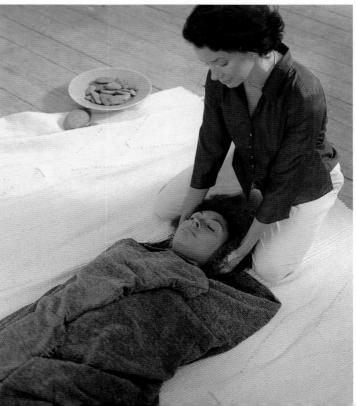

Reiki for common ailments

One of the simplest and most instantly effective ways of using Reiki is for the treatment of common, everyday ailments. Anyone attuned to Reiki will tell you how surprised they have been at the rapid relief a short self-treatment can bring from a common cold, headache or indigestion. On the one or two occasions I have had a cold since being attuned to Reiki, friends have taken the opportunity of experimenting and have sent me some Reiki from a distance. What has happened is nothing short of amazing – one minute I have been feeling lightheaded and sneezing, the next I have been trying to remember when exactly my symptoms disappeared without trace. Reiki energy is so quick, yet so subtle, that some ailments fade away almost imperceptibly, just as emotional hurts can whenever you send Reiki to a situation.

knowing ourselves through illness

Reiki treatments for common complaints can help us consider with calm insight the causes of our ailments. Reiki's greatest gift to us is empowerment to take responsibility for ourselves and our own healing, and that often means being able to recognize issues in our lives which, if not resolved, can make us ill. Many of us find that physical illness is the visible result of "dis-ease" created by negative belief systems that are causing conflict in our lives. Sometimes the mental and emotional origins of an illness can be hard to see, and even harder to accept, especially if we feel judged and vulnerable. But recognition of the causes of illness is a blessing, and certainly no reason to be judgemental towards ourselves or others, which can bring no positive results. The way

in which many of us grow up competing with and comparing ourselves to others, nurturing fear rather than love, makes criticism a "normal" reaction, and a habit we must wish to leave behind as a beginning to healing ourselves. Criticism has never been found to help the healing process, but it can make us ill if our bodies hear enough of it.

some recommended reiki hand positions

All these hand positions can be held for as long as necessary or comfortable. You can also suggest to the recipient that distant healing sent to the source of the complaint will be very beneficial, and you can add this to a hands-on treatment if he or she agrees. In your mind, create the distant symbols (emotional, and power too if you wish) over their head or on the backs of your hands.

Menstrual pains   You can crouch down or your recipient may be willing to stretch out on a sofa, in which case you can slide one hand underneath her, which is very supportive. Place one hand on the lower stomach and the other on the lower back for relief from pain and stomach cramp. This will lighten and relieve the surrounding area, including the thighs.

Women who suffer from menstrual pains can use this Reiki time to celebrate the unity of females in the world and the expression of female energy, rather than something which "cramps your style" as a woman.

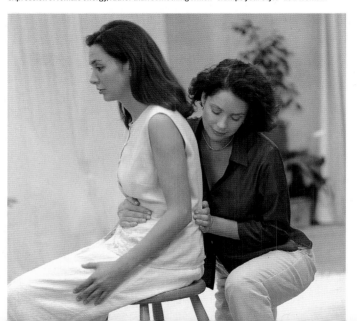

◁ Hands on the back and front of the abdominal area are a great way to relieve menstrual pains.

Backache

Ask your recipient to sit on a backless chair or to lie on his or her stomach, then place your hands together in the shape of T-cross between the shoulder blades and down the spine, to release tension and worry. Place your hands at the top and bottom of the spine to balance energy along the backbone.

Backache is often caused by worrying and feeling burdened. Lower back pain can indicate insecurity in material matters, such as worry about money. Trust in the Universe, which gives you everything, and know that your security will grow if you do.

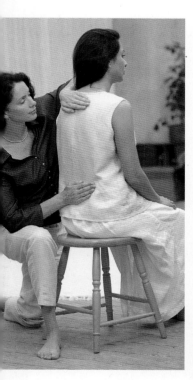

△ Back pains can be soothed away with the spirit level position.

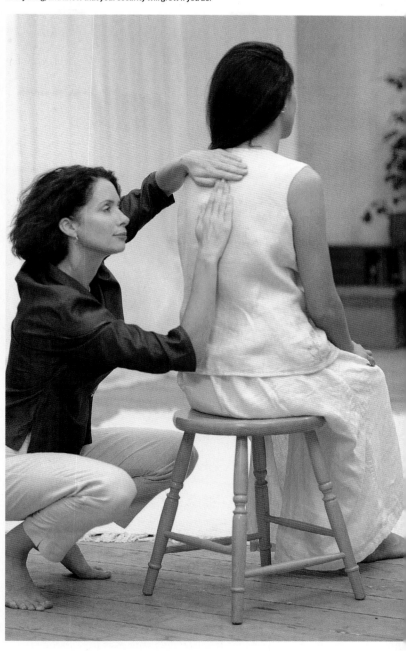

▷ A T-cross made with the hands will treat back and shoulder areas, and stimulate the heart chakra and surrounding organs.

Headaches

Stand behind the recipient and place your hands lightly on or over her eyes, your fingers meeting at the nose or overlapping. Placing both hands on the sides of the head at the back feels very supportive and dispels tension rising from the neck, balancing energy in the brain. Treating a headache by placing one hand on the forehead and one on the medulla, from the back and the front, is also effective.

Headaches have many possible sources, including eye strain, sexual tension, an exaggerated need for perfection, and issues relating to how we face the world and feel about ourselves.

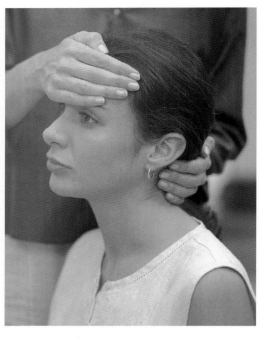

◁ Melt away tensions in the neck which can result in headaches with this supportive position.

▷▽ These two hand positions are very effective when relief is needed from migraine, eye strain or from stressful situations.

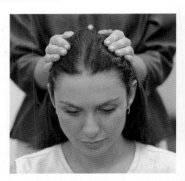

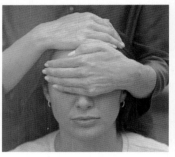

Toothache, neuralgia and earache

Standing behind the recipient, gently put both hands across the cheeks, your fingers meeting at the nose or overlapping. Sometimes hands over the head, ears and face can also be very helpful, easing tension caused by frowning and unnatural jaw pressure. Teeth problems and neuralgia may originate from trifling worries or may be the result of anger stored in the jaw, often originating from guilt surrounding communication issues. Placing your hands over the throat can therefore also be helpful.

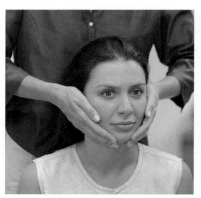

△ Cup your hands around the jaw area for toothache, and also for symptoms created by headcolds.

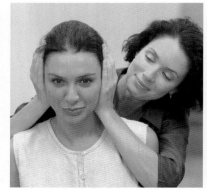

△ Hands over the ears are warming, lightening a painful earache.

Colds

Stand behind the recipient, and place one hand on the forehead and one hand on the centre of the chest. This will help to clear both and to bring relief from an aching neck and shoulders, stuffiness and coughing. It also covers the heart chakra, aiding self-nourishment. Both hands over the face will help to clear sinuses and ease irritation.

Someone who has received Reiki for a cold may find they want to explore the emotional origins of their exhaustion, or if the cold could be due to a cleansing process at this time.

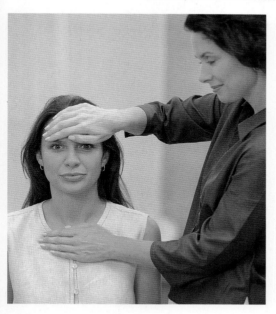

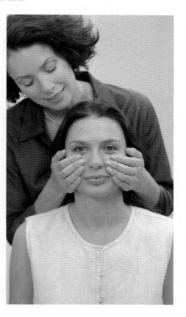

◁ ▷Heads and chests are often very uncomfortable when we have colds. Free blocked up, painful sinuses and relieve the effects of catarrh with these two hand positions.

Indigestion

Crouch beside the recipient and place one hand on the sternum and one on the solar plexus at the centre or bottom of the ribcage, to aid stomach acid and general digestion. Place one hand lower down in the region of the second chakra for a upset stomach, constipation or diarrhoea.

Most indigestion is obviously felt after meals, especially with certain dry foods. It is worth thinking about any emotions we are finding it hard to digest and process. If you are constipated, ask the Universe to help you release everything you no longer need. If you have diarrhoea, ask what you are fearing in life, or finding hard to carry?

◁ These hand positions aid the digestion of food and can also help to free any blockages that are caused by the tension of emotional problems – often a cause of bad digestion.

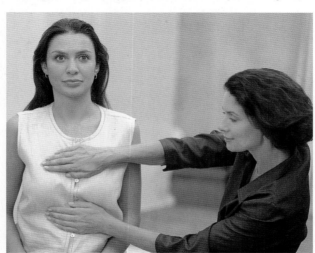

Reiki in pregnancy

Throughout pregnancy and during the birth, Reiki blesses mothers and their babies with universal love and healing. What could be better than to put your hands on yourself and know you are healing and giving love to yourself and your unborn baby? For a father-to-be, Reiki provides a unique opportunity to bond with the baby in its mother's womb, building a strong and spiritual relationship before this tiny new being enters the world and sees either parent for the first time.

Reiki can help an expectant mother in many ways with the miracle of carrying another human inside her and passing on life. Using Reiki in the early days of the pregnancy helps reduce exhaustion and nausea. It brings relief to every part of a stretched and aching body at various points up until and including the birth itself. Reiki will help to calm fear of the unknown and will soothe a woman who feels invaded and impatient to give birth. When she is feeling eager to reclaim her own body, Reiki is a gift she can give herself. Reiki can make a baby wriggle with pleasure in the womb, and can also have a calming effect.

reiki during birth

You can send Reiki to your baby and the birth itself throughout your pregnancy, if you or your partner practise. If you don't, get in touch with a Reiki practitioner who will be thrilled to do so. When the time to give birth arrives, Reiki can help to ease the pain and will create a peaceful atmosphere for the baby to be born into. If you have been attuned, you can give your baby Reiki whenever you hold and nurse it. Give yourself plenty of Reiki at the same time if you like, which will help your body to maintain its natural chemical and physiological balance.

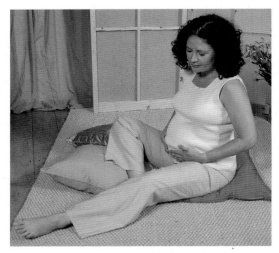

◁ What better way to communicate with your baby than to give both of you Reiki. This position is also good to use when you are lying in a warm relaxing bath.

▷ Reiki provides a wonderful way for the expectant father to bond with baby, and for all three of you to share the experience.

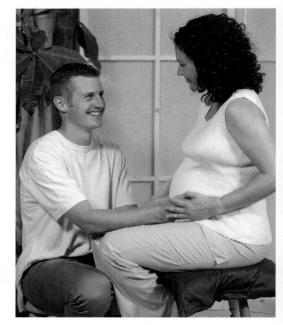

To be. No more. This is all.

This is the joy supreme.

Jorge Guillén

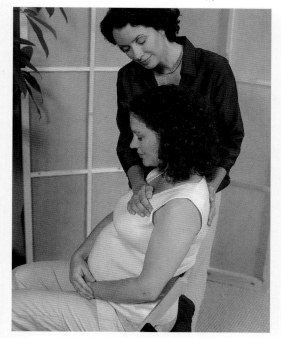

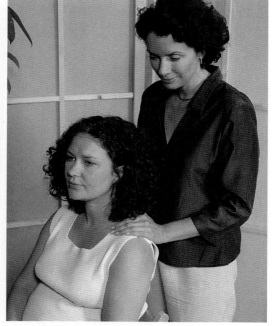

△ Reiki treatments during pregnancy help to refresh the body and the mind at a time when there is a lot happening.

△ Soothing hands on the shoulders and back can provide great relief from the baby's weight during the final weeks of the pregnancy.

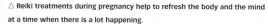

some suggested hand positions in pregnancy

- Place one hand on the centre of the sternum and one hand on the back, to treat the back and give healing to the love, or heart, chakra.
- The "spirit level" position is useful in pregnancy for general balance and well-being. Place one hand at the top of the spine/base of neck, and one at the coccyx at the base of the spine.
- Stand behind the recipient and place your hands on her shoulders for a few moments, to help relieve the tension created by carrying the extra weight.
- Treat the feet often, as they take a lot of the strain of a pregnancy..
- In late pregnancy, when the stomach begins to feel heavy, put both hands on either side of the base of the stomach. The mother or her partner may prefer to do this, and as long as the recipient is comfortable it will refresh and support this area.

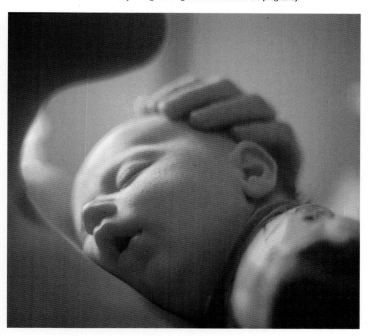

△ Holding your newborn baby in Reiki hands is a gentle and loving way to be together, and the skin-to-skin contact will make the baby feel safe and secure.

Reiki for children and babies

People love Reiki at any age, and for youngsters it is fun to experience the sensations of this healing energy while feeling better at the same time. Having given Reiki to a nine-year-old with a headache at a party, I found I was a source of entertainment, to be summoned whenever a grazed knee or stomach-ache presented itself, and I began to suspect that fake ailments were being concocted. Parents soon know that Reiki is safe for their children when they see, or in many cases hear about, the positive effects it has.

Reiki sessions with babies and children take much less time than those for adults. Generally, the younger the child, the quicker the Reiki is absorbed into the system and the swifter the results. As a guideline, allow ten minutes or less with babies, and about 20–30 minutes with children, but don't worry, you can never do harm with Reiki or overdo it. Children move away or become distracted when they have had enough.

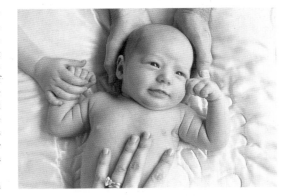

◁ **Reiki is gentle enough for all living things, no matter how new to the world they are.**

a treat for parents

Being empowered to help heal your own children, by touch or over distance, must be one of the best feelings in the world. Most youngsters are keen and curious to feel the Reiki once they trust you, but I always ask parents if they would like to be able to do it for their children themselves. They can then also give a child the comfort only a parent can bring, especially when he or she is unwell or feeling miserable. Reiki given to children by their parents creates a subtle bond between them and enriches their understanding of one another. Reiki encourages children and grown-ups to grow, nurtured by the feeling of infinite love, experienced in a tangible, tactile way. A child who knows this love will surely be able to play a part in creating a loving world.

children can do reiki too

Sometimes a child will ask, "Do I have to come to you if I want Reiki?" Maybe you will see them one day with their palms flat against themselves, concentrating on whether they can feel the Reiki energy flowing as when you do it. Sometimes, when you are giving Reiki to a parent, a child will want to take part. Children often get

sympathetic symptoms if their parents are in distress and they want to be able to help. For legal reasons, always ask the parent before attuning a youngster, and also so that you know the child will get the support needed in any healing process.

The youngest Reiki practitioner I know is Jo, aged 11, who wanted to do Reiki himself after being amazed at his own speedy recovery from hay fever. Two years after his attunement to First Degree, he still loves to use Reiki on himself and his family.

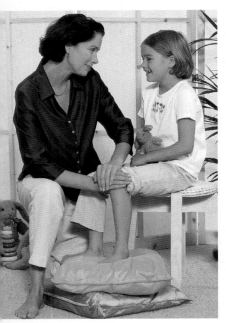

◁ **Children have great fun feeling the sensations that come from magic Reiki hands.**

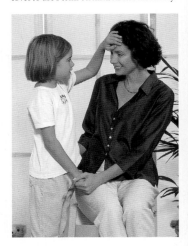

△ **Children often need no encouragement to try Reiki out on adults and on themselves.**

some suggested hand positions for treating children

- For a stomach-ache or emotional upset, gently place your hands level on the child's stomach and her back while she is standing, or sitting next to you on a sofa.

- For coughs, wheezy colds and hay fever, place your hands level on the child's chest and back. This position is easy to practise when you are both seated on a sofa.

- For a headache, give the child water to drink, and place your hands gently over her head.

Remember, children will let you know when Reiki has done the trick. Don't be alarmed if they look flushed after a few minutes – they can get very hot quickly when you are giving them Reiki, on the head or neck in particular.

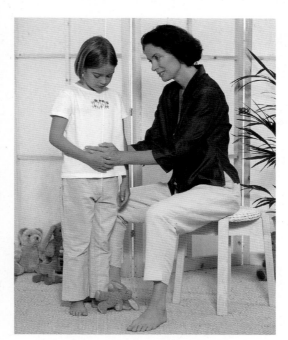

◁ Children take much less time to benefit from Reiki because they are smaller, with faster metabolisms. Try these hand positions to ease a stomach-ache.

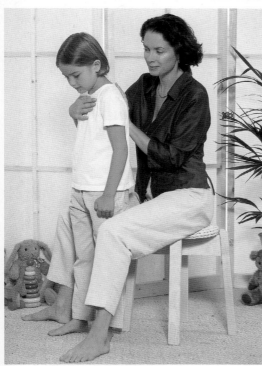

△ Any tightness caused by a chest infection or a painful, irritating cough can be eased with this position.

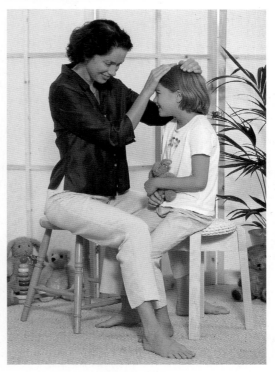

△ A gentle Reiki touch will ease a child's headache and coax a smile.

Reiki for the dying

We and every living thing on our planet are connected in a cycle of life, a cosmic web extending through and beyond our own Universe. In birth and death, transformation occurs, forming, changing, continuing.

healing and curing

Sometimes, especially in the Western world, we confuse curing with healing, but they are not the same thing. Though we may have struggled to find the cure for a physical disease, anyone who has been present at a peaceful departure from this world will have witnessed the pervading presence of wholeness, and will know the value of holistic healing at the point of transition. Even as we learn more about the human potential to attain greater longevity in the future, sooner or later we all go with the flow from the river to the ocean. Perhaps subconsciously, we choose to confuse curing and healing to mask our fear of dying, seeing ourselves as losing our loved ones and being lost in a void – isolated, rather than returning to love and life in another state of being. True healing creates a safe space in which an awareness of unity with the infinite is rekindled. This spiritual reunion, at-one-ness with our life-giving Universe, allows a peaceful transition from this world to the next, which is healing in a true sense. Healing allows people to leave this life at peace with

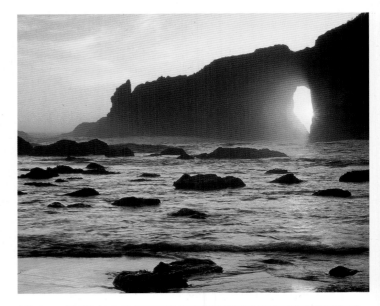

△ The love and light that emanate from a Reiki session remind us that curing a physical illness is not the same as healing the person mentally and spiritually.

themselves, open to transformation without fear or struggle, so that even when an illness is not cured, the person can be healed emotionally and spiritually.

Ancient spiritual teachings and new physics expand our faith and our concepts of finite life but, whatever our beliefs, at the point of death it is possible for us to be without fear. We are bombarded by images of violent, painful death on television and in newspapers. This is negative and disempowering when we feel we cannot do anything about it, and it perpetuates fearfulness. Reiki can help the dying and their loved ones to create a passing-over which is joyful, a surrender to something greater than ourselves, a transformation made without fear and with love.

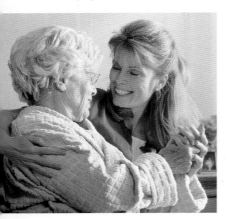

◁ The healing feeling is one of the best things we can give to someone when they are close to leaving the physical world.

If someone has been suffering and is afraid, hands-on Reiki from one or more people can be a great comfort in itself. The loving touch engenders love in the recipient; it facilitates peace and the knowledge that we are all part of the divine plan. For the family and friends of the person about to leave this life, it can be a wonderful experience to participate in this healing, which celebrates life, aids inner peace and therefore swifter recovery from the sense of individual loss. Giving and receiving healing helps us to celebrate the transition of a soul from one place to another, and to sense one more natural, joyous progression in the Universe. Relatives and friends of terminally ill people who have received Reiki healing often notice great beneficial changes in their state of mind.

During this quiet and reflective time, we see how someone can be happier than ever during the last phases of earthly life. Issues

some suggested hand positions

If the person is in pain, you may prefer to hold your hands over them instead of on the body itself. You can also channel Reiki in shifts, and in other ways such as beaming and distant healing. Use the methods that are most appropriate for you both – Reiki is a gift from our Creator to all of us and you can never pass it on badly. Wherever the recipient wants to feel the healing power of Reiki will be the right place. Remember how we explored the power of prayer, and how all spiritual disciplines regard prayer as nourishment for the soul, just as food nourishes and sustains the physical body. Even when a person has left their earthly body, you can continue to love and bless them in this way.

• Place both hands on or near the third (solar plexus) chakra, or under the back and on the front of the third chakra. This is the place where we store all our emotions. After, or instead of, placing one hand underneath the recipient, you may like to place one hand on the heart chakra. This will help heal fear and transform it into love.

• Standing at the person's head, visualize drawing the mental/emotional healing symbol on your palms and in the air above the recipient's head. Then place both your hands under the back of the head, gently rolling it on to one hand and then the other, so that you are both balanced and comfortable. This position is very comforting at any time and facilitates mental healing and peace of mind. If you have not learned how to use the symbols, say a prayer instead.

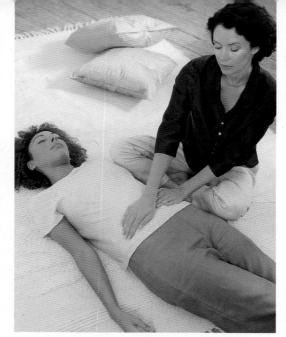

◁ These positions are also comforting to anyone feeling isolated from their source at any time of their life.

▽ Reiki can relieve pain and anxiety of all kinds. Use these caring positions for people in particularly stressful times.

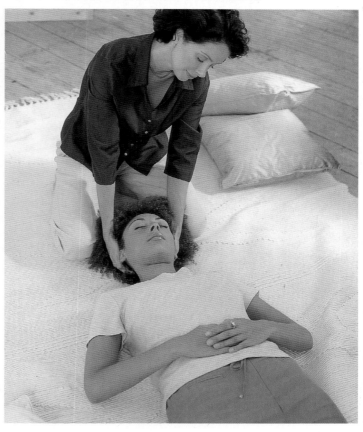

that may have been difficult for the person to live with for years, preventing them from loving themselves and others, may be resolved at last. When we make this emotional transition, our physical bodies can follow with ease. Reiki creates positive change in us at any time, and often gratitude, forgiveness, love and peace are found at this most special and sacred stage of life.

therapeutic reiki treatments

Reiki for animals

Animals and plants enjoy receiving Reiki just as much as we do. A great many people feel the healing power of animals, which express love unconditionally and often comfort us when we are fearful. Those who have hugged trees and given them healing also experience a strong reciprocal healing response. It is a wonderful experience to share Reiki with the plant and animal kingdom, strengthening and reminding us of our connection to all life.

treating animals

All animals can be treated with Reiki as a tonic or to ease suffering. I have tried it with beetles and dogs, and it works. With a pet, you can place your hands on or over an injury or wound, and you will generally know when it has had enough. It will move

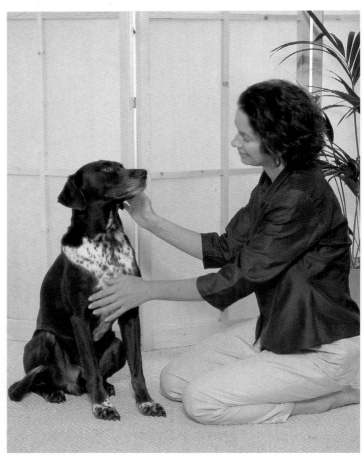

△ You can give pets a daily Reiki treatment, helping to maintain their general health and happiness. Spend a few moments calming and settling your pet before you begin.

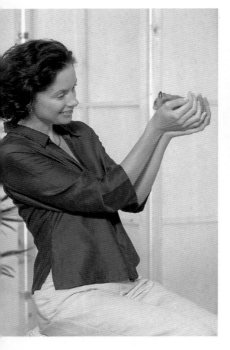

△ No matter how great or small, all creatures yield to healing hands.

away, become distracted, or begin to preen or wash itself. With an energetic pet, it may be more successful to send healing, perhaps programmed for every alternate hour during the night while it sleeps. The results can be seen the following day, and this technique would be suitable for a hamster or other nocturnal animal. Small animals, such as weak or injured birds found in the garden, will benefit from being held in Reiki hands

for ten minutes, which will probably be enough. Reiki is also very beneficial to animals who are emotionally upset.

The Reiki will swiftly and safely reach wherever it is required, so it is always healing. You can also complement your hands-on healing with distant healing, sent to the local stable or veterinary surgery for example, but don't send Reiki while the animal is under general anaesthetic.

some suggested hand positions for treating animals

The following positions are for pet-sized creatures, so adapt as necessary.

• Hold your hands either side of the ribcage, with the animal seated on your lap or on the floor. This will treat the whole body and the Reiki will reach central parts immediately.

• Put one hand on the head of your pet as though you are going to stroke its ears, and one very lightly on the middle of its back.

• Hold the animal in your hands, with one hand at the top of the spine and one by its tail at the base of the spine.

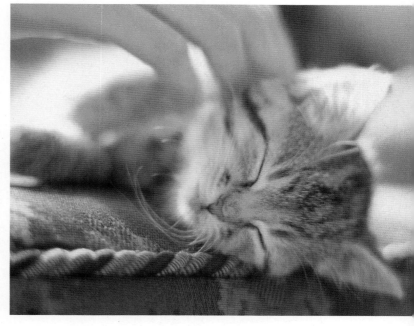

△ Cats are particularly sensitive to touch and will show their pleasure when you are giving them affection. When you use Reiki hands, they will enjoy it even more.

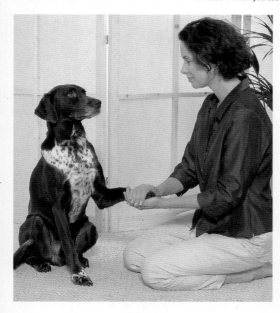

△ Specific injuries or wounds can be helped quickly and easily by placing your hands directly on the injured limb.

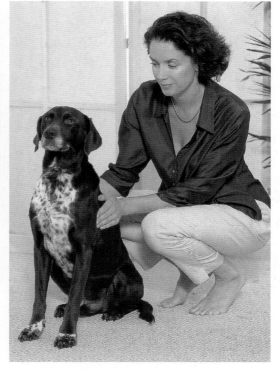

▷ If it is difficult to know exactly where the problem is, just place your hands where it is comfortable for you and your pet, and let Reiki do the rest.

Relaxation through Meditation

During an experience of meditation we are calm, aware, focused, happy and loving. We let go of the burden of ourselves and enter into a wider state of consciousness. Having achieved this wonderful state, we can then learn to transfer these same attitudes to all our interactions. It is possible, through the regular practice of meditation, to live each moment untroubled by negativity and the stress that inevitably builds up.

Finding your inner self

Human beings have many levels: our physical bodies, energy flow, instinctive responses, thinking processes and wisdom each play a vital part in our overall functioning, and all need to be in balance to ensure health and wellbeing. All too often, however, a hectic modern lifestyle can unbalance these levels, making us feel jaded in body, mind and spirit. The regular practice of meditation helps us to rebalance ourselves so that all the levels are able to work together in harmony.

Meditation has three aspects: the regular practice of techniques that enable us to reach the meditative state, the experience of the state of meditation, and recreating this state in daily life. There are traditional meditation techniques appropriate to all temperaments and levels of attainment. They all involve symbolically "going up into the solitude of the mountains" so that we can then "return to the bustle of the marketplace" and live a changed life as a result of our experience.

We practise meditation because we believe (with Robert Browning) that:

There is an inmost centre in us all,
Where Truth abides in fullness…and to know
Rather consists in opening out a way
Whence the imprisoned splendour may escape.

Meditation allows us to experience that splendour for ourselves and live our lives in the glow of our own inner radiance.

"Only the present moment exists."
Traditional wisdom

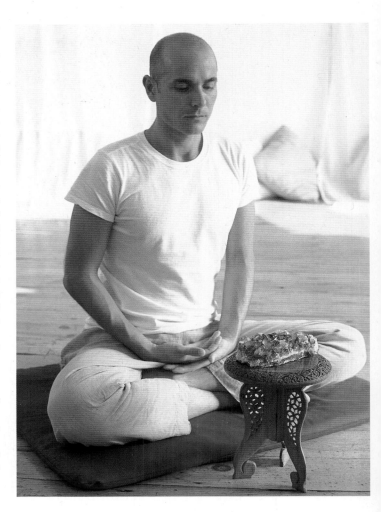

△ Meditation is practised with the spine erect and the body motionless. The mind is still but alert, vibrant and focused inward.

removing inner obstructions

The path to and from our "inmost centre" may be obstructed by lack of awareness, self-obsession, the stress of an unbalanced lifestyle, or by negative attitudes and thought patterns.

Most of us try to crowd too much activity into our lives, and lack the stillness and silence that are necessary to rebalance the nervous system. Regular meditation practice establishes a healthy rhythm of activity and rest for both mind and body. Our minds are constantly active, mulling over current problems, planning anxiously for a future we cannot control, regretting past actions or creating personal doctrines

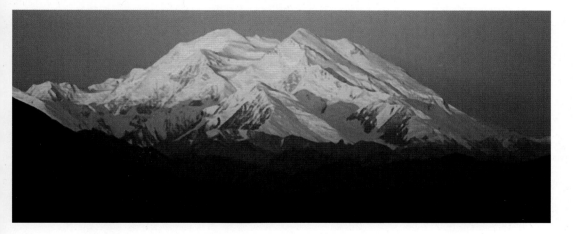

△ Symbolically compared with the solitude of the mountains, meditation involves a withdrawal from the bustle of human activity.

▷ These traditional clay figures in a circle of friendship represent the unity nurtured by the meditative way of life.

and dogmas, opinions and prejudices. These mental "games" draw us, like magnets, away from the present moment. Meditation teaches us to live in the moment, and grow through the experiences of here and now. When we are inclined to wallow in negative emotions such as anger or resentment, and to see insults and dangers where none exist, meditation helps us to replace defensive energy-sapping reactions with open and trusting responses that enable us to build loving relationships.

reducing stress

If you practise the meditation techniques outlined in this book regularly and with enthusiasm, you will soon start to feel the benefits, as both the causes and the effects of stress diminish.

Stress is a normal part of life, and a certain amount is essential to motivate and develop humans, but the pace and complexity of life in modern Western society can overburden our systems and block our natural ability to manage stress. Human beings are (as far as we know) the only animals with brains that are constantly

thinking – but the result may be that we allow ourselves to remain stuck in negative thought patterns, squandering our precious energy and unbalancing the nervous system.

Like that of any other animal, the human nervous system operates instinctively and is programmed to deal physically with threats to survival. Stress is a natural reaction that enables us to respond to danger, either by fighting or running away. Once the threatening episode is over the nervous system should rebalance itself as we return peacefully to our normal activities. Unlike other animals, however, humans are apt to remain in a state of arousal, because we go on feeling anxious about past and future events, as well as preferring to be continually active and stimulated in the present.

Because stress hormones make us feel excited, it is easy to become addicted to activities and challenges that trigger their release. This is why we want to watch exciting programmes on television and take part in testing activities. But if we remain in a constant state of arousal, we deny our bodily systems the chance to rest and renew themselves. Stress accumulates until the system reaches breaking point – and the result is illness and malfunctioning of the body or mind. By practising the techniques of meditation, we can reverse this build-up of stress by learning to stop and consciously clear the mind and emotions of negative attitudes the moment we become aware of them.

stress and your health

Meditation practice can help to reduce the unpleasant effects of prolonged stress, protecting you from symptoms such as:

- muscle tension and pain in the joints
- tension and migraine headaches
- the inability to concentrate or think clearly
- digestive problems, which may include diabetes
- interrupted sleep patterns
- breathing difficulties
- cardiovascular problems
- allergic reactions
- physical fatigue
- nervous exhaustion
- weakness of the immune system
- other auto-immune problems

▽ Regular meditation gives you the energy and clarity you need to deal with the multiple demands of daily life.

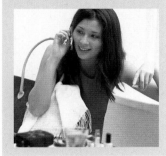

Basic body and breath awareness

The traditional position for meditation practice is to sit with the knees out to each side. This creates a pyramid with a firm triangular base so that it is difficult to topple over and easy to keep the spine erect, even when you are totally engrossed in inner experiences. However, in Western society we seldom sit in this position.

Although the hips, like the shoulders, are ball-and-socket joints, designed to turn freely in all directions, we normally move through a very narrow range of standing and sitting positions. Imagine how restricted you would feel if you could move your elbows only up or down in front of you but

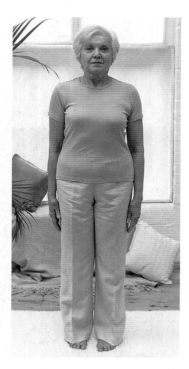

△ In Tadasana, the mountain pose, the body extends upward from a firm base, with the sides, front and back of the body aligned, creating a sense of equilibrium and repose.

not to the sides – yet this is what we do with our knees as we sit at a desk and in a car or armchair, while walking or running, and even when we are lying down. In ancient India it would have been as natural and comfortable to sit cross-legged on the floor as sitting in an armchair is for us, and with gentle practice and suitable props you can enjoy the benefits of this pose and also regain a more natural range of movement in your hip joints.

breath with posture and movement

In exercise, moving with the breath brings a new mental awareness and a feeling of both relaxation and energy flow, so it is important to develop the habit of leading every movement with a conscious slow breath either in or out, as directed.

Do the exercises suggested for just a few moments, as frequently as possible during the day. Relax and enjoy them, and never force your body into any position. You will be amazed how quickly you begin to shed the tightness that has been restricting your body for years. A relaxed body and mind creates a wonderful sense of wellbeing and makes meditation practice very rewarding.

Start by standing in the classical Tadasana pose – feet parallel and a little apart, ankles lifted, knees straight and springy (not locked), tailbone (coccyx) tucked under, waist pulled in and back, breastbone (sternum) lifted, chin parallel to the floor. The gaze is soft and straight ahead. Imagine a straight line down each side of your body. It should pass through your ankles, knees, hips, waist, shoulders and ears. Having located all these points, breathe in to stretch up, and out to bring them into line. You should feel as though you are hanging from the ceiling by a strong cord, with your limbs loose like a puppet. The same exercise – stretching up on the breath in and aligning on the breath out – can be practised while seated on a chair or on the floor.

using yoga poses

The classical yoga poses (asanas), are designed to promote strength, flexibility, balance, breath awareness, relaxation and focus. This makes them ideal exercises for all the koshas, and an excellent preparation for meditation. However, provided it is performed with the same awareness, any gentle stretching can also exercise all the koshas.

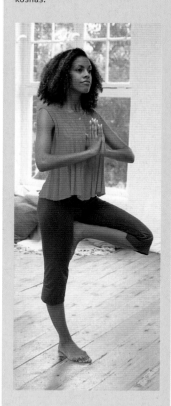

△ Vrksasana, the "tree" pose, is one of the classic yoga postures used in preparation for meditation practice.

swing a leg

This exercise, repeated frequently at odd moments during the day, releases muscular tension, improves balance and develops body awareness. At the end of the sequence, quietly observe everything you can feel in your body.

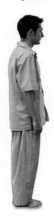 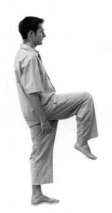 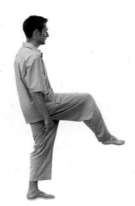 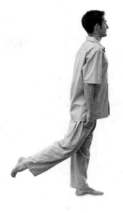

△ **1** Standing in Tadasana, become comfortable with your breath, awareness and posture, so that you can maintain them throughout the exercise. If your balance is shaky, stand where you can hold on to a table, the back of a chair, or a wall if you need to.

△ **2** Raise one leg, bending the knee, until the thigh is parallel to the floor. Balance on the other leg, using your breath to stretch up and align your body, and to hold the position. When you are balanced, shake your raised ankle gently and rhythmically.

△ **3** After a moment, change the movement so that you are swinging the lower part of the raised leg, from the knee, with the ankle relaxed. Continue to focus on the breath, and maintain the Tadasana pose.

△ **4** Now swing the whole of the raised leg from the hip, forward and back, keeping it relaxed and maintain the Tadasana pose. Take a deep breath in, then breathe out, as you lower your leg and stand on it. Breathe in to raise the other thigh parallel to the floor and repeat the sequence.

deep standing squat

This exercise brings awareness and strength to the legs and back. Loosen the muscles around the hip, knee and ankle joints by practising a few squats frequently.

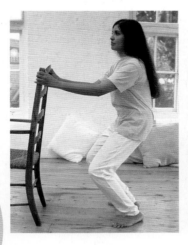 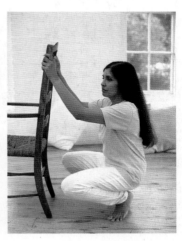

> "The physical postures should be steady and comfortable. They are mastered when all effort is relaxed and the mind is absorbed in the Infinite."
> *From A. Shearer's translation of Patanjali's Sutras, Ch2*

△ **1** Stand at arms' length in front of a stable object, such as a chair or table, and grasp it firmly for support as you squat. Your feet should be comfortably apart and turned out at 45 degrees, so that your ankles, knees and hips are in alignment when you sink down into the squat. Keep your spine erect and your gaze forward.

△ **2** Breathe in and stretch up through your spine and neck, then breathe out to squat down as low as you are able. Keep your heels on the floor if you can, or raise them until your lower back becomes more flexible. Breathe in to rise and out again to repeat the squat.

Opening up the chakras

Gentle stretches and movements, working with the breath, help to release muscular tension in the physical body and also to free obstructions at the energy level. Breathing up through the body from the floor, and down from above the head, increases the energy in the spine, which flows through the chakras.

increasing vitality

The knees, hips and pelvis are all part of the "life" area of the body, where the centres that process vitality are located. The legs and the base of the spine are under the influence of the base chakra, and the hips and pelvis are under the influence of the sacral chakra. Seated stretches and bends energize these two chakras. If you add a twist to your movement you will be activating the navel chakra as well.

opening the chest

Exercises that open up the chest will foster improved breathing and better posture, and these can be done in a standing, kneeling or sitting position.

To start, the breath in is focused upon stretching up. If you are standing or kneeling, this stretch begins through the legs, then continues through the lower, middle and upper spine, and the neck. The upward stretch opens your chest to create space for deeper breathing and improves your posture by lengthening your spine to allow increased energy flow through the chakras, including the heart chakra in the chest and the throat chakra above. The breath out – done with the same relaxed attention – can be focused into movements involving the limbs, while still maintaining the strength and openness of the spine and neck.

By linking your breath with movement in these exercises, you are working from within, rather than making the correct "shapes" as seen from outside. In this way you can release physical tension and mental and emotional stress with every combined breath and movement. It is best to start with simple movements in order to focus on this co-ordination of mind and body with the rhythm of the breath.

Every nerve impulse that passes between the brain and the body has to travel through the neck, so it is very helpful to release any tension that has built up in this area. Continue the upward stretch of the spine through the neck and into the skull, and maintain the stretch during the movements to open the chest. At the same time, be aware of any tension in the throat and face and keep them relaxed.

wide-angled seated movements

The more you sit on the floor with your legs comfortably wide apart and practise these movements, the more quickly your hips, lower back and spine will release the muscular tension that is so restrictive and can also cause pain and malfunction.

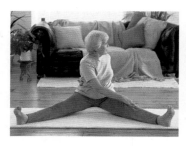

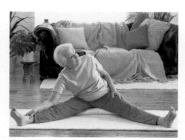

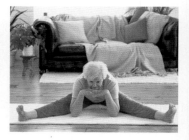

△ **1** Twist for navel chakra: sit on a cushion with your back straight and legs apart, toes pointing to the ceiling and the backs of your knees relaxed on the floor (though tight hamstring muscles may keep the legs bent to begin with). Breathe in and stretch the spine up. With your right hand on your left thigh, breathe out, twisting your trunk to the left and your left shoulder round behind you. Breathe in to return to the centre and stretch up. Breathe out to change sides. Repeat several times.

△ **2** Side bend for sacral chakra: breathe in and stretch up. Place one hand on each thigh. As you breathe out, slide your right hand down your right leg and look up to the left, bringing your left shoulder back to open the left side of the chest area. Breathe in to straighten up and repeat on the other side. Repeat several times.

△ **3** Forward bend for base and sacral chakras: place your fingertips on the floor in front of you and gently "walk" them forward, keeping your spine stretched. Avoid rounding your back and jutting your chin forward to reach further than is comfortable, as this causes tense muscles, whereas relaxation loosens them. Breathe in to stretch right through your spine. As you breathe out, sink forward a little more. As you relax deeply, you may want to rest your head in your hands with your elbows on the floor and smile. Come up again gently and slowly.

opening the book

This can be done standing, seated or kneeling. It is important to keep the chest open and the breastbone (sternum) lifted. The upper spine and neck are stretched up, strong and unmoving, and the elbows are at shoulder level as you move the arms.

▷ **1** Stand "tall", stretching through the spine, with palms joined in front of your body and elbows at shoulder height. Breathe out for this "closing" position, stretching your ribcage at the back.

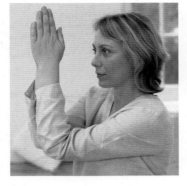

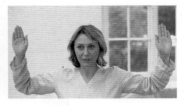

△ **2** Breathe in to "open the book", bringing your elbows (still at shoulder height) to the sides, palms facing forward. The spine and neck should not move at all as you press the elbows right back. Repeat the movement several times.

elbow rotations

As with all arm movements, the spine and neck are not involved and need to be held firmly in position throughout.

▷ **1** Place your fingertips on your shoulders and, keeping your breastbone lifted, bring your elbows in front of your body, as high as possible. Breathe out for this "closing" position, stretching your ribcage at the back.

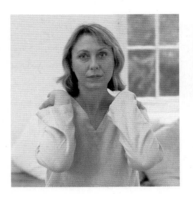

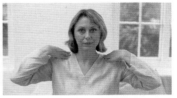

△ **2** Breathing in, rotate your elbows up, round and back, squeezing your shoulderblades together and stretching your ribs at the sides. Your spine and neck should remain stretched up and unmoving. Repeat several times, then circle your elbows the other way.

chest expansion

It is important to keep the spine and neck stretched up and unmoving as the arms are raised and lowered. This is an isometric exercise (developing muscle strength without moving) for the spine and neck and an isotonic exercise (stretching and moving) for the arms and the pectoral muscles in the chest.

"Open the window in the centre of your chest and let spirit move in and out."
Rumi, 13th century

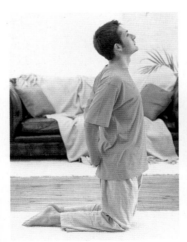

△ **1** Clasp your hands behind your back, keeping the palms firmly pressed together all the time. As you breathe in, push your clasped hands down toward the floor, squeezing your shoulderblades together.

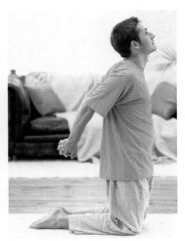

△ **2** As you breathe out, raise your straight arms up behind you, keeping the palms firmly pressed together. Repeat several times. Even if only a little movement is possible at first, this is a powerful exercise, and you will find that your range of movement will increase with practice.

Learning to let go

The combination of relaxed stretching and deep, slow breathing is a quick and effective way to settle the "bodymind" in preparation for meditation. You can practise the following stretches and breathing techniques at any time of the day – preferably several times during each day. The resulting reduction in your stress levels will be gradual but cumulative. The practice leads to a calmer mind, clearer thinking, a more comfortable, relaxed body and a more open-hearted acceptance of the way things are – including the inadequacies of other people and of yourself.

active preparation

Of the eight limbs in Patanjali's system of raja yoga, the yoga of meditation, five are "outer" (*bahir*) or active limbs. All five physical aspects are to be practised together, and all are necessary to remove tensions from the body, emotions and mind, in order to experience the meditative state.

If we are angry with someone, or discontented with ourselves, or unable to sit still, or struggling with unhealthy breathing patterns and high stress levels, or if our minds are distracted by outer sensory stimuli and constant inner chatter, it is impossible to give our full attention to meditation practice. Patanjali's first two limbs reinforce an attitude of respect and care for others through social restraint (yama) and for ourselves through purification (niyama). These are followed by a firm, comfortable seated position (asana) for meditation practice, breathing exercises (pranayama) to balance and increase energy, and finally relaxation and "switching off" (pratyahara). Only then are we ready to practise the three "inner" (*antar*) limbs that make up samyama (these are concentration, meditation and absorption/ecstasy).

skiing

This exercise stretches and flexes all the muscles that hold the spine, releasing tension and tightness that may be restricting blood flow, nerve communications and energy flow. It also opens the front of the chest and makes the breastbone more flexible, for better breathing.

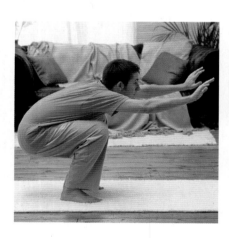

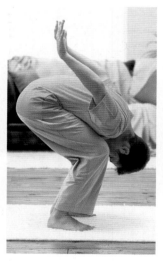

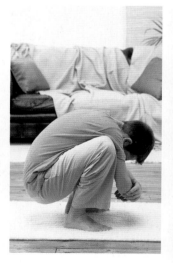

△ **1** Stand with your feet comfortably apart and parallel. Bend your knees and squat right down, stretching your arms out in front of you for balance. Lift your arms, opening your chest, as you breathe in. Imagine you are holding two ski poles and plant them firmly in the snow ahead of you.

△ **2** Breathing out, sweep your arms down and back, reaching as high behind you as you can to wave your imaginary ski poles in the air after they have propelled you forward. Repeat this movement several times. The visualization of the movement should make you feel flushed with exertion and enjoyment.

△ **3** When you feel you have done enough skiing, squat down with your arms and trunk between your knees and rest. Breathe naturally and feel the weight of your body stretching your lower back and legs.

easing the spine and neck

When you exercise lying down, gravity supports and cradles you, so these exercises are very soothing – especially if you feel stiff or have painful twinges in your lower back, hips or neck. You may feel more comfortable lying on your back if you place a small cushion under your head (not your neck) to lengthen your neck and bring your chin down toward your chest. Keep your neck area free, so that it can stretch.

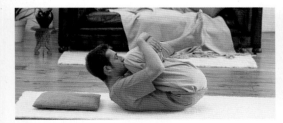

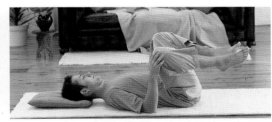

△ **1** Bend your knees on to your chest and clasp your hands around your shins (or the backs of your thighs). Breathing out, curl up your spine to bring your nose or forehead (not your chin, as this constricts your neck) to touch your knees. Breathe in to replace your head on the cushion, with your chin tucked in. Breathe out to begin the sequence again and repeat several times.

△ **2** To ease your lower back and hips, lie with your bent knees comfortably apart and one hand on each knee, with your elbows resting on the floor if possible. This is an open and relaxed pose that can ease pain from trapped nerves (such as sciatica). Breathing deeply and naturally, use your hands to circle your knees in toward each other then out to the sides in slow circles, really relaxing all your back and leg muscles.

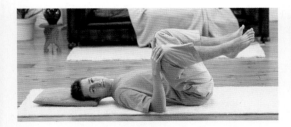

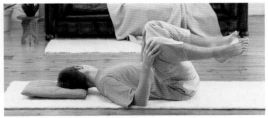

△ **3** Keeping your spine relaxed and knees wide and supported by your hands, with elbows resting on the floor, take your full attention to your neck. Breathing out slowly, turn your head to one side and turn your eyes to look at the floor.

△ **4** Breathe in to raise your head and eyes to the centre and out to turn them to the other side. Repeat several times, focusing on awareness and relaxation of all your neck muscles. Keep your spine, legs, arms and jaw completely relaxed throughout.

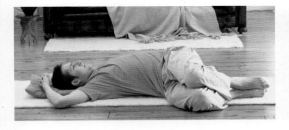

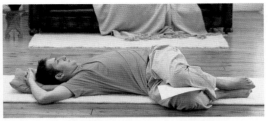

△ **5** Bring your arms overhead, clasping your hands loosely if you can, or simply bringing your bent arms as high as possible – your elbows should be relaxed on the floor. This position stretches the front of your body. Place your feet together on the floor close to your buttocks, and relax your upper body, neck and jaw. You will move only from the waist down. Breathe in and, as you breathe out, drop your knees (keeping them pressed together) to the floor on your right side. Breathe in to raise your knees and out to lower them to the left.

△ **6** For extra strengthening of the upper inner thighs – essential for good posture – press a sheet of paper between your knees and hold it there as you move your knees from side to side.

Breathing techniques

Focusing on the breath is a universal technique for enlightenment and healing, and many traditions use breathing practices either as a way to prepare for meditation or as meditation techniques in themselves. Conscious control of the breath, or pranayama, is the fourth limb of Patanjali's system. The technique of holding the breath – either in or out – is beyond the scope of this book, as accomplishing it safely requires one-to-one teaching, but becoming aware of the breathing process and directing the flow of the breath is within the capacity of everyone.

Slowing down the breathing and lengthening the breath out (which is what happens when we sing or chant) switches the nervous system into its peaceful happy mode, allowing stress to be dissolved and rest, digestion, absorption and healing to take place at every level of the five koshas.

Patanjali's path to enlightenment

This use of the breath fits in perfectly with Patanjali's philosophy. He describes three vital steps (which have been called "preliminary purificatory practices") that

encapsulate his path to enlightenment. The steps are as follows (quote marks refer to the translation of Patanjali's *Sutras* by Alistair Shearer, Ch2, v1/2):

"Purification" [through self-discipline]
"Refinement" [through self-awareness]
"Surrender" [through self-surrender and continual letting-go]
"These are the practical steps on the path of yoga."
They nourish the state of samadhi *[absorption/ecstasy/expansion]*
"And weaken the causes of suffering."

The whole process of self-development starts with taking conscious control over our own nervous system, so that we experience more "expansion" and joy and less stress and unhappiness. Our circumstances influence the outcome of events far less than our own basic attitudes, and these can be changed from negative to positive by the simple act of changing our breathing pattern.

The breath forms part of the energy system and the physiological processes in the energy kosha, while nervous energy runs the mental computer in the kosha of unconscious programming. All the koshas

meet and blend in the chakra system in the energy kosha and all can therefore be consciously influenced through the practices of breathing and meditation.

Although some translations of the *Yoga Sutras* describe Patanjali's three "purificatory steps" as "preliminary", there is really no end to our need of them. We always have to maintain our discipline and keep our attention focused - and we never stop needing to let go of something or other.

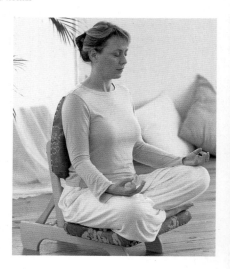

"Those who see a glass as half empty feel deprived, whereas those who see it as half full feel blessed."
Traditional wisdom

viloma: focusing on the breathing muscles

This useful focusing technique can be practised anywhere, sitting with the spine erect and the hands and eyes still.

▷ **1** Place your hands on your knees, palms either up or down, with thumb and index fingers touching to close the energy circuits. As you breathe in deeply, feel your ribs expand and your diaphragm contract downward against your stomach. Notice how these movements cause air to flow into your lungs.

2 As you breathe out, count "One and two and...", then stop your breath in mid-flow for the same count. Repeat until you have slowly and comfortably expelled enough air, then repeat this cycle four times more and rest. Then reverse the cycle, breathing in counting "One and two and..." and out slowly for five breaths. Use the fractional breath in to start your day or whenever you need energy, and the fractional breath out to relax before meditation.

watchpoints for breathing practice

Regular practice will calm the mind and raise your energy levels. As the lungs strengthen, their capacity will be increased. Practise little and often – a few rounds of the breathing exercises now and then throughout the day will prepare you for longer sessions during meditation practice.

- Avoid any breathing practices after meals – when your stomach is full it presses against your diaphragm, constricting your lungs.
- Keep your spine stretched and as straight as possible (allowing for its natural curves) whether you are standing, sitting, kneeling or lying down to practise breathing. This allows maximum lung expansion and helps the free flow of both air and energy.
- Keep your breastbone lifted to open your chest and give your diaphragm room to move freely. Keep it lifted even when breathing out, letting your diaphragm and rib muscles do all the work.
- Always breathe in through your nose, as it is the filter that protects your lungs from cold, dust and infections from outside. Breathe out through your nose unless you are making sounds.
- Develop your focus on, and conscious awareness of, your breathing patterns, so that you constantly monitor their effects upon you. Develop the habit of watching yourself breathing.
- Slow your breathing down – especially your breath out – whenever you feel agitated or anxious, in order to gain conscious control over your autonomic nervous system.
- Stop your breathing practice and rest for a few natural breaths the instant you feel breathless. Start again when your nervous system has settled down and relaxed. It is not used to being watched and controlled, as breathing is usually an unconscious process.

alternate nostril breathing

This universally popular exercise quickly balances the nervous system, so that you feel calm and centred after just a few rounds – ready either for meditation practice or to get on with your day refreshed.

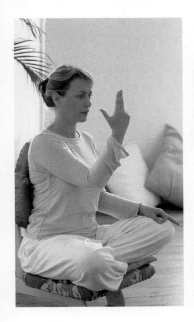

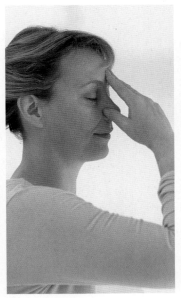

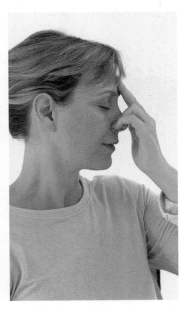

△ **1** Sit erect with your left hand on your knee or in your lap. Raise your right hand to place it against your face. Your thumb will close your right nostril, your index and middle fingers will rest aginst your forehead at the brow chakra and your ring finger will close your left nostril.

△ **2** Your eyes may be closed, or open and gazing softly ahead. Keep your eyeballs still, as quiet eyes induce a quiet mind. Close your right nostril with your thumb. Breathe in through the left nostril.

△ **3** Release the right nostril and close the left with your ring finger. Breathe out slowly, and then in again, through your right nostril. Then open the left nostril, close the right and breathe out. This is one round. Do five rounds, breathe naturally to rest, then repeat a few times.

double breathing

This exercise fosters your self-awareness and observation. It also tones the muscles that give you "core strength" and support your spine, giving you increased energy and stamina for self-discipline, and improving posture and energy flow. Start each round by breathing in from your feet up (if you are standing), or from the base of your spine if you are sitting.

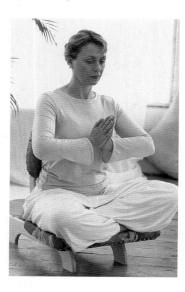

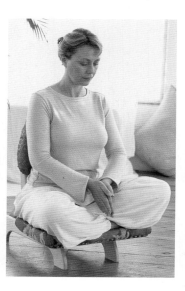

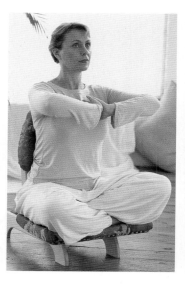

△ **1** Bring your palms together at chest level with elbows wide, lifting your breastbone and drawing your spine erect. Breathe slowly and deeply a few times to settle yourself.

△ **2** Point your fingers downward and focus on the base of your body. As you breathe in, tighten the muscles of your upper inner thighs and pelvic floor, and at the same time draw your lower abdominal muscles back toward your spine. This movement lifts your life energy upward.

△ **3** As you breathe out, turn your hands so your fingers point toward your collarbones, at the base of your throat, lifting your elbows to shoulder level. At the same time draw your energy up from the base, through the waist as you tighten your abdominal "corset muscles", and up to your head as you lift your chin. In this position breathe in, opening your ribs at the back of your chest by pressing your palms firmly together, as you bring spiritual energy down into your heart centre. Breathe out as you lower your fingertips and take your energy to the floor. Repeat the cycle twice more, then rest.

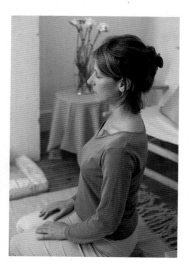

◁ Breathing practices can be done in a kneeling position if you find this comfortable. The pose creates a strong, stable base and helps to keep the spine erect to maximize the flow of energy. When you are kneeling or sitting, start the upward breath in from the base of your spine.

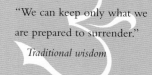

"We can keep only what we are prepared to surrender."
Traditional wisdom

grounding ritual

This is an essential step at the end of your meditation, so that you clear your mind of all you have experienced and go back to daily life refreshed and in "active mode", rather than "heady" and "spaced out". It is an exercise in self-surrender, as you give to the earth all the relaxation and joy you feel as a result of your meditation practice. This is one reason why we meditate – to share positive energy with those with whom we interact.

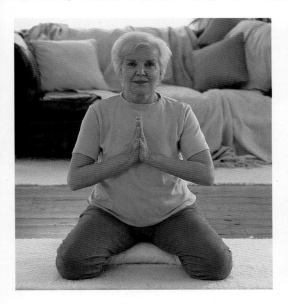

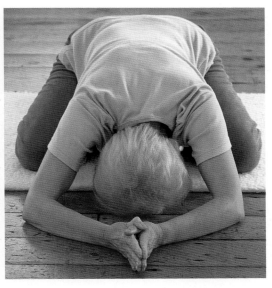

△ **1** At the end of your visualization or other meditation practice, bring your palms together and breathe in, mentally giving heartfelt thanks for the experience, whatever it was like for you.

△ **2** As you breathe out, fold forward to ground yourself by placing your hands on the floor – and your head also if you can reach – giving to the earth all the experience and benefit you have received.

bee buzzing breath

This technique uses sound to begin extending the length of the breath out. It induces instant relaxation and reduction of stress, and is an exercise in "letting go".

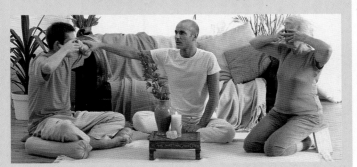

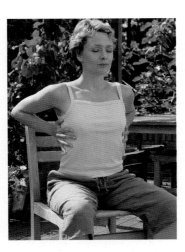

△ **1** Sit erect, placing your thumbs in position ready to close your ear flaps, and your fingers ready to close your eyelids and lips.

2 Breathe in deeply. As you breathe out, "close down" and make a humming sound like a bee. Feel this sound vibrating through your body, loosening tightness and tension. Before you run out of breath, open your eyes and ears to breathe in and repeat.

△ **Explore the physical effects of your breath on your abdominal organs by placing your hands on the sides of your ribs, then on the front and finally on your lower abdomen.**

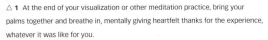

Posture principles

Meditation practices are traditionally performed sitting with the spine erect so that energy flows between the "heaven" (light) and "earth" (life) poles of our being. Energy needs to flow smoothly up and down through the physical spine and the energy channels of the subtle body, so that the brain and breathing function optimally and the chakras are balanced and full of vitality. An erect spine is quite easy to maintain if the right props are used to begin with and the right exercises are performed regularly to strengthen the muscles that hold the spine erect and open the hip joints. Remember to keep the shoulder blades down.

meditation and relaxation

Relaxation is quite different from meditation. It is part of the fifth limb of Patanjali's system – pratyahara, or withdrawal of the senses from outer stimuli. Relaxation practices are done lying down in as comfortable a position as possible. Western psychotherapists usually favour a reclining position because their techniques require the client to be relaxed as they follow a guided visualization or answer questions about their past. Meditation practice takes us deeper than this, with the mind quietly focused on a single object. Relaxation – like physical stretching and awareness of breathing – is very useful as a preparation for meditative practice but should not be confused with it.

sitting on a chair

When starting to practise meditation, most Westerners find it easiest to sit upright on a firm chair. Your thighs should be parallel to the floor – in order to achieve this you may need to raise your feet (without shoes) by resting them on a cushion. Sit erect with your hands, palms down, resting on your thighs, hands and feet parallel and pointing forward. This posture is known as the "Egyptian position". If you lean back at all you will quickly develop a backache, so sit

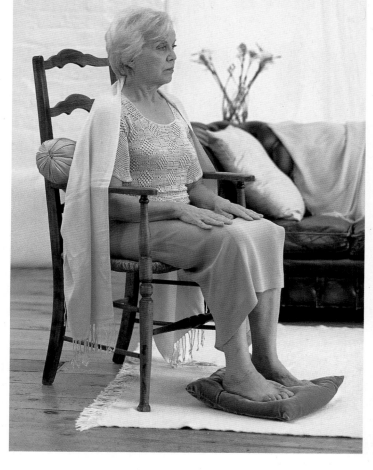

erect with the base of your spine pressed against the chair back or a firm cushion.

Once you are settled in this position you can gradually increase the time you can comfortably remain motionless. Spend up to ten minutes watching your natural breath or practising breathing exercises to centre your energies along the axis of the spine. You will feel energized and relaxed as a result. Later you may wish to sit motionless for half an hour or longer while you practise

△ **If you choose to sit in a chair for meditation practice, make sure it gives firm support and is a suitable height. Your spine should remain erect, with your head and neck aligned.**

your meditation techniques. If the seated position suits you, you may decide always to practise meditation seated on a particular chair, or you may want to try out a variety of positions as your hips become more flexible through regular stretching exercises.

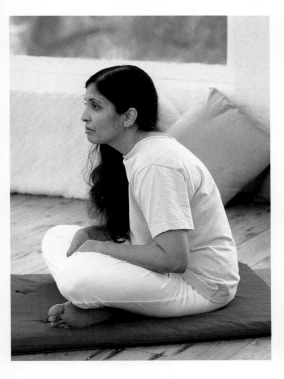

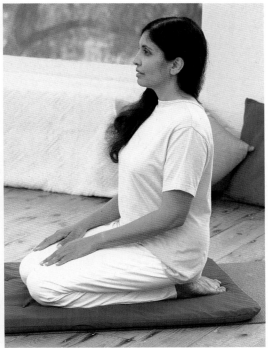

△ Lack of spinal strength and the right support result in poor posture, with the head jutting forward and the spine rounded. The neck automatically shortens and tenses when the back is humped in this way, constricting the flow of energy, and it is impossible to maintain the position comfortably for the whole period of meditation practice.

△ Good posture results from choosing the right position. The head and neck are aligned and erect, and the spine is vertical. To prevent strain and help with alignment, the base of the spine can be supported on a firm cushion or a folded blanket positioned between the feet.

sitting on the floor

This is the traditional Eastern way to meditate, since chairs were not used in homes until very recently. As a result, people had very flexible hips, so sitting cross-legged on a cushion on the floor was easy and natural. Most Westerners first need to loosen up their hip joints – which has the additional benefit that it reduces the risk of developing arthritic hips in old age. Meanwhile, it is better to sit on a chair, or on your heels in the yogic Vajrasana pose, than with a slumped spine in an attempt to sit with crossed legs on the floor. Whatever position you adopt, do use support where it is needed until your muscles and joints have strengthened and loosened enough for you to be comfortable without support. Many excellent meditation stools and chairs are available, some of which are illustrated in this section.

where support may be needed

Your spine may need help in order to remain comfortably erect. You can sit supported by a cushion against a wall – if you are on the floor or in bed – or with a cushion against the back of a firm upright chair (not an armchair). Sitting on your heels may be the easiest way to learn to sit erect without support.

Your hips may not yet open freely enough to allow your knees to rest on the floor in a cross-legged pose. Cushions supporting your thighs will help you to stretch up through your lower back and a firm cushion under your tailbone will relieve pressure in the lower back by lowering your knees. Strategically placed cushions can make sitting on the floor the most comfortable option.

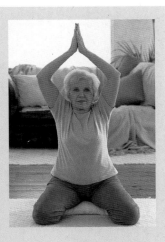

△ A cushion under the tailbone eases the lower back by lifting the hips.

Choosing a posture

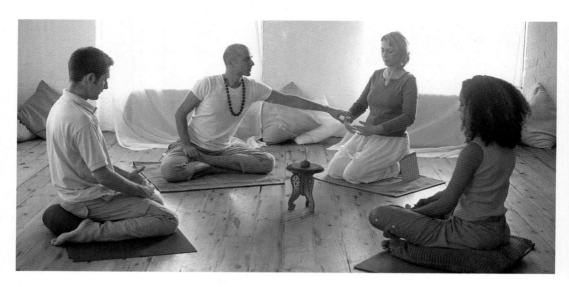

Regular practice is the best teacher, as your body quickly gets used to the new routine and settles into it more and more easily. When you find a position that is comfortable for you, practise sitting in it until you can remain motionless, relaxed yet alert, for half an hour or more. It is helpful to vary your position when you sit at home, or to change purposefully from one position to another without disturbing your inner focus whenever your muscles begin to ache. This is much better than focusing on the complaints coming from your body when you push it to sit too long without moving.

△ You may find it helpful to attend a meditation class, where you can be shown different ways to sit and try out the various props available before buying any of them for yourself.

easy cross-legged pose

This involves sitting erect with hips loose and knees wide. Each foot is tucked under the opposite thigh so that the weight of the legs rests on the feet rather than the knees. Place cushions under each thigh and/or under the buttocks if you feel pressure in the lower back. The tailbone (coccyx) should hang freely, letting the "sitting bones" take the weight of the trunk. Place your hands on your knees or rest them in your lap with palms facing up.

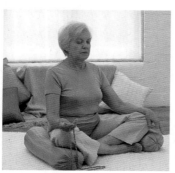

◁ If the hips are not sufficiently flexible for the knees to rest on the floor when sitting cross-legged, support them with a couple of cushions. Resting the hands palms up enables you to hold a mala, or rosary.

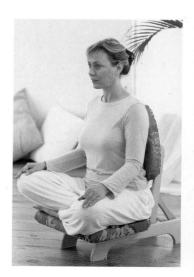

▷ This low chair, which folds for easy carrying, is specially designed for meditation. It supports the back when sitting in the cross-legged pose. The hands are in *gyana mudra*, with the tips of thumb and forefinger joined to complete the energy circuit.

Buddhist position

The yogic kneeling pose called Virasana is sometimes used for meditation. Buddhists often choose to sit on a very firm cushion that lifts the hips, with the knees resting on the floor on each side of the cushion and the shins and feet pointing back. Lifting the hips in this way helps to keep the spine correctly aligned, and this position can be very comfortable as long as your knees are fairly flexible.

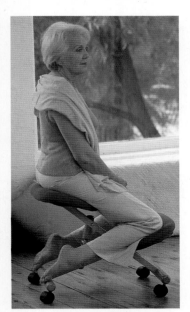

◁ Using a "kneeling" chair helps to keep the spine straight and gives a good, well-supported position that is similar to the Buddhist kneeling pose.

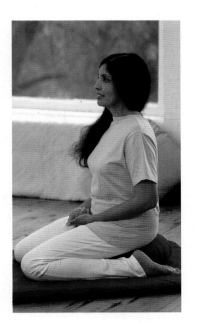

▷ While sitting on a firm cushion in Virasana, the knees and feet can also be supported on a larger cushion. The meditator sits between the feet, rather than on the heels. The hands are in the gesture called *bhairavi mudra*, to focus the energy for meditation.

early morning meditation

Many people like to meditate first thing every morning, while the mind is quiet and before the events of the day have a chance to distract it. If you meditate in bed, use a V-shaped pillow or ordinary pillows to support your back, so that you can sit erect in a cross-legged position. Wear a shawl round your shoulders and pull up the bedclothes so that you feel warm while you are doing your meditation practice. Choose a practice that energizes rather than relaxes you, such as chanting or repeating a mantra using a mala. You may prefer to keep your eyes open in a soft gaze.

▷ Your bed can be a haven of peace and warmth if you prefer to meditate on waking in the morning.

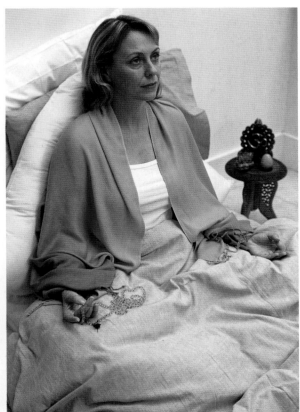

▽ A V-shaped pillow helps you to maintain an erect posture while meditating in bed. A mala, used for counting the repetitions of a mantra, is traditionally kept concealed in its special bag when not in use.

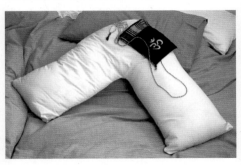

The time, the place

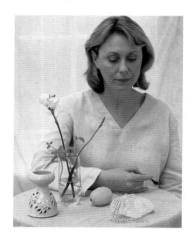

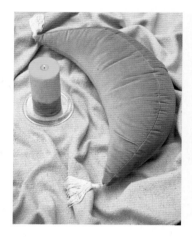

◁ Your "meditation corner" may contain a number of objects on which to focus: any object can act as a trigger to put you in the right frame of mind for your practice.

▷ A crescent-shaped "moon cushion" is often used as support when sitting for meditation.

meditating at a regular time

It is helpful to place your meditation practice in the context of long-established habits – such as before showering in the morning, or after cleaning your teeth, or before lunch or supper. Since you do all these things daily you will meditate daily as well. A good time is when you wake up or before a meal – after meals people are apt to feel sleepy – or in the evening after a brisk walk or listening to soothing music. You might read an uplifting book in bed and then meditate before going to sleep. Choose a time when you are normally alone and undisturbed – the fuller your day, the more rewarding and de-stressing your meditation session can be. Couples often meditate together at a mutually convenient time, or get up early before the household is awake. Whatever time you choose, stick to it to establish your meditation habit.

It takes determination to establish a new habit and to make room in your life for a new regular activity. It helps if you train your mind to meditate routinely at a specific time and place. You may still be tempted sometimes to skip your meditation slot and do something else instead, but you will begin to feel uncomfortable when you miss your practice. There will be days when you have to forgo your normal routine, but that will be a conscious decision rather than simply forgetting or procrastinating.

creating a meditation corner

If you always do your meditation in the same place this will also help to establish your meditation habit. Choose a quiet and uncluttered space so that the moment you sit there your mind becomes calm and focused. Make sure you will be warm enough, as body temperature drops when you relax and turn inward.

Your "meditation corner" might consist of a special chair in a peaceful part of your home, or perhaps you might sit on a

meditation in bed

If you practise meditation in the early morning your bed (with a warm shawl around you and the covers pulled up) can become your "meditation corner". Have a wash, a drink and a good stretch to really wake you up first – and make sure you sit with your spine erect.

If you regularly meditate in bed in the morning, and this is the place where you are in the habit of turning your mind inward, it can also be very soothing to perform simple meditation techniques before you go to sleep at night.

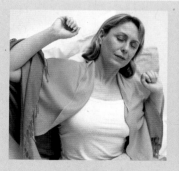

△ When you wake up, have a relaxed, "releasing" stretch before starting your early morning meditation.

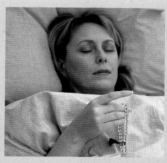

△ Last thing at night, relax with your mala and repeat a mantra or simple prayer before you go peacefully to sleep.

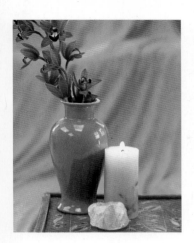

△ **If you choose to meditate sitting on the floor, a low table is useful for holding objects on which you wish to focus your gaze.**

favourite cushion, or spread out a lovely rug. The corner might contain a table holding a candle and flowers, or anything you find soothing and inspiring.

objects of devotion

The things you keep in your meditation corner can be used for the classic technique called *tratak* – or "gazing". This involves sitting erect and motionless while focusing your gaze upon an object.

The point of focus is often a lighted candle. If you practise this form of meditation, check that there are no draughts to move the candle flame, as this can give you a headache. (Epileptics and migraine sufferers should avoid gazing at a flame.) After gazing softly, without staring, for a while, close your eyes and keep the image in your mind's eye. When it fades, gaze at the candle again and repeat the visualization. Your mental image will gradually become firmer and your concentration deeper.

You may like to light a candle before starting meditation practice and blow it out with a "thank you" as a final gesture. A flame is a universal symbol for the presence of the divine, and you may like to develop a greater awareness of this presence dwelling within you and surrounding you.

There are different forms of tratak. A flower can be held and turned around in the hand, as you observe every detail of its

postural stretch

If you have been sitting all day in a car or at your desk, you may want to regain a strong upright posture before you start an evening meditation session. You could try standing with a weighty object on your head to strengthen the spinal column and improve your sense of balance. Previous generations learned "deportment" by walking around the room balancing piles of books on their heads, and porters the world over have strong straight backs, developed by carrying loads on their heads.

▷ Stretching your spine up against the weight of gravity makes your meditation pose "firm and comfortable", as Patanjali recommends.

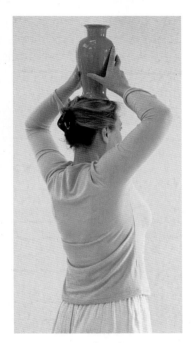

beauty and structure. Holding a crystal in your hands and feeling its contours and coolness is another form of tratak – in this case the eyes are closed throughout and the "gazing" is accomplished through the sense of touch. You could equally well choose to gaze at any object that inspires you.

relaxing horizontal stretch

Stretching out on your back is the perfect preparation for meditation. Ten minutes lying stretched out on the floor on your back, with your mind gently but firmly focused on the movement of your breath while your body relaxes, is an instant restorative.

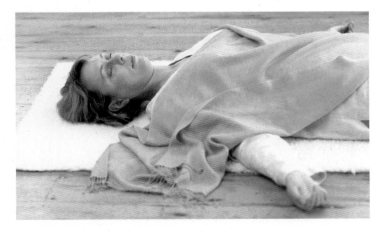

△ Keep alert and warm while you relax on your back. Stretching in this position prepares you for keeping your spine erect – the spine should always be as straight as possible when meditating. While you lie on your back and relax your body, many meditation techniques can be used to keep your mind alert and focused, such as counting your breaths from one to ten and back again, visualizing energy moving through the spine, repeating a mantra, or visualizing a tranquil scene in the country or by the sea. After your relaxation take a few deep breaths, move your fingers and toes, stretch and yawn and sit up very slowly. You are now ready for meditation practice.

The art of visualization

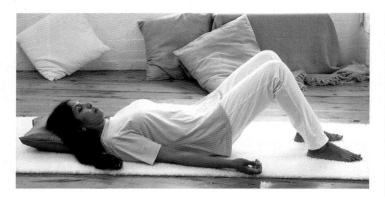

△ **For relaxation adopt a comfortable position lying on your back with your knees raised and feet flat on the floor. A cushion under your head keeps your neck from contracting at the back.**

▽ **Once you are deeply relaxed, focus your imagination and all your senses on being present in the place you want to be.**

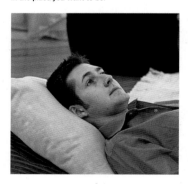

Visualization is a technique that brings the senses into full play, and enables us to build up a happy inner world. Relaxed visualization is a tool used in many different types of therapies. Its aim is to help us change our perception of the world by changing the way we feel inside ourselves. It can be done lying down or reclining just as well as sitting in an upright meditation pose. This means that we can help ourselves to feel better when we are tired and depleted, or ill in bed, or needing to create a calm and relaxed state to prepare for a peaceful night's sleep.

choosing an affirmation

You can use your relaxation time for your own greatest long-term benefit by using affirmations to create lasting change. The first step is to decide on an affirmation or resolve, known as a *sankalpa*, to repeat when you are in a state of deep relaxation.

You need to ask yourself what positive changes in your behaviour (life), perception (light) or attitude (love) would make you more like the person you would wish to be. The answer requires reflection and an honest appraisal of your personal qualities. Having decided on your sankalpa, you can set about creating a suitable visualization by using your imagination and all five senses to become fully present in a place of your choice where you feel naturally safe and relaxed. Once this scene is set you can go

deeper and reinforce the changes in attitude, outlook and purpose that you have already decided to adopt. The unconscious mind is happy to respond to the suggestions put to it by the conscious mind, provided your nervous system is in a thoroughly relaxed and trusting state and that you express your intention in the following ways:

- Phrase your affirmation as clearly and as briefly as possible, with no "ifs" and "buts", descriptions or qualifiers.

- Mention just one change. When that change has occurred you can replace your sankalpa because it will have become redundant.
- Describe the change you wish for in the present tense, such as "I am…[happy, healthy, confident, successful at…,.or forgiving of…]" or, "I am becoming more and more…day by day." The unconscious mind lives only in the present and ignores the past or future. Tomorrow never comes and is of no interest to it.
- Express your sankalpa in positive terms only, for the unconscious mind becomes confused by negative words such as "not" and "never".
- Avoid any words like "try" or "work at" or "difficult" because they immediately put the nervous system on guard and undo all the good relaxation you have achieved up to now
- Repeat your sankalpa three times slowly and decisively, so that your unconscious mind knows you mean business. In this way you are programming it to carry out your intentions all the time – even when the conscious mind is busy with other things. This is why the sankalpa has such a powerful effect.

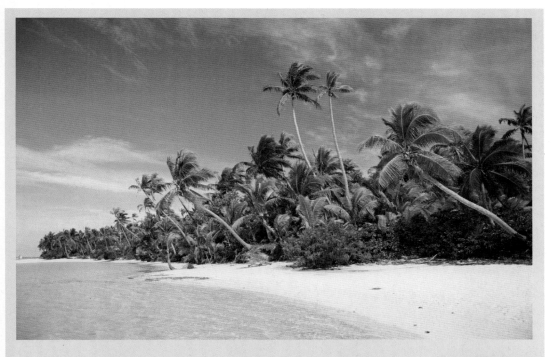

visualizing a beach scene

You have become deeply relaxed, perhaps after some stretching and deep breathing exercises. Sit or lie down in a comfortable position and start to imagine yourself reclining on a beautiful beach. You are lying on soft sand near the water's edge on a pleasant sunny day. Use all your senses to appreciate all the details of the scene, so that you experience it fully.

You can feel the texture and dampness of the sand beneath you, dig your toes into it and let it run through your fingers. Look at the scenery around you, the deep blue of the sea and sky, the pale sand, the distant horizon, a few fluffy white clouds, seagulls flying overhead. You can hear the seagulls calling, the wavelets lapping across the sand and the sound of a gentle breeze moving the leaves of the trees behind you. You can smell the salt air and taste it on your

△ The beauty, warmth and peace of a tropical beach make it pleasing to all the senses, so it is an ideal subject for a visualization to help you create your happy inner world.

▷ The more detailed your visualization the more completely you will be able to experience the scene. Taste and feel the coolness of an iced drink on a hot day.

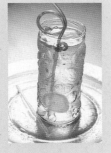

lips. What else can you feel, see and hear? Perhaps the air caressing your body, the intricate patterns of individual grains of sand and tiny shells, the sound of children laughing in the distance. Can you smell the sea, taste a half-eaten peach, feel the welcome coolness of the wind lifting your hair?

When you have built up all the details of this lovely scene, stay in it for a while feeling peaceful and contented, grateful and relaxed. The whole purpose of this visualization is to bring you to this inner place where you know that "all is well", now and always. Before you decide to leave the beach repeat your sankalpa (the affirmation or resolve you have already decided upon) slowly and clearly three times. Then gradually let the whole scene dissolve, knowing that it is always there for you to return to, no matter what is going on in the external world.

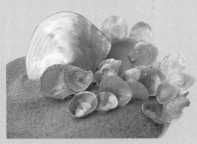

◁ Feel the sand between your toes and visualize the soft sheen of seashells.

Taking imaginary journeys

Visualizations while in deep relaxation are enjoyable and can reveal unexpected insights. They prepare for more structured traditional meditations.

The visualization described opposite takes you on a journey that starts with your everyday awareness and leads to a higher level of consciousness, as you walk slowly through the countryside and up a hill to your goal before returning more quickly by the same route. The Buddhist walking meditation, a practice in which the action of walking is itself the focus of awareness, can be a helpful preparation for your imaginary walk through the chakra fields. Remember to perform a grounding ritual at the end of your visualization to avoid feeling "spaced out" afterwards.

telling the story
You may wish to make a tape of the visualization described opposite so that your voice guides you gently through it, with frequent pauses to build up the scene in your mind. Or get a friend to read it aloud to you. It should take about 20 minutes.

walking meditation

This popular Buddhist meditation combines the senses of touch, sound and sight. Walking in slow motion requires focus and concentration. Synchronize your breathing and mantra repetitions with your steps.

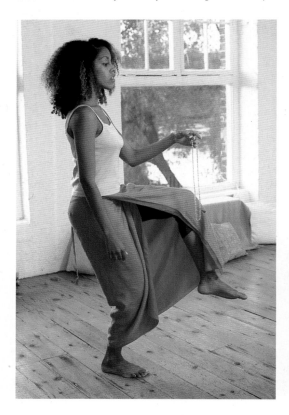

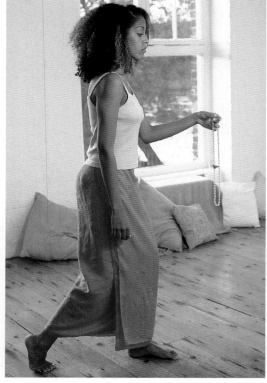

△ **1** Stand tall with your mala held in front of you at heart level. Very slowly raise one foot and step forward on to it, bending your back knee. As you step forward, keep your weight distributed evenly between both feet.

△ **2** Take your whole weight on to your front foot, lifting your back foot and standing as tall as you can. Gaze straight ahead all the time. Repeat the movements, saying your mantra with each step.

a walk through the chakra fields

Relax deeply, feeling your senses becoming very alert so that you notice every detail of your imaginary surroundings.

 Start by walking along a short lane that takes you to a stile giving access to a meadow. A sea of red flowers – perhaps poppies – grow in this field. They represent the vitality and growth of the base chakra. A footpath leads you gently uphill across this field to another stile. Follow this path, absorbing the vibrant redness, feeling the solid ground beneath you and the movement of your legs and feet as you walk. Inhale the natural earthy smell of living, growing plants.

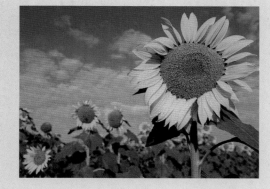

 The next stile takes you into a grove of orange trees laden with ripe fruit, representing the sensuality of the sacral chakra. Enjoy the abundance of nature and its glorious power to reproduce and sustain life. Eat some of the fruit, letting the delicious juices flow in your mouth. Dance your way along the path to the next stile.

 This leads you into a field of golden sunflowers, representing the light and heat of the navel chakra, which is often called the solar centre. Here we store our reserves of energy, or prana – just as the seeds of the sunflowers store the energy of life. Feast your eyes on the gold around you and let your skin soak up the warmth from the sun. Feel confident that your reserves of energy will always support whatever you set out to accomplish. At the end of the field is a gate in a wall.

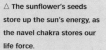

△ The sunflower's seeds store up the sun's energy, as the navel chakra stores our life force.

 This gate opens into a formal walled garden with a path that takes you under a long archway festooned with climbing roses in every shade of pink, luminous against their glossy green leaves and exuding heavenly scents. This beautiful garden represents your heart chakra, with its atmosphere of peace and joy. You touch the velvety petals and the roses lean down to share their beauty with you, inviting you to pick them. You take just one to keep as your constant companion, before passing through the gate at the end of the garden.

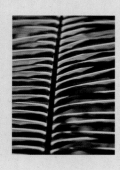

△ Notice every detail of the lush growth that fringes your path on your walk.

 You find yourself on high ground under a wide blue sky across which birds are flying and calling to each other. The sky is reflected in pools of blue water from melting snows, and vivid blue gentians open their faces to the warm sun. This scene represents the throat chakra and the energies of pure space and sound. You hear your name being called and walk trustingly toward a high pass ahead of you.

Someone comes to meet you, offering to guide you onward and representing your own higher wisdom, found in your brow chakra. This chakra is often called the third eye: the "all-seeing eye" of the higher mind that unites the two hemispheres of the brain – logical intellect and creative imagination – to create insight. Your guide may tell you something or give you something to ponder upon later, before leading you over the pass.

 Beyond is a grassy glade surrounded by trees. In the centre is a small white building – clearly a very special and spiritual place – that represents your crown chakra. Your guide gestures to you to enter alone, which you do very respectfully. There you sit and repeat your sankalpa, slowly and clearly, three times. You remain in this place, absorbing its spiritual energies, until you feel it is time to return to everyday awareness. You say "thank you" before rising and leaving to walk slowly back the way you have come, knowing that you can return here whenever you wish.

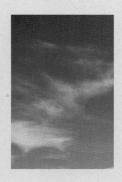

△ The endless blue sky represents the throat chakra, whose element is ether, or space.

Back in the lane where you started your journey you become aware once more of your physical body. Take a few deep breaths, move your fingers and toes, yawn and stretch. Perform your grounding ritual to end your session, then get up slowly.

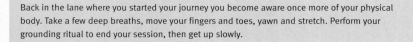

Meditation in daily life

Many people think of the meditative state as being rather "otherworldly", something that they can only achieve if they divorce themselves from daily life. Although regular meditation practice requires that we set time aside to turn the attention inward, it can also be woven into daily life. We can turn mundane chores into a form of meditation by practising "mindfulness" – focusing all our thoughts on them; we can experience a sense of spiritual enlightenment from appreciating the beauty of everything around us; we can use meditative practices when trying to engage with and understand our emotions; and we can introduce meditative elements into the ways in which we relate to others.

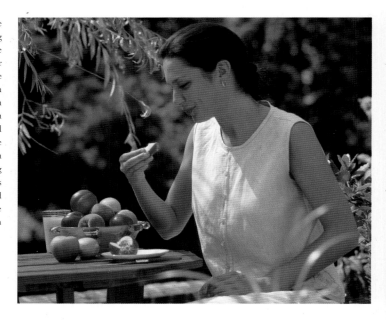

▷ **By focusing all your awareness on everyday activities such as eating, you can turn them into a form of meditation.**

key elements

There are many ways in which you can bring meditation into every aspect of your day-to-day life:

- Focus your mind and body entirely on what you are doing at this moment, letting distractions wash around you.

- Live in the present moment as much as you can.
- Try to perceive the beauty and worth in everything (and everyone) around you, and in everything you do, no matter how mundane the task.

- Learn to use your senses to the full.
- Develop self-awareness, and work with the interplay between your emotional and physical self – noticing how certain breathing practices and positions affect your mental state, for example.

working with your feelings

The following traditional technique, based on experiencing "opposites", allows you to become impartially aware of your feelings (many of which are usually below consciousness):

- Relax deeply – sitting, reclining or lying on your back.
- Imagine various "pairs of opposites" and notice the physical sensations that arise.
- Start with pairs that have little or no positive/negative emotional associations – such as hot/cold, hard/soft, light/dark – and observe

how you feel in your body while remaining deeply relaxed.
- Move on to a more emotionally challenging pair, starting with the positive side, and observe what feelings are evoked: birth/death, spacious/confined, happy/sad, delighted/angry and welcome/excluded are some examples.
- Still deeply relaxed, observe what feelings arise in your body as you contemplate the negative half of the pair – so that you can recognize and identify them from now on and

understand what "pushes your buttons" and how you feel out of sorts when your emotions are negative. You can then take appropriate action to make you feel better and defuse tension in and around you.
- Repeat the positive half of the pair before moving on to the next pair of opposites.
- End with your sankalpa and some gentle deep breathing before coming out of relaxation with a grounding ritual.

relating to others

This Buddhist "loving kindness" meditation helps you to relate better to those around you. Breathe in universal love and kindness to help and support yourself, then breathe it out, directing it to a specific person or group. Repeat this meditation often, until it becomes second nature both to receive and to give loving kindness. Make it part of your daily life: any part of it can be used in any situation to promote peace and harmony.

- Relax deeply in a seated position with your spine erect.
- Breathe in, drawing "loving kindness" from the universe into yourself.
- Breathe out, directing that loving kindness with gratitude toward a particular person, or to all those who have taught you (given you light in many ways). Breathe more loving kindness into yourself.
- Breathe out, directing loving kindness with gratitude toward a particular

person or to all those who have nurtured and nourished you (given you life in many forms). Breathe in...
- Breathe out, directing loving kindness with blessings toward a person or people you love dearly. Breathe in...
- Breathe out, directing loving kindness with blessings toward acquaintances, neighbours, people you work with. Breathe in...
- Breathe out, directing loving kindness with forgiveness to people who annoy or obstruct you, who are unkind or dismissive. Breathe in...
- Breathe out, directing loving kindness with forgiveness to anyone who has ever hurt or injured you in any way. Breathe in...
- Breathe out, radiating the prayer, "May all people everywhere be happy." Breathe in and give thanks for all the loving kindness you receive. Pause before coming out of your meditation and grounding yourself with a ritual.

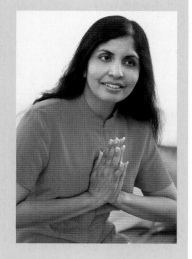

△ The traditional Indian greeting "Namaste", spoken with a bow while bringing the hands together at the heart chakra, acknowledges the presence of the divine in the heart of each person, conveying the sense that everyone is part of the unity of creation.

how are you feeling?

As a way of linking the physical and non-physical, it is important to get into the habit of noticing consciously what your senses are telling your mind. This makes it much easier to monitor your emotions as they arise, because you can feel them through your senses. In fact, there is no other way to feel how you are "feeling". For every emotion there is a corresponding physical sensation: we "see red" when angry, our legs "turn to jelly" when we are frightened, sadness makes the heart "ache" or we are "in the dark" when confused.

Once you learn to recognize how you are actually feeling you can avoid reacting negatively to everyday situations. Whenever you notice a negative feeling arising, pause for an instant (the proverbial "counting to ten"), relax and visualize the positive, opposite feeling. You can then respond in a positive manner instead, bringing what you have learned through the regular practice of meditation into your daily life.

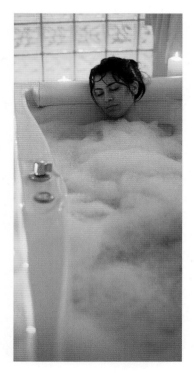

▷ Use the time you spend in the bath or shower each day to relax and enjoy the present moment.

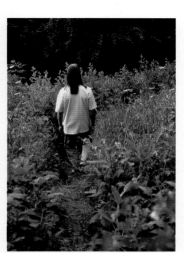

◁ When you take a walk among plants and trees, focus your whole mind and all your senses on the experience, noticing the beauty of everything you pass along your path. Plants teach us how to "just be".

Focusing the mind

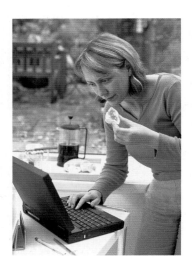

The demands of modern life can tempt you to attend to several things at once – with the result that nothing is done with full awareness, your attention is fragmented and you lose your sattvic outlook on life. Regular meditation practice helps you to recover a focused approach, dealing with each moment as it arises calmly and giving it your full attention.

pulling in opposite directions

According to the teachings of yoga the mind tends to function in two opposing ways: centrifugally and centripetally.

Centrifugal force is when energy is drawn away from the centre to the periphery, where it is dissipated and loses its force. This is what happens when you allow worldly attachments to grab and hold your attention, hang on to negative emotions and prejudices, or try to do everything at once. Spreading yourself too thinly without refocusing squanders your energies, letting them drain away like water being scattered across sand, so that you end up feeling depleted and unfulfilled. Wasting your vital forces in this way leads to stress, exhaustion and eventually to illness.

◁ Modern life is made even more complex by technology that allows us to do several tasks at once. Concentrate on one thing at a time.

▷ When the phone rings, focus on it briefly rather than grabbing it immediately, giving yourself time to settle and prepare your mind.

Centripetal force is energy that flows from the edges to the middle, as when you pick up sensations from the surface of the body and register them consciously in the brain. All the practices that prepare for meditation have the quality of drawing energies back into your central self, into a deep pool or store. Using this energy, you can respond richly to life in a sattvic, conscious, focused and loving manner, directing your full attention to each task.

directed attention

"Alternating current" flowing between a subject (me) and an object (you) is a simple way to describe all relationships. This current needs to be focused rather than dissipated

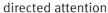

if relationships are to be nourishing and creative. The Sanskrit word for this is *ekagrata*. It means "one-pointedness" and refers to the process of gathering attention in from the periphery and then directing it on to a specific object. Ekagrata is a

▽ As you water a plant, focus on its beauty and the care you are giving it. Bringing the whole of your attention to each action is a form of meditation in itself, and makes any routine daily task more rewarding.

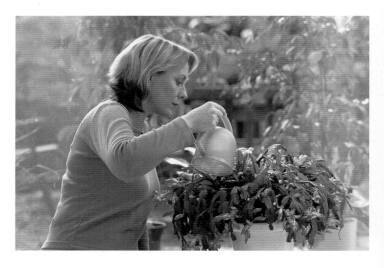

"time out" prevents "burnout"

Most of us need more time for ourselves and this can usually be achieved by following Patanjali's advice. Self-discipline enables you to say "no" and keep certain periods of the day sacrosanct for your own recharging and deep healing. With self-awareness, when you feel you are losing your focus you can stop to stretch, breathe, or repeat a mantra to bring you back into sattvic balance before proceeding. Self-surrender enables you to let go of all unnecessary or negative concerns, feelings or thoughts and to simplify your lifestyle, trusting in the divine guidance and support within yourself that is just waiting for you to draw upon it. Your "higher self" will never force its attentions upon you – it is up to you to seek within, to ask for help and to make time to be receptive to your inner voice through meditation.

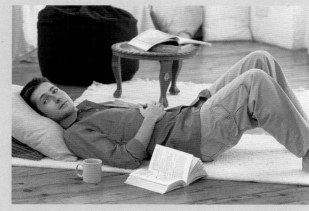

△ When taking time out, find a private space and don't let yourself be distracted by other people, near and distant noises or worrying about other demands on your time. Cultivating self-awareness will give you the confidence to take a break when you need one.

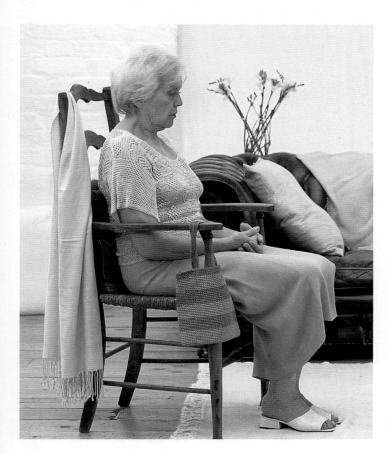

rhythmical two-way mental process similar to the physical process of breathing in and out, and the emotional process of receiving sensations and responding appropriately. We are seldom fully aware of how much energy is tied up in long-term attachments, hopes, fears, plans and resentments that bind us to the past or future and prevent us from living fully in the present.

coping with life's demands

Modern technology often makes it possible to do several tasks at once. In the office you may be listening to instructions, designing a spreadsheet on a computer and taking a telephone call, but it is all too easy to forget part of the instructions, mess up the spreadsheet and be unhelpful to the caller. Domestic situations can dissipate energy in the same way – absentmindedly answering a child's questions while driving a car in heavy traffic having left late for an appointment, then forgetting to pick up the cleaning. The more you can release energy tied up in supporting negative emotions and thought patterns, the more will be available to support your busy life instead.

◁ Before going out to keep an appointment, a short meditation will help you to centre your energy and clear your mind.

Glossary

analgesic reduces sensitivity to pain.

anti-allergic acts to reduce sensitivity to various substances.

antibacterial agent that kills bacteria.

anticoagulant stops blood from clotting.

antidiabetic prevents the development of diabetes.

antifungal prevents the development of fungus.

anti-inflammatory reduces inflammation.

antilactogenic prevents or slows down the secretion of milk in nursing mothers.

antimigraine reduces or helps to prevent migraines.

antiparasitic prevents the development of parasites.

antipruritis relieves itching.

antipyretic counteracts inflammation or fever.

antisclerotic anti-aging; prevents the hardening of tissues.

antiseptic prevents the development of bacteria.

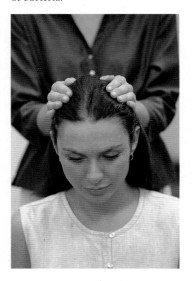

antispasmodic prevents muscle spasm, convulsion.

antitussive relieves or prevents coughing.

antiviral agent that prevents the development of viruses.

aphrodisiac arouses sexual desire.

astringent causes the contraction of living tissue.

balsamic fragrant substance that softens phlegm.

capillary dilator dilates the capillaries, and so aids circulation.

cardiotonic has a tonic effect on the heart.

carminative relieves flatulence (wind).

choleretic stimulates the production of bile in the liver.

cicatrizant healing; promotes scar tissue.

decongestant relieves congestion in the skin, digestive, circulatory and respiratory systems.

depurative purifying or cleansing.

diaphoretic see *sudorific*.

digestive stimulant stimulates a sluggish digestion.

emmenagogic induces or regularizes menstruation.

essential oil volatile plant oil obtained by distillation (exception: oil obtained by expression of the peel of citrus fruits).

febrifuge reduces temperature; antipyretic.

hypertensor increases blood pressure in hypotensive person.

hypotensor reduces blood pressure in hypertensive person

lactogen promotes the secretion of milk.

laxative loosens the bowel content.

lipolytic breaks down fat.

litholytic breaks down sand or small kidney or urinary stones.

mucolytic breaks down mucus.

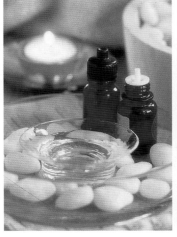

neurotonic stimulates and tones the nervous system.

oestrogenic stimulates the action of the female hormone, oestrogen.

phlebotonic improves or stimulates lymph circulation; lymph tonic.

prophylactic prevents disease.

rubefacient increases local blood circulation, causing skin redness.

stomachic stimulates secretory activity in the stomach.

styptic arrests haemorrhage by means of astringent quality; haemostatic.

sudorific induces or increases perspiration.

synergy the working together that occurs when two or more substances used together give a more effective result than the same substances used alone.

utertonic agent that improves the tone of the uterus (womb).

vasodilator causes blood vessels to increase in lumen (the hollow inside of the blood vessel).

vulnerary speeds up the healing process of wounds.